Sleisenger & Fordtran's

Gastrointestinal
and Liver Disease

Review and Assessment

Sleisenger & Fordtran's

Gastrointestinal and Liver Disease

Review and Assessment

To Accompany Sleisenger & Fordtran's
Gastrointestinal and Liver Disease, 6th Edition

Richard A. Weisiger, M.D., Ph.D.
Professor of Internal Medicine
University of California, San Francisco
School of Medicine
Chief, Gastroenterology Faculty Practice
San Francisco, California

Lyman E. Bilhartz, M.D., F.A.C.P.
Associate Professor of Internal Medicine
Director of Gastroenterology Clinical Services
University of Texas Southwestern Medical Center
Attending Physician
Parkland Memorial Hospital and
Zale-Lipshy University Hospital
Dallas, Texas

W.B. Saunders Company

A Division of Harcourt Brace & Company
Philadelphia   London   Toronto   Montreal   Sydney   Tokyo

W.B. SAUNDERS COMPANY
A Division of Harcourt Brace & Company

The Curtis Center
Independence Square West
Philadelphia, Pennsylvania 19106

SLEISENGER & FORDTRAN'S GASTROINTESTINAL AND LIVER DISEASE
REVIEW AND ASSESSMENT TO ACCOMPANY SLEISINGER & FORDTRAN'S
GASTROINTESTINAL AND LIVER DISEASE   ISBN 0–7216–7703–7

Printed in the United States of America.

Last digit is the print number: 9   8   7   6   5   4   3   2   1

*This book is dedicated to our respective children—
Alex, Beth, Chris, Jacob, Tess Marie and Nathaniel—
who through their energy and enthusiasm
continually remind us that anything is possible
and much is desirable.*

Contributors

Lyman E. Bilhartz, M.D., F.A.C.P.
Associate Professor of Internal Medicine, Director of Gastroenterology Clinical Services, University of Texas Southwestern Medical Center; Attending Physician, Parkland Memorial Hospital and Zale-Lipshy University Hospital, Dallas, Texas

Waldo P. Bracy, Jr., M.D.
Assistant Professor of Internal Medicine, University of Texas Southwestern Medical Center, Dallas, Texas (current practice in Arlington, Texas)

John J. Brandabur, M.D.
Clinical Instructor in Internal Medicine, University of Washington School of Medicine; Staff Gastroenterologist, Section of Gastroenterology and Therapeutic Endoscopy, Virginia Mason Medical Center, Seattle, Washington

Geri Brown, M.D.
Assistant Professor of Internal Medicine, University of Texas Southwestern Medical Center, Dallas, Texas

Mary F. Chan, M.D.
Assistant Professor of Internal Medicine, Division of Gastroenterology, Washington University Medical Center, St. Louis, Missouri

Byron Cryer, M.D.
Assistant Professor of Internal Medicine and Associate Dean, University of Texas Southwestern Medical Center; Staff Physician, Veterans Affairs Medical Center, Dallas, Texas

Marta L. Davila, M.D.
Assistant Professor of Internal Medicine, Division of Gastroenterology, Stanford University Medical Center, Palo Alto, California

Osvaldo Fajardo, M.D.
Assistant Instructor of Internal Medicine, University of Texas Southwestern Medical Center, Dallas, Texas (current practice in San Antonio, Texas)

Eddie Flores, M.D.
University of Texas Southwestern Medical Center, Dallas, Texas (current practice in Dallas, Texas)

Markus Goldschmiedt, M.D.
Assistant Professor of Internal Medicine, University of Texas Southwestern Medical Center, Dallas, Texas (current practice in Dallas, Texas)

Jay D. Horton, M.D.
Assistant Professor and Howard Hughes Postdoctoral Research Fellow, University of Texas Southwestern Medical Center, Dallas, Texas

Johannes Koch, M.D.
Assistant Clinical Professor of Internal Medicine and Radiology, University of California, San Francisco School of Medicine; Attending Physician, San Francisco General Hospital, San Francisco, California

Stephen W. Lacey, M.D.
Assistant Professor of Internal Medicine, University of Texas Southwestern Medical Center, Dallas, Texas

Steven Lidofsky, M.D., Ph.D.
Associate Professor of Internal Medicine and Pharmacology, Director of Hepatology, University of Vermont College of Medicine, Burlington, Vermont

Bruce A. Luxon, M.D., Ph.D.
Assistant Professor of Internal Medicine, St. Louis University Health Sciences Center, St. Louis University, St. Louis, Missouri

David, J. Magee, M.D.
Assistant Professor of Internal Medicine, University of Texas Southwestern Medical Center, Dallas, Texas

Carol S. Murakumi, M.D.
Staff Physician, Fred Hutchinson Cancer Center, Seattle, Washington

Don Rockey, M.D.
Assistant Professor of Internal Medicine, University of California, San Francisco School of Medicine, San Francisco, California

Neal Toribara, M.D.
Adjunct Assistant Professor of Internal Medicine, Veterans Affairs Medical Center, San Francisco, California

Anne H. Wang, M.D.
Assistant Clinical Professor of Internal Medicine, University of California, San Francisco School of Medicine; Associate Director, Gastroenterology Faculty Practice, Moffitt Long Hospital, San Francisco, California (current practice in Portland, Oregon)

Richard A. Weisiger, M.D., Ph.D.
Professor of Internal Medicine, University of California, San Francisco School of Medicine; Chief, Gastroenterology Faculty Practice, San Francisco, California

Robert Willenbucher, M.D.
Associate Clinical Professor of Medicine, Mt. Zion GI Faculty Practice, University of California, San Francisco School of Medicine, San Francisco, California

Preface

This edition of *Gastrointestinal and Liver Disease Review and Assessment* consists of 1045 multiple-choice questions and answers designed to provide a comprehensive and useful review of the broad fields of gastroenterology and hepatology. It is a companion study guide to the 6th edition of *Sleisenger & Fordtran's Gastrointestinal and Liver Disease.*

Gastrointestinal and Liver Disease Review and Assessment is designed to aid in the education of gastroenterology and hepatology fellows, practicing gastroenterologists and hepatologists, residents in internal medicine, internists, and other physicians who wish to improve their ability to solve clinical problems. It should be especially helpful to gastroenterology fellows and others preparing for the Subspecialty Examination in Gastroenterology of the American Board of Internal Medicine—a test which, in 1997, had a pass rate of only 62%.

The questions are in the format of a Board examination. Answers, often quite detailed, are provided in the second section and are linked to specific pages in *Sleisenger & Fordtran's Gastrointestinal and Liver Disease, 6th Edition* and often other pertinent references. By allowing 2½ minutes to answer each question, one can simulate time constraints of the Board examination.

Recognizing that not even the most recent 6th edition of *Gastrointestinal and Liver Disease* is fully up-to-date in all areas, we have included several hundred questions dealing with clinical problems in new and rapidly changing fields. These include treatment of *Helicobacter pylori* infection, interpretation of endoscopic ultrasound, diagnosis and treatment of viral heptitis A, B, C, D, and E, the genetics of colon cancer with implications of screening, appropriate use of laparoscopic surgery for gastrointestinal and biliary disease, treatment of the gastrointestinal complications of AIDS, the utility and complications of TIPS shunts, and the utility of new agents for treating inflammatory bowel disease. References to the most readily available, recent medical literature are included through early 1997.

This edition of *Gastrointestinal and Liver Disease Review and Assessment* was prepared in response to a number of requests. We hope that it will be useful; but we recognize that you may disagree with some of our answers. While every attempt has been made to identify errors of fact, it is impossible to be authoritative when a field is evolving rapidly. We welcome your comments and criticisms by letter or e-mail and will incorporate them when drafting the next edition.

Have fun with the questions, discuss them with your colleagues, and let us know what you think.

RICHARD A. WEISIGER, M.D., Ph.D. (dickw@itsa.ucsf.edu)
LYMAN E. BILHARTZ, M.D., F.A.C.P. (lyman.bilhartz@email.swmed.edu)

Contents

Stomach and Duodenum

S&F Section VI

1. A 34-year-old man presents to the emergency department with a two-week history of persistent epigastric pain, which has abruptly worsened over the past day. This morning he has had intractable nausea and vomiting and an episode of hematemesis. His only medical problem is chronic right shoulder pain, for which he has been taking ibuprofen. Physical examination reveals a well-nourished young man lying in bed on his left side, with legs flexed at the hips and knees. Vital signs show temperature of 38.1° C, blood pressure of 120/80 mm Hg, pulse of 110 beats per minute, and respirations of 24 breaths per minute. Abdominal examination reveals scant bowel sounds, tympany, and diffuse tenderness in all quadrants to deep palpation and to percussion. Rectal examination reveals brown, trace heme–positive stool. Which of the following is the MOST likely diagnosis?
A. Actively bleeding duodenal ulcer
B. Perforated duodenal ulcer
C. Penetrating duodenal ulcer with pancreatitis
D. Gastric outlet obstruction from pyloric channel ulcer
E. Bleeding prepyloric ulcer with pyloric channel obstruction

2. Referring to the previous question, which of the following tests is LEAST indicated?
A. Gastrografin upper gastrointestinal series
B. Plain abdominal films, supine and upright
C. Upper endoscopy
D. Peritoneal lavage
E. Serum amylase level

3. The diagnosis of perforated duodenal ulcer has been established and the patient is to undergo treatment. Which of the following treatment options is LEAST indicated?
A. Volume resuscitation
B. Continuous nasogastric suction
C. Exploratory laparotomy
D. Broad-spectrum antibiotics
E. Cautery of bleeding source

4. Match each of the following tests for *Helicobacter pylori* with the entity that is actually being measured when the test is positive.
1. Rapid urease test   A. *Helicobacter pylori*
2. Urea breath test   B. ^{13}C-carbon dioxide
3. Warthin-Starry stain   C. Urea
                          D. Ammonia

5. A patient with rheumatoid arthritis on chronic naproxen (Naprosyn) therapy relates that she has a previous history of a bleeding ulcer and wants to reduce the likelihood that she will have a recurrent ulcer related to her NSAID use. She takes no other medications. Which of the following therapies is currently approved by the U.S. Food and Drug Administration for the prevention of NSAID-induced ulceration?
A. Misoprostol
B. Omeprazole
C. Sucralfate
D. Ranitidine
E. None of the above

6. *Helicobacter pylori* is a frequent cause of chronic active gastritis. Each of the following statements regarding *H. pylori* gastritis is true EXCEPT:
A. Most patients are asymptomatic and have normal-appearing mucosa at endoscopy.
B. The most common histologic pattern is mild superficial gastritis.
C. Bacterial colony counts are higher in patients with atrophic gastritis.
D. It is associated with gastric and duodenal ulcer disease.

7. A patient with a previous history of documented duodenal ulcer presents for evaluation of a recurrence of her ulcer-like symptoms. Endoscopy is performed and reveals a duodenal ulcer. Rapid urease testing of an antral biopsy specimen is positive. She is given a two-week course of bismuth, tetracycline, and metronidazole along with an H_2 receptor antagonist that she continues to take until next seen. Her symptoms improve; however, four months after her last endoscopy, she has a recurrence of symptoms. Repeat endoscopy reveals a duodenal ulcer. Which of the following is MOST likely?
A. *Helicobacter pylori* was eradicated but she has been reinfected.
B. *H. pylori* was eradicated and she developed rebound gastric acid hypersecretion.
C. The urease test result gave a false-positive result.
D. Treatment of the *H. pylori* was unsuccessful.

8. A 52-year-old woman with newly diagnosed Zollinger-Ellison syndrome is referred for evaluation. Upper endoscopy reveals thickened rugal folds and multiple duodenal ulcers. Baseline gastrin level is

1050 pg/mL. Computed tomography of the abdomen reveals distinct 2- and 1-cm masses in the left lobe of the liver. Each of the following would be an appropriate treatment option EXCEPT:

A. Omeprazole to reduce acid hypersecretion
B. Exploratory laparotomy with left hepatic lobe resection
C. Hepatic artery chemoembolization
D. Exploratory laparotomy with duodenotomy and intraluminal examination

9. A patient has been taking an H₂ receptor antagonist for treatment of a duodenal ulcer found on an upper gastrointestinal barium study. After eight weeks of therapy he still has persistent symptoms. Upper endoscopy is performed that reveals a persistent duodenal ulcer. Which of the following would be a reasonable next step?

I. Obtain gastric secretory analysis
II. Advise patient to stop smoking
III. Switch therapy from cimetidine to ranitidine
IV. Obtain an antral biopsy for *Helicobacter pylori* during the endoscopy

A. I and III
B. II and IV
C. I, II, and III
D. All of the above

10. A 35-year-old man with no previous medical history presents with a complaint of dyspepsia unresponsive to H₂ receptor antagonists. Upper gastrointestinal series reveals a duodenal ulcer. *Helicobacter pylori* serology is positive, and he is treated with an H₂ receptor antagonist along with antibiotics to eradicate *H. pylori*. Two months later, he is asymptomatic and feels well. Which of the following is the MOST appropriate next step?

A. Upper gastrointestinal barium study
B. Repeat *H. pylori* serology
C. Upper endoscopy
D. Determination of serum gastrin levels
E. None of the above

11. Which of the following statements regarding acute infection with *Helicobacter pylori* are TRUE?

I. Characteristic symptoms include nausea, vomiting, and epigastric pain, usually lasting for one to four days.
II. Histologic examination reveals mild lymphocytic infiltration of the lamina propria.
III. The acute infection causes a hypochlorhydria lasting for several weeks.
IV. Seroconversion of the *H. pylori* antibody test occurs on average six months after the initial infection.

A. I and III
B. II and IV
C. I, II, and III
D. None of the above

12. Which of the following are TRUE statements about locating gastrinomas?

A. Eighty to 90 percent of gastrinomas can be localized by established diagnostic techniques, including exploratory laparotomy.
B. Selective angiography and computed tomography can detect 0.5- to 1.0-cm tumors.
C. Selective angiography can identify up to 65% of gastrinomas preoperatively.
D. Magnetic resonance imaging is superior to computed tomography in localizing small gastrinomas.

13. A 50-year-old woman is referred for evaluation of dyspepsia. She does not use NSAIDs and has no previous history of ulcer disease. A duodenal ulcer is seen on endoscopy, and antral biopsy specimens demonstrate *Helicobacter pylori*. Which of the following is the MOST appropriate next step in her management?

A. Urea breath test
B. Antibiotics for eradication of *H. pylori*
C. Six to eight weeks of treatment with an H₂ receptor antagonist
D. Four to six weeks of treatment with omeprazole
E. None of the above

14. Which of the following statements regarding *Helicobacter pylori* are TRUE?

I. *H. pylori* infection increases the risk of gastric lymphoma.
II. *H. pylori* is associated with mucosa-associated lymphoid tissue (MALT) lymphomas.
III. The incidence of gastric lymphoma correlates with the prevalence of *H. pylori*.
IV. The risk of nongastric lymphoma is higher in subjects infected with *H. pylori*.

A. I and III
B. II and IV
C. I, II, and III
D. All of the above

15. Which of the following patients would be the MOST appropriate to receive prophylactic therapy for the prevention of NSAID-induced ulcers?

A. An 80-year-old woman with no prior medical history is placed on ibuprofen, 800 mg t.i.d., for osteoarthritis. One day after starting ibuprofen, she develops dyspeptic symptoms.
B. A 50-year-old, nonsmoking man started ibuprofen, 600 mg t.i.d., two weeks ago for osteoarthritis. Since starting his NSAID, he has had no

symptoms. His medical history is remarkable for exercise-induced asthma and a bleeding duodenal ulcer.

C. A 55-year-old man has blood type O and negative serology for *Helicobacter pylori.* For the four years before being placed on an NSAID, he has had dyspeptic symptoms but has undergone two upper endoscopies two and three years ago that were unremarkable. He is about to be started on indomethacin, 50 mg t.i.d., for ankylosing spondylitis.

D. A 65-year-old woman with a history of rheumatoid arthritis for the last eight years is taking ibuprofen, 800 mg t.i.d., has positive serology for *H. pylori,* and a hematocrit of 29%.

16. In which of the following duodenal ulcer patients would *Helicobacter pylori* LEAST likely be eradicated? The dosing regimens are as follows: clarithromycin, 500 mg b.i.d.; amoxicillin, 1 g b.i.d.; bismuth (Pepto-Bismol), 8 tabs/day; metronidazole, 250 mg t.i.d.; omeprazole, 20 mg b.i.d.; tetracycline, 500 mg q.i.d.
    A. A patient given a 14-day combination of bismuth, metronidazole, and tetracycline
    B. A patient given a 14-day combination of clarithromycin, amoxicillin, and omeprazole
    C. A patient given a 14-day combination of bismuth, metronidazole, tetracycline, and omeprazole who earlier had received metronidazole for giardiasis
    D. A patient given a 14-day combination of omeprazole and amoxicillin

17. Treatment of *Helicobacter pylori* infection should cause improvement in which of the following conditions?
    I. Gastric and duodenal ulcers
    II. Gastric B-cell lymphoma
    III. Gastric and duodenal inflammation
    IV. Gastric adenocarcinoma

    A. I and III
    B. II and IV
    C. I, II, and III
    D. All of the above

18. Which one of the following is NOT an advantage of selective proximal gastric vagotomy?
    A. Postoperative diarrhea and dumping syndrome are uncommon.
    B. Leakage and small bowel obstruction are uncommon.
    C. The criminal nerves of Grassi, which stimulate acid secretion, are severed.
    D. Severing the nerves to the antrum prevents antral spasm.
    E. Laparoscopic proximal gastric vagotomy is possible.

19. A previously healthy 52-year-old man, taking no medications, is referred for upper endoscopy after an upper gastrointestinal series showed a gastric ulcer on the lesser curve. Which of the following diagnostic approaches would be MOST appropriate?
    A. Esophagogastroduodenoscopy (EGD) with biopsy of the ulcer margin
    B. Serologic test for *Helicobacter pylori* and treatment with antibiotics if positive
    C. EGD with biopsy of the ulcer margin and rapid urease test for *H. pylori* from antral mucosa
    D. EGD with biopsy of the ulcer margin and rapid urease test for *H. pylori* from antral mucosa and random biopsies of antral mucosa, submitted for histology only if rapid urease test is negative

20. Which one of the following statements regarding *Helicobacter pylori* and gastrin is TRUE?
    A. Normal subjects not infected with *H. pylori* have higher mean serum gastrin concentrations than infected subjects.
    B. Eradication of *H. pylori* causes a decrease in mean serum gastrin concentrations in both normal subjects and patients with duodenal ulcers.
    C. Normal subjects who are infected with *H. pylori* should have occasional checks of their serum gastrin concentrations.
    D. Normal subjects infected with *H. pylori* have basal and peak acid outputs that are generally higher than acid outputs in noninfected control subjects.

21. A 35-year-old man with no prior medical history presents for evaluation of dyspeptic pain for two weeks. He has no complaints of vomiting, dysphagia, or weight loss. His physical examination, serum chemistries, and blood cell counts are normal. Which of the following would be the MOST appropriate next step?
    A. Upper gastrointestinal barium study
    B. Abdominal sonogram
    C. Upper endoscopy
    D. H$_2$ receptor antagonist for six weeks
    E. Antibiotic therapy for *Helicobacter pylori*

22. A patient has been taking omeprazole, 40 mg/day, for the last three months for a large gastric ulcer. Before this diagnosis, the patient had been taking 650 mg of aspirin q.i.d. for back pain. At the first endoscopy, a 2-cm antral ulcer was observed and was believed to be related to aspirin use. Six biopsy specimens of the ulcer edge and one of the base were taken. On histologic evaluation of these specimens, no malignancy was observed. Aspirin use was discontinued, and omeprazole was taken for three months. On the follow-up endoscopy three months later, the gastric ulcer is still present but has de-

creased to 1 cm. Which of the following would be the LEAST reasonable step to take at this time?

A. At the next follow-up esophagogastroduodenos-copy (EGD), obtain six to eight specimens of the ulcer, preferably with jumbo biopsy forceps.

B. At the next follow-up EGD, obtain antral biopsy specimens for *Helicobacter pylori*. If the organism is present, add amoxicillin, 500 mg q.i.d., for two weeks, and continue the omeprazole, 40 mg/day, for another two months.

C. Refer the patient to a surgeon for a surgical excision of her ulcer.

D. Draw blood to test serum salicylate concentration.

---

23. Regarding the previous patient, which one of the following is MOST likely to occur during the three-month course of omeprazole treatment?

A. Carcinoid tumor
B. Enterochromaffin-like (ECL)-cell hyperplasia
C. Hypergastrinemia
D. Gastric adenoma
E. None of the above

---

24. A 25-year-old woman in her 20th gestational week is diagnosed with duodenal ulcer. She is referred for selection of the most appropriate medication. Which of the following ulcer healing medications can be safely given to this patient?

I. Sucralfate
II. H_2 receptor antagonists
III. Antacids
IV. Omeprazole

A. I and III
B. II and IV
C. I, II, and III
D. All of the above

---

25. Which of the following statements about the natural history of chronic *Helicobacter pylori* infection are TRUE?

A. Most individuals remain asymptomatic throughout their lives.

B. Over their lifetime, approximately 3% of infected patients eventually develop duodenal ulcers.

C. Atrophic gastritis is a late development in *H. pylori* infection, with the prevalence increasing 1% to 3% per year after infection.

D. Chronic *H. pylori* infection is epidemiologically linked to adenocarcinoma of the gastric body and cardia, but not the antrum.

---

26. Which of the following statements concerning peptic ulcer in childhood are TRUE?

I. *Helicobacter pylori* is found in less than 25% of children with duodenal ulcers.

II. Children with peptic ulcers often have other family members who are affected.

III. In childhood, gastric and duodenal ulcer occur with similar frequencies.

IV. Peptic ulcers in children frequently present as atypical symptoms.

A. I and III
B. I and IV
C. I, II, and III
D. All of the above

---

27. Match the following causes of gastritis or gastropathy with one of the three general types of gastritis/gastropathy it is most associated with:

1. *Helicobacter pylori*
2. Aspirin
3. Alcohol
4. Cytomegalovirus
5. Parietal cell antibodies

A. Erosive and hemorrhagic gastritis/gastropathy
B. Nonerosive gastritis
C. Distinctive (specific) gastritis

---

28. Hemorrhagic and erosive gastritis can be diagnosed endoscopically. Each of the following is a potential cause of hemorrhagic and erosive gastritis EXCEPT:

A. Stress in critically ill patients
B. Aspirin and other NSAIDs
C. *Helicobacter pylori*
D. Ischemia
E. Corrosive ingestion

---

29. The optimal treatment regimen for *Helicobacter pylori* infection remains to be established; nonetheless, all of the following generalizations about treatment for *H. pylori* are true EXCEPT:

A. Emerging resistance to metronidazole and clarithromycin has made them second-line agents for the treatment of *H. pylori*.

B. One-week regimens require three or four agents.

C. Two-week regimens require at least two agents.

D. All successful regimens include metronidazole and/or clarithromycin.

---

30. Match each consequence with the pH that is most appropriate to achieve the desired effect. Each answer is used only once.

1. pH at which greatest ionization, parietal cell trapping, and concentration of omeprazole will occur
2. pH at which the granules within orally administered omeprazole capsules will begin to dissolve
3. For optimal duodenal ulcer healing, gastric pH should be at or above this value for the majority of each 24-hour period
4. Lowest desirable continuous gastric pH for prevention of gastric bleeding in patients in intensive care units

A. pH 2
B. pH 3
C. pH 4
D. pH 6

---

31. Which of the following statements regarding *Helicobacter pylori* gastritis are TRUE?

I. *H. pylori* frequently colonizes areas of intestinal metaplasia within the stomach.

II. For the detection of *H. pylori* gastritis, the highest diagnostic yields at endoscopy are from antral biopsy specimens near the pylorus.

III. *H. pylori* antibodies are insensitive but specific markers for the presence of the associated gastritis.

IV. *H. pylori* organisms are noninvasive and generally reside in gastric mucus overlying the gastric surface and gastric pits.

A. I and III
B. II and IV
C. I, II, and III
D. All of the above

32. Which of the following statements are TRUE regarding *Helicobacter pylori*?

I. In the United States, there is an age-related increase in prevalence of *H. pylori*.

II. *H. pylori* infection is usually acquired during childhood.

III. *H. pylori* is found in more than 90% of patients with duodenal ulcer and in 60% to 80% of patients with gastric ulcer.

IV. *H. pylori* is more frequently associated with giant (>2 cm) gastric ulcers than with smaller gastric ulcers.

A. I and III
B. II and IV
C. I, II, and III
D. All of the above

33. Match each clinical indication with an appropriate medication.

1. Treatment of NSAID-induced gastric ulcer while NSAID use continues
2. Treatment of recurrent duodenal ulcers not related to NSAIDs
3. Prevention of recurrent bleeding duodenal ulcers
4. Prevention of NSAID-induced gastric and duodenal ulcers

A. Sucralfate
B. Ranitidine
C. Misoprostol
D. Omeprazole
E. Bismuth, metronidazole, and tetracycline

34. Nonerosive gastritis requires histologic confirmation. Each of the following is a potential cause of nonerosive nonspecific gastritis EXCEPT:
A. *Helicobacter pylori*
B. Postgastrectomy status
C. Pernicious anemia
D. Alcoholic gastritis
E. Autoimmune atrophic gastritis

35. Which of the following, when given as monotherapy, would be expected to eradicate *Helicobacter pylori* in at least 80% of infected patients?
A. Amoxicillin, 500 mg q.i.d.
B. Bismuth (Pepto-Bismol), two tablets q.i.d.

C. Omeprazole, 20 mg b.i.d.
D. Clarithromycin, 500 mg b.i.d.
E. None of the above

36. The surgical procedure associated with the LOWEST postoperative ulcer recurrence rate is:
A. Proximal gastric (highly selective) vagotomy
B. Truncal vagotomy with pyloroplasty
C. Truncal vagotomy with antrectomy
D. Subtotal gastrectomy without vagotomy

37. A 60-year-old woman with abdominal pain who has been taking indomethacin for osteoarthritis undergoes an upper endoscopy that shows a 1-cm duodenal ulcer. Rapid urease testing of an antral biopsy specimen is negative. She agrees to stop her NSAID use. At this point, which of the following drugs offers the MOST reasonable therapy?
A. Misoprostol
B. Cimetidine
C. Ranitidine, metronidazole, and amoxicillin
D. Cisapride
E. None of the above

38. A 60-year-old woman with abdominal pain who also has been taking indomethacin for osteoarthritis undergoes an upper endoscopy that shows a 1-cm duodenal ulcer. Rapid urease testing of antral biopsy specimen taken at the time endoscopy is negative. The patient states that she is unwilling to stop indomethacin. At this point, which of the following drugs offers the MOST reasonable therapy?
A. Misoprostol
B. Cimetidine
C. Cisapride
D. Omeprazole
E. None of the above

39. Match the infectious agent with its endoscopic and histologic features.

1. Tuberculosis
2. Syphilis
3. Cytomegalovirus
4. Herpes simplex
5. *Histoplasma*

A. Rarely seen in the stomach
B. Multiple bleeding gastric ulcerations with granulomas
C. Prominent pyloroduodenal involvement, gastric outlet obstruction, with caseating granulomas
D. Thick gastric folds may mimic linitis plastica; diagnosed by silver stain
E. Thick gastric folds in the fundus and body; intranuclear inclusion cells involving deep layers of the mucosa

40. Antral G-cell hyperplasia is associated with each of the following EXCEPT:
   A. Gastric acid hypersecretion
   B. Elevated fasting serum gastrin concentration
   C. Exaggerated gastrin release in response to feeding
   D. Exaggerated rise in serum gastrin levels after intravenous administration of secretin

41. Each of the following features is common to pernicious anemia and severe atrophic gastritis without pernicious anemia EXCEPT:
   A. Achlorhydria
   B. Vitamin B_{12} deficiency
   C. Atrophic gastric mucosa
   D. Hypergastrinemia
   E. Autoimmune antibodies

42. Match each drug with an associated side effect.
   1. Cimetidine   A. Gynecomastia
   2. Sucralfate   B. Milk-alkali syndrome
   3. Misoprostol   C. Gastric carcinoids
   4. Antacids   D. Increased uterine bleeding
                    E. Increased serum aluminum

43. All of the following statements regarding the saline load test for the diagnosis of gastric outlet obstruction are true EXCEPT:
   A. A nasogastric tube is used to instill 750 mL of saline into the stomach.
   B. After 60 minutes, the gastric contents are aspirated and measured.
   C. Under normal conditions (i.e., definitely no outlet obstruction) no more than 200 mL of fluid is obtained.
   D. The saline load test may be employed sequentially to determine if the outlet obstruction is resolving.

44. Which of the following statements regarding the pharmacokinetics of H_2 receptor antagonists are TRUE?
   A. Famotidine can be administered once daily in situations in which other agents cannot.
   B. Cimetidine and ranitidine may cause a slight elevation of serum creatinine level.
   C. Bioavailability of intravenously administered H_2 receptor antagonists is close to 100%.
   D. H_2 receptor antagonists can increase plasma alcohol concentrations.

45. Factors associated with increased mortality in patients undergoing surgery for bleeding peptic ulcer disease include each of the following EXCEPT:
   A. Age younger than 60 years
   B. Onset of bleeding in hospital
   C. Gastric ulcer
   D. Coexisting cardiac disease
   E. Presence of shock

46. Clinical manifestations of Zollinger-Ellison syndrome include each of the following EXCEPT:
   A. Diarrhea
   B. Steatorrhea
   C. Abdominal pain
   D. Pyrosis
   E. Urticaria

47. Each of the following is associated with the Zollinger-Ellison syndrome EXCEPT:
   A. Gastric carcinoid
   B. Peptic ulcer disease
   C. Enterochromaffin-like (ECL)-cell hyperplasia
   D. Expanded parietal cell mass
   E. Chief cell hyperplasia

48. Match the endoscopic ultrasound image to the appropriate diagnosis.

1.

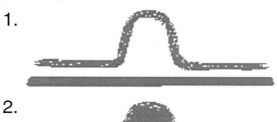

2.

3.

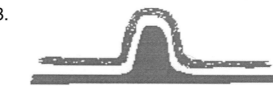

   A. Leiomyosarcoma
   B. Gastric varix
   C. Pancreatic pseudocyst
   D. Lipoma
   E. Leiomyoma

49. Match each patient profile with the pathophysiologic mechanism that is believed to be responsible for gastroduodenal ulceration in that situation.
   1. Patient after acute "crack" cocaine usage
   2. Head trauma patient
   3. Patient who has received parenteral ketorolac

   A. Prostaglandin depletion
   B. *Helicobacter pylori*
   C. Gastric acid hypersecretion with a normal serum gastrin concentration

4. Majority of duodenal ulcer patients
5. Patients with multiple endocrine neoplasia–1

D. Gastric acid hypersecretion with an elevated serum gastrin concentration
E. Gastroduodenal ischemia

---

50. Which one of the following characteristics on an upper gastrointestinal barium study is MOST reassuring that a gastric ulcer is benign?
  A. Mucosal folds that do not radiate to the edge of the ulcer crater
  B. An ulcer that is located within a mass
  C. A radiolucent line that rims the mouth of the ulcer crater
  D. Negative filling defects within the ulcer crater

---

51. Which of the following are associated with an increased risk of peptic ulcer?
  I. Renal transplantation
  II. Hepatic cirrhosis
  III. Chronic pulmonary disease
  IV. Multiple endocrine neoplasia–2

  A. I and III
  B. II and IV
  C. I, II, and III
  D. All of the above

---

52. Increased histamine release is associated with:
  I. Mast cell stimulation
  II. Basophilic leukemia
  III. Enterochromaffin-like (ECL) cell stimulation
  IV. NSAIDs

  A. I and III
  B. II and IV
  C. I, II, and III
  D. All of the above

---

53. Match the following statements with the conditions with which they are associated.
  1. Equal male-to-female ratio
  2. Bilious vomiting
  3. Abdominal films show "double bubble" sign
  4. Surgery usually curative

  A. Hypertrophic pyloric stenosis
  B. Congenital duodenal obstruction

---

54. Which of the following statements regarding bismuth are TRUE?
  A. Bismuth toxicity is very unusual in patients taking five to eight tablets of Pepto-Bismol daily.
  B. Bismuth darkens stools by converting colonic hemoglobin to hematin or other hemachromes.
  C. Bismuth, when given as monotherapy, can heal duodenal ulcers.
  D. Bismuth is more likely to cause toxicity in patients with renal failure.

---

55. Which of the following statements regarding basal gastric acid secretion are TRUE?
  I. The highest secretory rates are between 2 and 11 P.M.
  II. The lowest secretory rates are between 5 and 11 A.M.
  III. Basal gastric acid secretion is generally higher in men.
  IV. Basal gastric acid secretion correlates with basal serum gastrin levels.

  A. I and III
  B. II and IV
  C. I, II, and III
  D. All of the above

---

56. Which of the following statements regarding "giant" ulcers (ulcers >2 cm in diameter) are TRUE?
  I. NSAID use is commonly associated with giant gastric and duodenal ulcers.
  II. Postbulbar narrowing is frequently associated with giant duodenal ulcers.
  III. The risk is increased in end-stage renal failure.
  IV. Patients with giant duodenal ulcers tend to have higher rates of acid secretion than those with smaller duodenal ulcers.

  A. I and III
  B. II and IV
  C. I, II, and III
  D. All of the above

---

57. Match each drug with the appropriate pharmacokinetic association.
  1. Cimetidine
  2. Antacid
  3. Omeprazole
  4. Pepto-Bismol

  A. Increased serum procainamide concentrations
  B. Decreased serum phenytoin concentrations
  C. Increased vitamin B_{12} absorption
  D. Increased serum salicylate concentration
  E. Decreased efficacy if administered through nasogastric tube

---

58. Each of the following stimulates gastric acid secretion EXCEPT:
  A. Gastrin
  B. Somatostatin
  C. Acetylcholine
  D. Histamine

---

59. Which of the following stimulates gastric acid by increasing intracellular calcium?
  A. Histamine
  B. Peptide YY
  C. Secretin

D. Acetylcholine
E. None of the above

C. Somatostatin
D. Secretin

---

60. Which of the following statements regarding the characteristics of peptic ulcer pain are TRUE?
  I. Pain is usually epigastric.
  II. Pain usually resolves before the ulcer is completely healed.
  III. Many ulcers are asymptomatic.
  IV. Pain rarely awakens one from sleep.

  A. I and III
  B. II and IV
  C. I, II, and III
  D. All of the above

---

61. Which of the following statements regarding dosing of H_2 receptor antagonists are TRUE?
  I. Concomitant administration of antacids will reduce absorption of orally administered H_2 receptor antagonists.
  II. Patients with severe to moderate renal failure should have their H_2 receptor antagonist dose reduced by about 50%.
  III. In patients with liver failure, the half-life of cimetidine is prolonged.
  IV. Patients receiving hemodialysis and peritoneal dialysis should have their H_2 receptor antagonist dose increased about 50% to compensate for the amount removed during dialysis.

  A. I and III
  B. II and IV
  C. I, II, and III
  D. All of the above

---

62. Which of the following are TRUE statements regarding serum gastrin and provocative testing for Zollinger-Ellison syndrome?
  A. Gastrin levels of more than 1000 pg/mL are virtually diagnostic of Zollinger-Ellison syndrome.
  B. Marked hypergastrinemia (>1000 pg/mL) is specific for gastrinoma.
  C. A rise in gastrin level by 200 pg/mL after intravenous secretin administration is diagnostic of Zollinger-Ellison syndrome.
  D. Serum gastrin response to secretin infusion can aid in differentiating Zollinger-Ellison syndrome from hypergastrinemia due to common duodenal ulcer disease or antral G-cell hyperplasia.
  E. A dramatic decrease in serum gastrin with calcium infusion is diagnostic of Zollinger-Ellison syndrome.

---

63. Gastric acid hypersecretion in systemic mastocytosis is due to increased levels of:
  A. Gastrin
  B. Histamine

---

64. A 63-year-old man presents to the hospital with massive hematemesis. His past medical history is remarkable for mild congestive heart failure that is well controlled on captopril and digoxin. He denies any NSAID, tobacco, or alcohol use. Physical examination reveals a pale elderly man with a supine blood pressure of 100/70 mm Hg and a pulse of 100 beats per minute; these signs change to 80/60 mm Hg and 140 beats per minute on sitting up. Initial hemoglobin level is 8.1 g/dL. Nasogastric lavage shows coffee grounds material. Upper endoscopy after fluid resuscitation reveals a duodenal ulcer with a visible vessel and active oozing. Electrocoagulation therapy is applied, and cessation of bleeding is achieved. The patient is transfused with 4 units of whole blood. The following day, he is noted to have a pulse of 110 beats per minute, blood pressure of 100/70 mm Hg, and a hemoglobin level of 10 g/dL. He has passed three maroon stools, and nasogastric lavage is grossly bloody. A decision to perform emergency surgery is made. Each of the following is a true statement about this case EXCEPT:
  A. Direct suture of the bleeding vessel will be important to achieve hemostasis.
  B. Vagotomy and antrectomy is preferred over vagotomy and pyloroplasty because the perioperative morbidity is lower.
  C. The risk of perioperative complications is greater than for elective ulcer surgery.
  D. Wound infection, duodenal stump leakage, and bile duct injury are more likely in this case than with elective ulcer surgery.
  E. Proximal gastric vagotomy with ulcer oversew would be an option in this case.

---

65. Which of the following are TRUE statements about surgery for perforated ulcer?
  A. Simple, direct suture closure of the perforation without omental patch or an acid reduction procedure is sufficient.
  B. Delaying surgery more than 48 hours is associated with increased perioperative mortality.
  C. For gastric ulcer perforations, resection of the ulcer is desirable to lessen the risk of ulcer recurrence.
  D. Ideal candidates for medical management alone (nasogastric suction, antibiotics) are elderly patients with comorbid conditions.

---

66. Regarding the use of prokinetic agents in the treatment of gastric stasis, which of the following statements are TRUE?
  A. Intravenous erythromycin (3 mg/kg q8hr) may be helpful in "jump starting" the stomach.
  B. Parenteral metoclopramide has both antiemetic and prokinetic properties.

C. Orally administered cisapride accelerates gastric emptying of both liquids and solids.

D. In refractory cases, a combination of erythromycin and cisapride may be warranted to induce gastric emptying.

---

67. Which of the following findings increase the likelihood that a gastric ulcer is associated with a gastric adenocarcinoma?

  I. Larger size

  II. Gastric metaplasia

  III. Nodular folds in the adjacent mucosa that do not radiate to the edge of the ulcer crater

  IV. Simultaneous coexistence of a duodenal ulcer

A. I and III

B. II and IV

C. I, II, and III

D. All of the above

---

68. Which of the following factors are associated with an increased risk of gastric cancer?

A. Male sex

B. Whole milk

C. Smoked foods

D. *Helicobacter pylori* infection

---

69. Which of the following statements regarding gastric metaplasia within the duodenum are TRUE?

  I. It may be found in subjects who do not have a history of ulcer.

  II. It is common in patients with atrophic gastritis.

  III. Duodenal *Helicobacter pylori* infection is always associated with it.

  IV. It is always associated with duodenal *H. pylori* infection.

A. I and III

B. II and IV

C. I, II, and III

D. All of the above

---

70. Each of the following factors is associated with increased mortality in bleeding peptic ulcer disease EXCEPT:

A. Coexisting medical illness

B. Ulcer located in the duodenum

C. Transfusion requirement of more than 5 units

D. Age older than 60 years

E. Presence of shock

---

71. Which of the following are TRUE statements regarding multiple endocrine neoplasia (MEN) syndrome and gastrinomas?

A. Gastrinomas are present in 60% of patients with MEN-1 syndrome.

B. Gastrinomas associated with MEN are more commonly extrapancreatic.

C. Gastrinomas associated with MEN-1 are malignant in approximately 10%.

D. Hyperparathyroidism in MEN-1 may mask a gastrinoma by suppressing gastrin release.

E. Gastrinomas associated with MEN-1 are usually solitary.

---

72. The mechanism of steatorrhea in patients with Zollinger-Ellison syndrome involves which of the following?

  I. Precipitation of conjugated bile acids

  II. Inhibition of pancreatic lipase

  III. Decreased micellar formation

  IV. Ileal dysfunction with resulting disruption of the enterohepatic circulation of bile acids

A. I and III

B. II and IV

C. I, II, and III

D. All of the above

---

73. A radiologist asks your opinion regarding an upper gastrointestinal barium examination that has as its only abnormality multiple ulcers in the postbulbar duodenum. Which of the following patients would be LEAST likely to have this radiographic abnormality?

A. A 27-year-old man with intermittent abdominal pain and diarrhea whose barium enema reveals cecal and ileal ulcers

B. A 60-year-old man with a gastrin level of 1200 pg/mL, substantial increase in serum gastrin in response to secretin infusion, and gastric pH of 5 after pentagastrin injection

C. A 55-year-old woman taking ibuprofen for the last year who has no dyspeptic symptoms

D. A 60-year-old patient with adenocarcinoma of the colon with liver metastases who has received hepatic artery infusions of 5-fluorouracil

---

74. Which of the following are TRUE statements regarding the role of chemotherapy in the treatment of metastatic gastrinoma?

A. It should not be administered to patients with lymph node involvement.

B. Reduction in tumor size causes less acid secretion.

C. Reduction in tumor size improves symptoms due to tumor invasion or mass effect.

D. Hepatic artery chemoembolization is superior to conventional chemotherapy.

75. Match the endoscopic ultrasound image to the appropriate cause of extramural gastric wall compression.

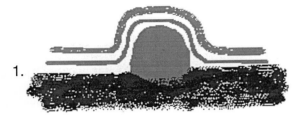

1.

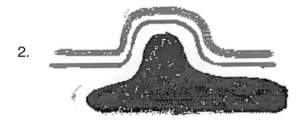

2.

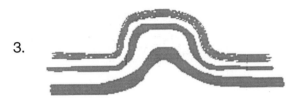

3.

A. Leiomyosarcoma
B. Enlarged spleen
C. Aberrant splenic artery
D. Lipoma
E. Pancreatic pseudocyst

76. A 53-year-old man undergoes endoscopy for evaluation of epigastric symptoms. During esophagogastro-duodenoscopy, a 1 × 2-cm polypoid mass is noted in the proximal stomach. Which of the following is the MOST appropriate next step?
A. Resection with snare cautery
B. Biopsy followed by abdominal computed tomography
C. Endoscopic ultrasonography
D. Fine-needle aspiration
E. Transabdominal ultrasonography

77. In the same patient as in question 76, biopsy samples are obtained and indicate a normal gastric mucosa. Which of the following is the LEAST likely diagnosis?
A. Leiomyoma
B. Gastric carcinoid
C. Adenoma
D. Lipoma
E. Pancreatic rest

78. Which one of the following conditions is associated with DECREASED gastric acid secretion?
A. Extensive small bowel resection
B. Systemic mastocytosis
C. Head injury
D. Acquired immunodeficiency syndrome
E. Retained antrum syndrome

79. Penetrating peptic ulcer may result in each of the following fistulous complications EXCEPT:
A. Gastrocolic fistula
B. Gastroesophageal fistula
C. Choledochoduodenal fistula
D. Gastroduodenal fistula
E. Cholecystoduodenal fistula

80. Which of the following are TRUE statements regarding truncal vagotomy with antrectomy for the treatment of ulcer disease?
A. It is contraindicated in duodenal ulcer disease with severe inflammation.
B. It has a higher rate of ulcer recurrence than truncal vagotomy with pyloroplasty.
C. It is not indicated for duodenal ulcer associated with G-cell hyperplasia.
D. It is the procedure of choice for bleeding duodenal ulcer.

81. The MOST common cause of anemia in patients who have undergone gastric surgery is
A. Iron deficiency
B. Folate deficiency
C. Vitamin B_{12} deficiency
D. Chronic disease

82. A 46-year-old man presents three weeks after truncal vagotomy and antrectomy with Billroth II gastrojejunostomy for a nonhealing duodenal ulcer. He complains of intermittent postprandial abdominal pain and fullness relieved after vomiting of bilious material. Physical examination is remarkable for a normally healing abdominal incision, active bowel sounds, and minimal tympany on percussion. Which of the following is the LEAST likely diagnosis?
A. Marginal ulcer
B. Angulation or kinking of the jejunal loop
C. Duodenal stump leakage
D. Small bowel adhesions

83. In the patient in question 82, which of the following would be the preferred treatment?
A. Oversewing of the perforated ulcer with an omental patch and selective vagotomy if stable at the time of surgery
B. Vagotomy and antrectomy
C. Subtotal gastrectomy
D. Nasogastric suction, intravenous fluids, and antibiotics

84. In biopsy of the stomach to confirm a suspected diagnosis of chronic atrophic gastritis, the BEST site to sample is:
    A. Prepyloric area
    B. Body of stomach, lesser curve
    C. Body of stomach, greater curve
    D. Antrum, greater curve

85. Which of the following are TRUE statements regarding gastric outlet obstruction due to peptic ulcer disease?
    A. Obstruction is more common than perforation or hemorrhage.
    B. A saline load test is diagnostic for gastric outlet obstruction when at least 250 mL of the original 750 mL of normal saline instilled is recovered after 30 minutes.
    C. The majority of patients with gastric outlet obstruction due to peptic ulcer disease will require surgery despite initial successful medical management.
    D. Initial management of gastric outlet obstruction should be endoscopic dilation of the obstruction.
    E. Nocturnal vomiting and emesis containing food ingested more than 12 hours previously is highly suggestive of gastric outlet obstruction.

86. Which of the following statements regarding the risks of cigarette smoking are TRUE?
    I. Active cigarette smokers are at increased risk for both gastric and duodenal ulcers.
    II. Continued cigarette smoking delays ulcer healing.
    III. Compared with nonsmokers, smokers have more frequent recurrences of acute ulceration.
    IV. More than 50% of duodenal ulcer patients who continue to smoke after *Helicobacter pylori* eradication have a recurrent ulcer within one year.

    A. I and III
    B. II and IV
    C. I, II, and III
    D. All of the above

87. Which one of the following types of gastritis is MOST likely to be seen following a severe alcoholic binge?
    A. Hemorrhagic and erosive gastritis/gastropathy
    B. Nonerosive gastritis
    C. Specific (distinctive) gastritis

88. Which of the following are TRUE statements regarding the origin and location of gastrinomas?
    A. Gastrinomas arise from ectodermal tissues in the pancreas.
    B. The most common location of gastrinomas is the tail of the pancreas.
    C. Extrapancreatic gastrinomas occur in up to two thirds of patients with Zollinger-Ellison syndrome.
    D. Duodenal wall gastrinomas are easily identified by upper endoscopy.
    E. More than 90% of all gastrinomas are found in the "gastrinoma triangle."

89. A 35-year-old woman was noted to have chest pain and transient ischemic changes on electrocardiogram (ECG) while having a vaginal delivery under spinal anesthesia. After delivery she is alert, is normotensive, and is observed in the intensive care unit (ICU) while serial ECGs and cardiac enzyme levels are obtained. Which of the following would be appropriate prophylactic therapy to prevent development of ulcers while she is in the ICU?
    A. Misoprostol
    B. Omeprazole
    C. Intravenous H_2 receptor antagonists
    D. Sucralfate slurry
    E. None of the above

90. The MOST common islet cell tumor of the pancreas in multiple endocrine neoplasia–1 (MEN-1) syndrome is:
    A. Insulinoma
    B. Gastrinoma
    C. VIPoma
    D. Glucagonoma
    E. GRFoma

91. Anemia after partial gastrectomy is MOST commonly due to:
    A. Folate deficiency
    B. Iron deficiency
    C. Vitamin B_{12} deficiency
    D. Erythropoietin resistance
    E. Hemolysis

92. Which one of the following gastrinoma patients has a particular requirement for the MOST complete reduction of gastric acid secretion?
    A. A patient with residual unresected gastrinoma
    B. A patient with hypercalcemia secondary to parathyroid tumor
    C. A patient with severe acid reflux disease
    D. A patient who has developed refractoriness to H_2 receptor antagonist treatment
    E. A patient with basal acid output levels greater than 150 mEq/hr

93. Match each peptic ulcer complication with its associated clinical feature.
    1. Gastrocolic fistula   A. NSAID use
    2. Perforation   B. Succussion splash
    3. Intractability   C. Bacterial overgrowth
    4. Gastric outlet obstruction D. Peritonitis
    5. Hemorrhage   E. Shock

94. Concurrent administration of an H_2 receptor antagonist might result in decreased absorption or decreased efficacy of which of the following?
 I. Ketoconazole
 II. Phenytoin
 III. Omeprazole
 IV. Theophylline

 A. I and III
 B. II and IV
 C. I, II, and III
 D. All of the above

95. Omeprazole inhibits gastric acid secretion by:
 A. Decreasing gastrin production
 B. Decreasing histamine production
 C. Increasing prostaglandin secretion
 D. Increasing bicarbonate secretion
 E. None of the above

96. Ménétrier's disease is a hypertrophic gastropathy characterized by each of the following EXCEPT:
 A. Giant gastric folds in the fundus and body
 B. Hypochlorhydria, hypoalbuminemia
 C. Histologic evidence of foveolar hyperplasia
 D. Increased risk of gastric lymphoma
 E. Higher incidence in males with usual onset in middle age

97. Match each characteristic with the type of gastric cancer with which it is associated.
 1. Female predominance
 2. Antecedent metaplasia
 3. Signet ring cells
 4. Atrophic gastritis
 5. Better prognosis

 A. Intestinal type gastric carcinoma
 B. Diffuse type gastric carcinoma

98. Each of the following statements regarding the effects of vagotomy on gastric acid secretion is true EXCEPT:
 A. Vagotomy does not affect gastrin-mediated acid secretion.
 B. Sham feeding will stimulate less than 10% of the peak acid output after successful vagotomy.
 C. Gastric distention stimulates gastric acid secretion to a lesser degree after vagotomy.
 D. Maximal acid output decreases by 50% to 60% after truncal vagotomy.

99. Diagnostic tests that may aid in diagnosis of Zollinger-Ellison syndrome include each of the following EXCEPT:
 A. Upper gastrointestinal barium study
 B. Upper endoscopy
 C. Serum gastrin level
 D. Calcium infusion test
 E. Pepsin stimulation test

100. Which of the following are characteristics of postgastrectomy syndrome?
 A. Postprandial nausea and vomiting
 B. Exacerbated by complex carbohydrates
 C. Tachycardia, sweating, palpitations, and dizziness
 D. Worse after eating solids

101. Which of the follow are TRUE statements regarding truncal vagotomy?
 A. Vagotomy decreases acid secretion by parasympathetic denervation of parietal cell mass
 B. Vagotomy decreases neurogenically mediated release of gastrin.
 C. Vagotomy decreases parietal cell responsiveness to gastrin.
 D. Vagotomy increases antropyloric motility, thus contributing to the dumping syndrome and diarrhea.

102. Causes of recurrent duodenal or gastric ulcerations after ulcer surgery include each of the following EXCEPT:
 A. Retained distal antrum
 B. NSAID or aspirin use
 C. Gastrin level greater than 1000 pg/mL
 D. Retained proximal antrum
 E. Gastric cancer

103. A patient comes in for evaluation of dyspepsia. She tells you that aspirin, coffee, tea, and spicy foods aggravate her symptoms. She has taken no medicines in the past month. An upper gastrointestinal barium study reveals a duodenal ulcer. You start her on a course of therapy to heal her ulcer. Which of the following should be eliminated from her diet to reduce her risk of recurrent ulcer?
 I. Spicy foods
 II. Caffeinated beverages
 III. Foods with a high calcium content
 IV. Alcohol

 A. I and III
 B. II and IV
 C. I, II, and III
 D. IV only
 E. None of the above

104. Which of the following are TRUE causes of diarrhea or steatorrhea in Zollinger-Ellison syndrome?
 A. Direct secretory effect of circulating gastrin on the small bowel mucosa
 B. Inactivation of pancreatic enzymes at low pH
 C. Increased luminal flow rates due to hypersecretion
 D. Precipitation of bile salts at low pH

105. The completeness of vagotomy may be assessed by each of the following EXCEPT:
A. Sham feeding
B. Secretin stimulation test
C. Endoscopic application of Congo red dye
D. Insulin-induced hypoglycemia

106. A patient with known cancer of the gastric antrum undergoes endoscopic ultrasonography (EUS) for staging. EUS depicts a 2-cm hypoechoic mass extending into the muscularis propria. A single 3-cm round, well-demarcated node is noted at the gastroesophageal junction. Based on this information, the MOST appropriate TNM classification for this tumor is:
A. T2N1M0
B. T2N2M0
C. T2N3M0
D. T3N1M0
E. T3N2M0

107. The enteroendocrine cells, located in the crypts of the small bowel mucosa, are:
A. A homogeneous cell population by histochemical and morphologic criteria
B. Responsible for the production of a variety of gastrointestinal hormones
C. Primarily responsible for absorption of a variety of nutrients
D. Responsible for secreting mucus into the intestinal lumen
E. Involved in secreting digestive enzymes such as lactase and maltase into the lumen

108. Each of the following factors is associated with intractability of ulcer disease EXCEPT:
A. Smoking
B. NSAID use
C. *Helicobacter pylori*
D. Gastrin level greater than 1000 pg/mL
E. All of the above are associated with intractable ulcer disease.

109. Which of the following are TRUE statements regarding gastric cancer?
A. Patients younger than age 40 have a better prognosis.
B. Depth of invasion is the primary prognostic indicator.
C. Survival rates are similar for men and women.
D. Early gastric cancer is defined as penetrating only up to the muscularis propria.
E. Serum carcinoembryonic antigen levels greater than 5 ng/mL are found in nearly 50% of patients with resectable gastric cancer.

110. The MOST common site of peptic ulcer perforation is:
A. Anterior wall of the duodenal bulb
B. Antrum of the stomach
C. Body of the stomach, greater curve
D. Body of the stomach, lesser curve
E. Pyloric channel

111. Regarding the epidemiology of peptic ulcer, which of the following statements are TRUE?
   I. Lifetime prevalence of peptic ulcer is 5% to 10%.
   II. Lifetime prevalence of peptic ulcer is higher for females than for males.
   III. There is a familial clustering of peptic ulcers.
   IV. Prevalence of peptic ulcer increases with advancing age for females but not for males.

A. I and III
B. II and IV
C. I, II, and III
D. All of the above

112. Each of the following is an appropriate surgical therapy for gastrinoma EXCEPT:
A. Total gastrectomy with proximal vagotomy for patients with biochemical evidence of gastrinoma but no tumor at the time of surgery
B. Enucleation of solitary gastrinomas present in the head or body of the pancreas
C. Duodenal resection for multiple gastrinomas in the duodenal wall
D. Partial hepatic resection for a single hepatic metastasis

113. Match each substance with the gastric mucosal cell from which it is secreted.
1. Gastrin   A. Parietal cell
2. Somatostatin   B. Enterochromaffin-like (ECL)
3. Histamine   cell
4. Glucagon   C. D cell
5. Acid   D. G cell
6. Intrinsic factor   E. A cell

114. A 64-year-old woman has upper endoscopy to evaluate epigastric pain and weight loss. Markedly abnormal rugal folds are noted without frank ulceration. Multiple biopsy specimens, obtained using large biopsy forceps, show no malignancy. Endoscopic ultrasonography shows marked thickening of the third (middle) layer of the mucosa. The muscularis propria is intact. Which of the following are potential diagnoses?
A. Melanoma

B. Ménétrier's disease
C. Lymphoma
D. Gastritis
E. Metastatic breast cancer
F. Gastric cancer

---

115. Which of the following statements regarding gastroduodenal secretion in duodenal ulcer patients are TRUE?
 I. On average, maximal acid output is greater in duodenal ulcer patients than in nonulcer subjects.
 II. On average, nocturnal acid secretion is greater in duodenal ulcer patients than in nonulcer subjects.
 III. On average, proximal duodenal bicarbonate secretion is lower in duodenal ulcer patients than in nonulcer subjects.
 IV. Elevated gastric acid secretion in duodenal ulcer patients is a consequence of *Helicobacter pylori* infection.

 A. I and III
 B. II and IV
 C. I, II, and III
 D. All of the above

---

116. Which of the following nutrients is the MOST potent stimulator of gastric acid secretion?
 A. Fats
 B. Ethanol
 C. Carbohydrates
 D. Proteins
 E. Saline

---

117. A 60-year-old man is referred for evaluation of three months of upper abdominal discomfort and mild weight loss. An upper gastrointestinal series reveals thickened gastric folds involving the fundus and body of the stomach. Which of the following is the LEAST likely diagnosis?
 A. Ménétrier's disease
 B. Lymphoma
 C. Adenocarcinoma
 D. Zollinger-Ellison syndrome
 E. Granulomatous gastritis

---

118. Gastric hamartomas are associated with all of the following inherited disorders EXCEPT:
 A. Gardner's syndrome
 B. Peutz-Jeghers syndrome
 C. Familial polyposis
 D. Cronkhite-Canada syndrome
 E. Cowden's disease

---

119. Which of the following are TRUE statements regarding serum gastrin?
 A. A level of more than 200 pg/mL is virtually diagnostic of Zollinger-Ellison syndrome.
 B. An increase to more than 300 pg/mL after protein-meal ingestion is diagnostic of antral G-cell hyperplasia.
 C. Levels may be modestly elevated after vagotomy.
 D. Basal levels are higher after truncal vagotomy with pyloroplasty than after truncal vagotomy with antrectomy.

Stomach and Duodenum

━━━*Answers*

(1–B)   **(S&F, p. 669)**

The patient has peritoneal signs, including fever, abdominal pain, and rebound tenderness, suggesting a perforation. Peritoneal irritation is also suggested by the preferential flexion at the hips and knees. Contributing factors include a history of NSAID use. Nausea and vomiting may be due to ileus. Hematemesis may be secondary to continuous nausea and vomiting and resultant Mallory-Weiss tear. The patient has no evidence of actively bleeding peptic ulcer or gastric outlet obstruction.

(2–C)   **(S&F, pp. 668–669)**

Plain abdominal films may demonstrate free air or ileus. Gastrografin upper gastrointestinal series may demonstrate the site of perforation. Peritoneal lavage may demonstrate bile-stained fluid with low glucose concentrations or bacteria. An elevated serum amylase level may be present, which reflects absorption of salivary and pancreatic amylase through the peritoneum. Upper endoscopy is contraindicated in the presence of a perforation.

(3–E)   **(S&F, p. 705)**

Volume replacement and correction of electrolyte abnormalities is essential for successful treatment of perforated ulcers. Continuous nasogastric suction decreases fluid output through perforation and relieves symptoms relating to paralytic ileus. Broad-spectrum antibiotics are important for preventing bacterial peritonitis after soilage by gastric contents. In the very ill patient, exploratory laparotomy is warranted to identify the site of perforation and for repair. Because endoscopy is contraindicated, severe bleeding should be treated with surgical exploration.

(4–1-D, 2-B, 3-A)   **(S&F, pp. 611–612)**

If bacterial urease is present in a mucosal biopsy specimen, incubation in a medium containing urea will liberate ammonia and carbon dioxide. The ammonia raises the pH of the medium and changes a pH-sensitive indicator (phenol red) from yellow to red. In the urea breath test, urea labeled with either carbon-13 (a stable isotope) or carbon-14 (a radioactive isotope) is ingested with a liquid meal to retard gastric emptying. If urease is present, ingested urea is metabolized to ammonia and labeled carbon dioxide. The labeled carbon dioxide is absorbed into the circulation and expired into the breath where it is detected by mass spectrophotometry in the case of carbon-13 or scintillation counting in the case of carbon-14. A variety of histologic stains will directly identify *Helicobacter pylori* on mucosal biopsy. These include the hematoxylin and eosin, Giemsa, and Warthin-Starry silver stains.

━━━**Reference**

Brown, K. E., Peura, D. A. Diagnosis of *Helicobacter pylori* infection. Gastroenterol. Clin. North Am. 22:105, 1993.

(5–A)   **(S&F, pp. 663–664)**

At this time, misoprostol at a dose of 200 μg q.i.d. is the only agent demonstrated to prevent NSAID-induced gastric and duodenal ulcers. H₂ receptor antagonists can prevent NSAID-induced duodenal ulcers but not NSAID-induced gastric ulcers. Omeprazole is being evaluated for this use, but reports have yet to be published.

(6–C)   **(S&F, pp. 608–609)**

Most patients with *Helicobacter pylori* infection are asymptomatic with normal endoscopic findings. Endoscopic biopsy typically shows chronic superficial gastritis and the presence of organisms. An association with gastric and duodenal ulcer disease is present, but the majority of infected persons have no ulcers. Although patients with atrophic gastritis may have immunologic evidence of prior *H. pylori* infection, the atrophic mucosa is inhospitable to *H. pylori* and organisms are rarely demonstrated.

(7–D)   **(S&F, pp. 655–656)**

Ten to 20 percent of patients fail to respond to "triple therapy" for *Helicobacter pylori* infection, and failure rates are higher after recent antibiotic use or prior treatment attempts. Reinfection rates are 0.5% to 3% per year or less. Rapid urease testing of antral biopsy specimens and urea breath tests have a sensitivity and specificity that is approximately 95%. Thus, within the first year after eradication therapy, a positive urease test is more likely a reflection of failure to cure the infection than of reinfection or of a false-positive test. After eradication of *H. pylori* in duodenal ulcer patients, gastric acid secretion does not increase and often decreases.

━━━**References**

Borody, T. J., Andrews, P., Manusco, N., et al. *Helicobacter pylori* reinfection rate in patients with cured duodenal ulcer. Am. J. Gastroenterol. 89:529, 1994.

Brown, K. E., Peura, D. A. Diagnosis of *Helicobacter pylori* infection. Gastroenterol. Clin. North Am. 22:105, 1993.

Cutler, A., Shubert, T. T. Long-term *Helicobacter pylori* recurrence after successful eradication with triple therapy. Am. J. Gastroenterol. 88:1359, 1993.

McColl, K. E. L., Fullarton, G. M., Chittajalu, A. M., et al. Plasma gastrin, daytime intragastric pH and nocturnal acid output before and at one and seven months after eradication of *Helicobacter pylori* in duodenal ulcer subjects. Scand. J. Gastroenterol. 26:339, 1991.

Moss, S. F., Calam, J. Acid secretion and sensitivity to gastrin in patients with duodenal ulcer: Effect of eradication of *Helicobacter pylori*. Gut 34:888, 1993.

(8–C)   *(S&F, pp. 687–690)*

Omeprazole is the treatment of choice for acid hypersecretion and its complications in patients with Zollinger-Ellison syndrome. Isolated hepatic metastases may be resected successfully with cure in selected patients with metastatic gastrinoma. Because the majority of extrapancreatic gastrinomas are in the duodenal wall, all exploratory surgeries should include duodenotomy and careful examination of the duodenal wall. Hepatic artery embolization has no established role in the treatment of metastatic gastrinoma.

(9–B)   *(S&F, pp. 653–656)*

Refractory ulcers may result from a hypersecretory state such as a gastrinoma. In cases of refractory duodenal ulceration not related to gastrinoma, evidence has been presented for and against a role for basal and nocturnal acid hypersecretion or an increased maximal acid output. In patients suspected to have gastrinoma, measurement of serum gastrin is a more sensitive and specific method than gastric secretory analysis to identify such patients and, therefore, is the preferred initial test when this potential diagnosis is being evaluated. Cigarette smoking may impair ulcer healing while on therapy, and cessation of smoking is probably useful in assisting ulcer healing. Although the available H_2 receptor antagonists vary in potency and duration of action, when evaluated in controlled trials, there have been no clear advantages of one agent over another. Eradication of *Helicobacter pylori* will enhance healing of ulcers refractory to conventional therapy; thus testing for *H. pylori* or, with duodenal ulcers, empirical antimicrobial therapy would be reasonable.

(10–E)   *(S&F, p. 643)*

Once the diagnosis of duodenal ulcer has been made, a follow-up study is not necessary to establish healing in patients who become symptom free. With giant duodenal or gastric ulcers or with ulcers involving complications, particularly in medically frail patients, a follow-up study may be warranted to establish healing.

After successful eradication of *Helicobacter pylori* there is a slow decline of IgG antibody titers with time. However, serologic studies do not become negative until 6 to 12 months after eradication, making *H. pylori* serum antibodies an unsuitable test for evaluation of *H. pylori* eradication. The least invasive method of confirming eradication of *H. pylori* in patients who have continuing symptoms after treatment is the ^{13}C-urea breath test.

■■■■ Reference

Cutler, A., Schubert, A., and Schubert, T. Role of *Helicobacter pylori* serology in evaluating treatment success. Dig. Dis. Sci. *38*:2262, 1993.

(11–A)   *(S&F, p. 606)*

Acute infection with *Helicobacter pylori* is rarely detected clinically, and most of what is known about the initial stages of the infection is from deliberate or accidental exposure in research settings. Nausea, vomiting, and moderate epigastric pain followed by profound hypochlorhydria lasting for many weeks is typical. Acute infection with *H. pylori* causes an intense neutrophilic gastritis, not mild lymphocytic infiltration; and seroconversion is rapid, as would be expected by a brisk inflammatory response in the mucosa.

(12–None are true)   *(S&F, pp. 686–687)*

Despite clinical and laboratory evidence suggesting the presence of a gastrinoma, 40% to 45% of patients have no identifiable tumor at exploratory laparotomy. Computed tomography is successful in identifying gastrinoma in only 30% of cases later found surgically and is unable to detect tumors smaller than 1 cm. Selective angiography is able to identify up to 33% of tumors identified at surgery, with poor detection of tumors smaller than 2 cm. Magnetic resonance imaging is considerably less sensitive than computed tomography, and tumors larger than 3 cm are detected successfully only 50% of the time.

(13–B)   *(S&F, pp. 655–666)*

Prior to 1994, there were ample data to recommend any of the four H_2 receptor antagonists, antacids, sucralfate, or omeprazole as initial therapy for the first presentation of duodenal ulcer. However, since that time, the NIH Consensus Development Panel on *Helicobacter pylori* in Peptic Ulcer Disease has recommended that "all patients with gastric or duodenal ulcers who are infected with *H. pylori* should be treated with antimicrobials regardless of whether they are suffering from the initial presentation of the disease or from a recurrence." Antibiotics should be combined with an antisecretory drug in this case.

■■■■ Reference

National Institutes of Health Consensus Development Panel on *Helicobacter pylori* in Peptic Ulcer Disease. NIH Consensus conference: *Helicobacter pylori* in peptic ulcer disease. JAMA *272*:65, 1994.

(14–C)   *(S&F, pp. 749–750)*

In a nested case-control study, patients with gastric non-Hodgkin's lymphoma had higher rates of positive serology for *Helicobacter pylori* than did matched controls without lymphoma. In the same study, patients with nongastric lymphomas did not have a higher rate of *H. pylori* infection. MALT lymphomas are low-grade B-cell lymphomas that arise from lymphoid aggregates in the gastric lamina propria. Lymphoid tissue is normally absent in gastric tissue not infected with *H. pylori* but is acquired in response to *H. pylori* gastritis. Almost all cases of MALT lymphomas are associated with an *H. pylori* infection, and some will regress when the infection is treated. Gastric lymphoma is rare in western countries. A region in Europe with a high incidence of gastric non-Hodgkin's lymphoma also had a higher rate of *H. pylori* infection than a region with low incidence of this lymphoma.

■■References

Doglioni, C., Wotherspoon, A. C., Moschini, A., et al. High incidence of primary gastric lymphoma in northeastern Italy. Lancet *339*:834, 1992.
Parsonent, J., Hansen, S., Rodriguez, B. S., et al. *Helicobacter pylori* infection and gastric lymphoma. N. Engl. J. Med. *330*:1267, 1994.
Wotherspoon, A. C., Ortiz-Hidalgo, C., Falzom, M. R., et al. *Helicobacter pylori*–associated gastritis and primary B-cell gastric lymphoma. Lancet *338*:1175, 1991.

(15–B)   (S&F, pp. 663–664)

A previous history of peptic ulcer disease is associated with a markedly increased risk of NSAID-induced ulcers. When NSAIDs must be used in this population, concurrent prophylactic therapy is prudent. Neither smoking, alcohol, nor *Helicobacter pylori* infection has been shown to increase the risk of developing NSAID-induced ulcers. The clinical impression that NSAID ulcers occur more commonly in the elderly probably reflects increased exposure, because elderly people take more NSAIDs than younger people. The presence or absence of dyspeptic symptoms does not predict with any degree of certainty which NSAID users are at risk for development of NSAID-induced ulcers. Although there is an association of blood group O with duodenal ulcers, this blood type has not been shown to increase risk for NSAID-induced ulceration.

(16–D)   (S&F, pp. 614–615)

Traditional triple therapy with bismuth, metronidazole, and tetracycline with or without a proton pump inhibitor has an acceptable eradication rate, as does the combination of clarithromycin, amoxicillin, and omeprazole. Although metronidazole resistance is common, the drug seems to still be effective if given with the other agents. Dual therapy with omeprazole and amoxicillin is ineffective in half of patients.

■■References

Graham, D. Y., Lew, G. M., Klein, P. D., et al. Effect of treatment of *Helicobacter pylori* infection on the long-term recurrence of gastric or duodenal ulcer: A randomized controlled study. Ann. Intern. Med. *116*:705, 1992.
Labenz, J., Gyenes, E., Ruhl, G. H., Borsch, G. Amoxicillin plus omeprazole versus triple therapy for eradication of *Helicobacter pylori* in duodenal ulcer disease: A prospective, randomized, and controlled study. Gut *34*:1167, 1993.
Labenz, J., Gyenes, E., Ruhl, G. H., Borsch, G. Omeprazole plus amoxicillin eradicates *Helicobacter pylori* in gastric ulcer disease. Am. J. Gastroenterol. *88*:491, 1993.
Tygat, G. N. J. Treatments that impact favorably upon the eradication of *Helicobacter pylori* and ulcer recurrence. Aliment. Pharmacol. Ther. *8*:359, 1994.

(17–C)   (S&F, pp. 655–656)

Duodenal ulcer healing in response to H_2 receptor antagonists is slightly accelerated when ulcers are also treated with antimicrobial agents directed against *Helicobacter pylori*. When *H. pylori* infection is cured, the active polymorphonuclear (PMN) component of gastric and duodenal inflammation clears. When *H. pylori* is not cured, the active PMN gastroduodenal inflammation is not affected. MALT lymphomas, a subgroup of B-cell lymphomas that arise from lymphoid aggregates, have been observed to regress in response to treatment of *H. pylori* infection. Although *H. pylori* is associated with gastric adenocarcinoma, there are no similar data to suggest that *H. pylori* eradication will cause regression of this cancer.

■■Reference

Wotherspoon, A.C., Doglioni, C., Diss, T. C., et al. Regression of primary low-grade B-cell gastric lymphoma of mucosa-associated lymphoid tissue type after eradication of *Helicobacter pylori*. Lancet *342*:575, 1993.

(18–D)   (S&F, pp. 698–700)

Because proximal vagotomy preserves normal innervation and function of the antrum, dumping syndrome and postoperative diarrhea are significantly less common (2%–3%) when compared with truncal vagotomy with antrectomy or drainage procedure (12%–23%). Also, the absence of resection or a drainage procedure eliminates complications due to anastomotic leakage or jejunal limb obstruction. A laparoscopic approach to proximal gastric vagotomy is feasible and greatly reduces time in hospital. The criminal nerves of Grassi represent small branches of the vagus nerve that originate near the distal esophagus and branch to innervate the cardia and greater curvature. Failure to interrupt these nerves may result in ulcer recurrence.

(19–D)   (S&F, p. 613)

In this age range, the presence of a gastric ulcer warrants histologic examination to exclude a malignancy. Because an endoscopy is already being done, the least expensive means of establishing the presence of *Helicobacter pylori* would be with a rapid urease test. Because the sensitivity of the rapid urease test is not 100%, it is easy to obtain antral biopsy speciens from normal-appearing mucosa and hold those specimens until the results of the urease test are known. If the results are negative, then the antral biopsy specimens should be submitted for histologic examination to exclude a false-negative rapid urease test.

(20–B)   (S&F, pp. 624–626)

Helicobacter pylori infection increases serum gastrin concentrations in both normal subjects and duodenal ulcer patients. This has been demonstrated by assessing gastrin concentrations in the same person before and after eradication. Serum gastrin concentrations in normal *H. pylori*–infected subjects, although higher than those in noninfected subjects, are still generally within the normal range for serum gastrin (5 to 80 pg/mL). The magnitude of *H. pylori*–induced hypergastrinemia in most normal and duodenal ulcer subjects is not sufficient to enhance acid secretion.

(21–D)   (S&F, pp. 641–643)

In patients with simple dyspepsia, especially in those younger than 40 years old, most experts now recommend deferring diagnostic procedures and giving an initial trial of antiulcer therapy as the most cost-effective option. Diagnostic evaluation can be reserved for those who fail empirical treatment.

(22–C) **(S&F, pp. 659–660)**

Most gastric ulcers heal with 8 to 12 weeks of treatment with an H₂ receptor antagonist. When ulcers prove refractory to medical management, attention should be directed to patient compliance, possible malignancy, NSAID use, continued smoking, unusual infections, inflammatory processes, and gastrinoma. Even with a recent negative aspirin history, salicylate levels should be checked to exclude aspirin use. Previous benign biopsy specimens do not fully exclude a malignant gastric ulcer; thus biopsy of multiple specimens should be repeated. Regardless of biopsy results, surgical excision is a reasonable approach for refractory gastric ulcer in patients who can tolerate surgery. However, surgical excision is not warranted until at least another 6 to 8 weeks of high-dose acid-suppressive therapy has been given and until *Helicobacter pylori* infection has been treated, if present.

(23–C) **(S&F, pp. 647–649)**

Normally, gastrin secretion from the antral mucosa is inhibited by gastric acid. The absence of feedback inhibition by acid leads to hypergastrinemia. With two to four months of omeprazole therapy, serum gastrin concentrations rise three-fold to four-fold on average. A possible consequence of hypergastrinemia is hyperplasia of enterochromaffin-like (ECL) cells located in the oxyntic mucosa of the stomach and, of greater concern, carcinoid tumor formation. Carcinoid tumor formation has only been observed in patients with hypergastrinemia due to pernicious anemia or gastrinoma. With short courses of omeprazole (two to four months), no carcinoid tumors nor changes in ECL-cell density have been observed. The greater density of gastric bacterial flora that develops during omeprazole therapy may also create problems. Studies suggest that aspiration is much more likely to lead to severe pulmonary infection if the patient is taking antisecretory drugs. The gastric flora may also convert dietary nitrate to N-nitroso compounds, which are known carcinogens in animal models. However, no evidence exists in humans to suggest a causal relationship between antiulcer therapy and gastric cancer.

(24–A or C) **(S&F, pp. 657–658)**

Sucralfate and antacids appear to be safe during pregnancy. Animal studies show no teratogenic effects from constant ingestion of antacids during pregnancy. Adverse effects of antacids during pregnancy include interference with iron absorption and, with sodium bicarbonate, metabolic alkalosis and fluid overload in both the fetus and mother. H₂ receptor antagonists cross the placenta and are excreted in breast milk. There are reports of cimetidine and ranitidine being used in pregnancy; however, controlled studies in pregnant humans are not available. The H₂ receptor antagonists as a group are category B with respect to

pregnancy, and, thus, these agents should not be used as first-line ulcer therapy in pregnancy. Omeprazole, when given in very high doses to pregnant animals, produces dose-related fetal toxicity. There are no human data on use of omeprazole during pregnancy, and it is listed as a category C drug with respect to pregnancy and thus should be considered unsafe for use in pregnancy.

■ **Reference**

Baron, T. H., Ramirez, B., and Richter, J. E. Gastrointestinal motility disorders during pregnancy. Ann. Intern. Med. *118*:366, 1993.

(25–A, C) **(S&F, pp. 608–609)**

Most individuals with *Helicobacter pylori* infection remain asymptomatic, but the natural history is not as benign as stated because one sixth (not 3%) eventually develop duodenal ulcers. Chronic *H. pylori* infection has been epidemiologically linked to adenocarcinoma of all parts of the stomach except the cardia.

(26–B) **(S&F, p. 631)**

Helicobacter pylori infection is found in more than 80% of children with duodenal ulcer. A positive family history is common and reflects familial clustering of *H. pylori*. Childhood gastric ulcer is very unusual. Childhood duodenal ulceration is often manifested as nocturnal pain without classic dyspepsia.

(27–1-B, 2-A, 3-A, 4-C, 5-B) **(S&F, pp. 712–713)**

All types of gastritis or gastropathy can be classified as (1) erosive and hemorrhagic gastritis/gastropathy, (2) nonerosive gastritis, or (3) distinctive (specific) gastritis. Stress, physical trauma to the stomach, corrosives, alcohol, and some drugs such as NSAIDs cause erosive and hemorrhagic gastritis/gastropathy. Generally, the endoscopic and histologic appearance is indistinguishable as to etiology. *Helicobacter pylori* gastritis and atrophic gastritis (as seen in pernicious anemia) are examples of nonerosive gastritis.

(28–C) **(S&F, p. 712)**

Hemorrhagic and erosive gastritis is most often diagnosed on the basis of the endoscopic appearance. These findings can be seen in a variety of clinical settings. Stress lesions, aspirin and NSAIDs, ischemia, and corrosive ingestion produce a variety of endoscopic findings, including multiple ulcerations, hemorrhage, petechiae, and erosions. In contrast, *Helicobacter pylori* does not ordinarily produce a hemorrhagic or erosive gastritis. The gastritis of *H. pylori* infection is generally nonspecific and requires histologic confirmation.

(29–A) **(S&F, p. 613)**

Despite emerging resistance to both metronidazole and clarithromycin, these agents remain mainstays of therapy; indeed, all successful regimens use one or both of these drugs. It is true that as of now, all proposed one-week regimens that actually work require three or four drugs, usually two antibiotics and one or two adjunctive agents such as bismuth, a proton pump inhibitor, or an H_2 receptor antagonist.

(30–1-A, 2-D, 3-B, 4-C) (S&F, pp. 624–625, 649)

Omeprazole is a weak base that is concentrated in the acid compartments of the parietal cell. With a pKa of 4.0, omeprazole rapidly permeates plasma membranes as an uncharged molecule at neutral pH. When it encounters the acidic compartments within the parietal cell that contain the proton pump, however, it ionizes, becoming trapped and concentrated. The best choice is the lowest pH listed of 2.0. Because omeprazole is acid labile, it can be inactivated if permitted to dissolve in the acidic gastric juice. Thus, oral preparations are packaged in enteric-coated granules that do not dissolve until they encounter a pH above 6 in the intestine. Through meta-analysis, a correlation has been demonstrated between ulcer healing and (1) the magnitude of acid suppression, (2) the duration of acid suppression, and (3) the length of therapy. In ordinary duodenal ulcer healing, there is little further increase in healing rate when gastric pH is elevated above pH 3 or when acidity is suppressed for more than 18 hours each day. Thus, the best answer for optimal ulcer healing was a pH of 3.0. Early studies with antacids indicated that gastric bleeding in patients in intensive care units was reduced when the gastric pH was maintained at more than 3.5, a pH level above which gastric pepsin activity is markedly reduced. Thus the best answer for the prophylaxis of stress ulcers is a pH of 4.0.

(31–B) (S&F, pp. 604–619)

Colonization with *Helicobacter pylori* has been demonstrated on ectopic gastric mucosa found in Barrett's esophagus, Meckel's diverticulum, and duodenal metaplasia, but not in areas of intestinal metaplasia of the stomach. Biopsy specimens taken from the antral mucosa immediately proximal to the pylorus have the highest yield unless the patient is taking proton pump inhibitors. In this case, samples from the gastric body are more sensitive. Serologic markers for *H. pylori* are both sensitive and specific for the presence of the infection in previously untreated individuals, exceeding 90% for both. The organisms are noninvasive and ordinarily reside within the gastric mucus on the gastric surface and in the gastric pits.

(32–C) (S&F, pp. 622–624, 633–634)

In developed countries such as the United States, the prevalence of *Helicobacter pylori* infection in asymptomatic individuals is 10% to 20% and increases by about 1% per year to more than 50% by age 60. The higher rate in older persons may reflect a cohort phenomenon because there is a higher rate of exposure and infection at younger ages. Ulcer size is unaffected by *H. pylori* infection.

(33–1-D, 2-E, 3-B, 4-C) (S&F, pp. 661–665)

When NSAID-induced ulcers are treated with omeprazole, NSAID treatment may be continued without slowing ulcer healing. The natural history of untreated duodenal ulcer is for intervals of exacerbation and remission. Greater than 90% of these ulcers are associated with *Helicobacter pylori*. Eradication of *H. pylori* drastically reduces recurrences of duodenal ulcer. Misoprostol will effectively prevent NSAID-induced gastric and duodenal ulcer.

(34–D) (S&F, p. 712)

Nonerosive gastritis is a histologic diagnosis that can be classified by topographic location and by level of mucosal involvement. The endoscopic findings are generally nonspecific and thus require both clinical and histologic information for diagnosis. Severe atrophic gastritis, with or without associated pernicious anemia, postgastrectomy gastritis, and *Helicobacter pylori* gastritis all have the same appearance endoscopically. "Alcoholic gastritis" is a misnomer because little inflammatory infiltrate is present with the erosions or subepithelial hemorrhages. Gastric lesions due to alcohol are classified as erosive or hemorrhagic gastritis/gastropathy.

(35–E) (S&F, pp. 655–656)

No monotherapy has a cure rate high enough to be acceptable for treating *Helicobacter pylori* infection. A treatment regimen can be considered useful if it cures the infection in 80% or more of infected patients. Bismuth or amoxicillin alone are effective in only 20%, whereas clarithromycin, 500 mg q.i.d., eradicates the organism in up to 50% of *H. pylori*-infected subjects. The lower dose of clarithromycin in this question, 500 mg b.i.d., is associated with only a 15% cure rate. Omeprazole, when given alone, appears to suppress but not eradicate the bacteria.

References

Peterson, W. L., Graham, D. Y., Marshall, B., et al. Clarithromycin as monotherapy for eradication of *Helicobacter pylori*: A randomized, double-blind trial. Am. J. Gastroenterol. 88:1860, 1993.

Tygat, G. N. J. Treatments that impact favorably upon the eradication of *Helicobacter pylori* and ulcer recurrence. Aliment. Pharmacol. Ther. 8:359, 1994.

(36–C) (S&F, p. 706)

Truncal vagotomy with antrectomy has the lowest postoperative ulcer recurrence rate (0%–2%), with proximal gastric vagotomy having the highest postoperative recurrence rate (10%–17%, depending on the skill of the operator).

(37–B) (S&F, pp. 662–663)

This patient's duodenal ulcer is most likely NSAID-induced, because urease testing was negative for *Helicobacter pylori*. When NSAID use can be discontinued, NSAID-induced ulcers will heal readily when treated with an H_2 receptor antagonist with a healing rate similar to that of ulcers not related to NSAID use. Limited data exist on the use of misoprostol to heal NSAID-induced ulcers.

(38–D)   **(S&F, pp. 662–663)**

As in the previous case, this patient most likely has a NSAID-induced gastric ulcer. When NSAID therapy must be continued, healing of gastric and duodenal ulcers can occur with H_2 receptor antagonists, but the rate of healing is slower than if NSAID use had been discontinued. In such cases, treatment of NSAID-induced ulcers with omeprazole (at a dose of 40 mg/day) results in healing rates of gastric ulcer that are the same as those seen when NSAID use is discontinued. Hence, omeprazole at a dose of 40 mg/day would be the treatment of choice.

(39–1-C, 2-D, 3-E, 4-A, 5-B)   **(S&F, pp. 719–722)**

Herpes simplex virus infection rarely involves the stomach alone but may occur as part of a disseminated process in immunocompromised patients.

(40–D)   **(S&F, p. 692)**

Like Zollinger-Ellison syndrome, antral G-cell hyperplasia causes elevated serum gastrin levels and gastric hypersecretion. Unlike gastrinoma, however, antral G-cell hyperplasia is not associated with an exaggerated increase in serum gastrin levels after secretin administration.

(41–B)   **(S&F, pp. 718–719)**

Both pernicious anemia and severe atrophic gastritis without pernicious anemia are characterized by achlorhydria, atrophic gastric mucosa, and hypergastrinemia. Autoimmune antibodies, prominent in pernicious anemia, are also frequently present in severe atrophic gastritis, suggesting that pernicious anemia may develop with time. The major difference is whether damage is sufficient to block release of intrinsic factor required for vitamin B_{12} absorption.

(42–1-A, 2-E, 3-D, 4-B)   **(S&F, pp. 645–651)**

Cimetidine can produce gynecomastia and impotence. However, gynecomastia is rare with less than eight weeks of therapy at normal doses of cimetidine. With sucralfate at the usual dose of 4 g/day, serum and urine aluminum levels increase. Aluminum is readily excreted by normal kidneys. Thus, any body burden of aluminum is normally eliminated within a few weeks after discontinuation of therapy. However, significant retention can occur with renal failure, resulting in possible neurotoxicity and brain deposition of aluminum. The most frequent side effects of prostaglandin analogs are crampy abdominal pain and diarrhea, both of which are dose dependent and more common at the start of therapy. This class of drugs also has uterotropic effects and may result in uterine cramping, bleeding, or spontaneous abortions. With calcium carbonate antacids, ingestion of large amounts of calcium and absorbable alkali can lead to hypercalcemia, alkalosis, and renal impairment—the milk-alkali syndrome.

(43–B)   **(S&F, p. 666)**

All of the statements are correct except for the timing of the aspiration, which should be done 30 minutes after instillation of the saline. The test is indeed useful to follow patients for response to medical therapy.

(44–B, C, D)   **(S&F, pp. 645–647)**

Famotidine has the longest serum half-life of the H_2 blockers available in the United States, but all H_2 blockers have similar efficacy when given once daily. The half-life of each of the H_2 receptor antagonists falls within the one-to four-hour range. Cimetidine and ranitidine compete with creatinine for renal tubular secretion. With oral administration, bioavailability is reduced 30% to 60% by first-pass hepatic metabolism. With intravenous administration, there is no first-pass effect. Thus, the intravenous dose of cimetidine, famotidine, and ranitidine is smaller than the orally administered dose. Because orally administered nizatidine undergoes little hepatic metabolism, its bioavailability after oral dosing is 100%. H_2 receptor antagonists inhibit gastric mucosal alcohol dehydrogenase, thereby increasing plasma concentrations of alcohol.

(45–A)   **(S&F, pp. 703–704)**

Age greater than 60 years is associated with increased mortality from hemorrhage and from postoperative complications but is not an independent risk factor. Most complications reflect coexisting disease. Chronological age is less important than cardiovascular condition.

(46–E)   **(S&F, pp. 683–684)**

Most clinical manifestations of Zollinger-Ellison syndrome reflect excess gastric acid secretion. Diarrhea reflects the large volume of gastric secretions, malabsorption due to inactivation of pancreatic enzymes and bile acids at low pH, and direct inhibition of small bowel absorption by gastrin. Abdominal pain often reflects active peptic disease of the duodenum or jejunum. Pyrosis due to acid reflux into the esophagus is common. Urticaria is not associated with Zollinger-Ellison syndrome. Its presence suggests systemic mastocytosis, a disease in which gastric hypersecretion is due to increased histamine levels.

(47–E)   **(S&F, pp. 679–680)**

Peptic ulcer disease due to hyperacidity is one of the hallmarks of Zollinger-Ellison syndrome. The trophic effect of hypergastrinemia results in a greatly expanded parietal cell mass, enterochromaffin-like (ECL)-cell hyperplasia, and an increased risk of gastric carcinoid.

(48–1-D, 2-B, 3-E)   **(S&F, pp. 744–745)**

Endoscopic ultrasonography has emerged as an important tool for evaluating gastric mass lesions. An important feature is the specific histologic wall layer involved. A lipoma is an abnormal growth within the submucosa, the middle, hyperechoic (white) layer. A gastric varix is a vascular (hypoechoic-dark) structure located within the first dark layer of the gastric wall (the deep mucosa). Leiomyoma arises from the muscularis propria, the outer dark layer.

(49–1-E, 2-C, 3-A, 4-B, 5-D)   *Cocaine (S&F, p. 630)*
NSAIDs (S&F, p. 629)
Helicobacter pylori (S&F, p. 623)
MEN-1 (S&F, p. 682)

Acute cocaine toxicity and other forms of stress cause ulcers primarily by compromising mesenteric blood flow. Reduced blood flow not only may cause ischemia but may also interfere with delivery of bicarbonate and removal of acid absorbed across the mucosal barrier. Central nervous system injury appears to cause gastric acid hypersecretion by a vagally mediated phenomenon independent of gastrin levels. Systemically administered NSAIDs produce ulcers through suppression of gastroduodenal mucosal prostaglandin synthesis, which is necessary to maintain normal bicarbonate and mucus secretion, blood flow, and regeneration. Gastrinoma is the most common pancreatic tumor in patients with multiple endocrine neoplasia (MEN) type-1. A gastrinoma produces hypergastrinemia and typically elevates gastric acid secretion. A common presentation of gastrinoma in patients with MEN-1 is peptic ulceration.

(50–C)   **(S&F, pp. 639–640)**

Even when a gastric ulcer appears benign by radiography, up to 7% prove to be malignant. Mucosal folds that are effaced, interrupted, fused, or nodular as they approach the margin of the ulcer crater suggest malignancy. A fairly reliable but insensitive radiographic feature that suggests benign disease is Hampton's sign, a radiolucent line about 1 mm in width that rims the mouth of the ulcer crater and results from undermining of normal mucosa. Negative, irregular filling defects in the ulcer crater indicate malignancy. However, an irregular ulcer base may also result from blood clots, granulation tissue, or debris.

(51–C)   **(S&F, pp. 634–635)**

An increased risk of duodenal, but not gastric, ulcers has been reported after renal transplantation. Peptic ulcer in uremia is not linked to *Helicobacter pylori*. The frequency of antibodies to *H. pylori* is similar in renal failure patients with and without peptic ulcer. There is an increased incidence of both gastric and duodenal ulcers in cirrhosis. Peptic ulcers occur in up to 30% of patients with chronic pulmonary disease, and the frequency of chronic lung disease in peptic ulcer patients is increased two- to threefold. This association may be, in part, related to cigarette smoking. Increased risk of peptic ulcers is associated with multiple endocrine neoplasia (MEN)–1 (which includes gastrinomas) but not MEN-2.

(52–C)   **(S&F, p. 630)**

In the oxyntic mucosa, histamine is present and released from both mast cells and enterochromaffin-like cells. An increased rate of peptic ulcer disease has been reported in myeloproliferative disorders associated with basophilia.

Cases of basophilic leukemia and chronic myelogenous leukemia with marked basophilia have been reported in association with increased gastric acid secretion and increased serum or urine histamine concentrations. Increased risk of peptic ulcer and increased acid secretion and histamine concentrations are also found in systemic mastocytosis. There is no known association of NSAIDs with increased histamine release.

(53–1-B, 2-B, 3-B,   **(S&F, pp. 566–569)**
4-A and 4-B)

Hypertrophic pyloric stenosis causes obstruction of the gastric outlet and is the most common disorder requiring abdominal surgery during the first six months of life. Males are affected three to four times as often as females. The typical infant begins to have nonbilious vomiting when three to four weeks old. Abdominal plain films indicate a distended stomach with a paucity of intestinal gas.

Congenital duodenal obstruction can be caused by either atresia or stenosis. Unlike pyloric stenosis, there is no sex difference. Patients with partial obstruction may not present for weeks, months, or years. Vomiting is usually the presenting symptom and is bile stained in 75%. Abdominal plain films usually show gaseous distention of the stomach and duodenum, the so-called double bubble sign. Surgery is curative for both conditions.

(54–A, C, D)   **(S&F, pp. 650–651)**

Bismuth absorption varies with the specific form of bismuth; absorption is much greater with colloidal bismuth subcitrate (CBS) than with bismuth subsalicylate (BSS) or bismuth subnitrate. Furthermore, co-administration of H_2 receptor antagonists increases bismuth absorption from CBS but not from BSS or bismuth subnitrate. Despite transient increases in serum bismuth concentrations, significant toxicity has not been reported in clinical trials or with intermittent use of CBS or BSS. In the colon, bismuth salts react with hydrogen sulfide to form bismuth sulfide, which blackens stools without causing a positive test for occult blood. Treatment with CBS heals duodenal ulcers at a rate greater than placebo and comparable to healing rates with H_2 receptor antagonists. The ulcer healing effects of CBS may be independent of bismuth's effects on *Helicobacter pylori* infection because bismuth monotherapy will usually only suppress rather than eradicate *H. pylori*. Because renal failure interferes with bismuth excretion, bismuth should be avoided or serum bismuth levels should be monitored in patients with renal disease.

(55–C)   **(S&F, p. 594)**

Gastric acid secretion follows a circadian pattern, with the lowest secretory rates from 5 to 11 A.M., and the highest from 2 to 11 P.M. Basal gastrin levels do not correlate with basal gastric acid secretion or these circadian changes.

(56–C) **(S&F, p. 643)**

NSAIDs impair ulcer healing, allowing normal acid peptic activity to cause persistent ulceration. The explanations that underlie the postbulbar narrowing seen with giant duodenal ulcers and the high incidence of giant ulcers in end-stage renal disease are uncertain. Acid secretion in patients with giant duodenal ulcers does not differ from that of the overall duodenal ulcer patient population except in the rare patient with gastrinoma.

(57–1-A, 2-B, 3-E, 4-D) **(S&F, pp. 645–651)**

H_2 receptor antagonists interfere with renal excretion of cationic drugs. By competing for renal tubular secretion, cimetidine and ranitidine increase serum concentrations of lidocaine, procainamide, and theophylline. Antacids decrease absorption of a number of drugs through intraluminal binding. Some of these drugs include tetracycline, ciprofloxacin, isoniazid, warfarin, digoxin, phenytoin, quinidine, cimetidine, ranitidine, ferrous sulfate, and theophylline. Omeprazole is dispensed as coated granules within a capsule. When administered through nasogastric or gastrostomy tubes, the capsule must be opened, thus exposing the active, acid-labile medication to gastric acid, which reduces the bioavailability of the drug. Pepto-Bismol (bismuth subsalicylate) is metabolized to salicylate and bismuth oxychloride at acidic pH, and the salicylate is absorbed.

(58–B) **(S&F, pp. 588–589)**

Although a number of endogenous peptides such as secretin, glucagon, neurotensin, gastric inhibitory peptide, and calcitonin gene–related peptide are capable of inhibiting acid secretion when infused intravenously, their physiologic significance in humans is uncertain. Available evidence supports a role for somatostatin and secretin as physiologic inhibitory regulators of gastric acid secretion. The other agents listed all stimulate acid secretion.

(59–D) **(S&F, pp. 588–592)**

Both acetylcholine from vagal nerve endings and gastrin from the blood stimulate the parietal cell to secrete acid by increasing the intracellular calcium concentration. Histamine activates the proton pump by increasing intracellular cyclic adenosine monophosphate. Peptide YY and secretin are inhibitors of gastric acid secretion.

(60–C) **(S&F, pp. 635–638)**

Epigastric pain is a primary complaint in about two thirds of ulcer patients. Other less common locations are the right and left hypochondrium. It is not uncommon to have a dissociation between pain and ulceration. The disappearance of symptoms does not guarantee ulcer healing. Ulcers frequently produce no symptoms. Asymptomatic ulceration is more common in NSAID users and the elderly. The pain experienced by ulcer patients is not simply due to acid bathing an ulcer crater. Night-time pain, which reflects the circadian rhythm governing acid secretion, occurs in about half of duodenal ulcer patients but may also occur in gastric ulcer patients and in patients with nonulcer dyspepsia.

(61–C) **(S&F, pp. 645–647)**

Absorption of H_2 receptor antagonists is inhibited 10% to 20% by concomitant antacids, whereas food does not reduce absorption. All H_2 receptor antagonists are eliminated by a combination of hepatic metabolism, glomerular filtration, and renal tubular secretion. Doses should be reduced by 50% in patients with moderate to severe renal failure. The half-life of cimetidine is increased in liver failure. However, it remains controversial as to whether a dose reduction is indicated in these patients. Because only small amounts of H_2 receptor antagonists are removed by peritoneal dialysis and hemodialysis, replacement doses are not necessary.

(62–A, C, D) **(S&F, pp. 684–686)**

A fasting serum gastrin concentration of more than 1000 pg/mL in combination with compatible clinical features of gastric acid hypersecretion is diagnostic of Zollinger-Ellison syndrome. Patients with pernicious anemia may occasionally have gastrin levels above 1000 pg/mL but lack the symptoms of hypersecretion. Clinical states associated with lesser elevations in gastrin levels are common duodenal ulcer disease, antral G-cell hyperfunction, renal insufficiency, diabetes mellitus, and rheumatoid arthritis. In normal subjects or patients with common duodenal ulcer disease, intravenous secretin has little effect on gastrin levels. In contrast, patients with Zollinger-Ellison syndrome have dramatic increases in serum gastrin levels after secretin infusion, with an increase of more than 200 pg/mL within ten minutes being diagnostic. Similarly, intravenous calcium infusion results in an exaggerated release of gastrin in Zollinger-Ellison syndrome, with an increase of more than 400 pg/mL.

(63–B) **(S&F, p. 691)**

Gastric acid secretion by parietal cells reflects stimulation by gastrin, histamine, and the vagus nerve. Increased levels of histamine originating from infiltrating mast cells may stimulate acid secretion in the presence of normal or low gastrin levels.

(64–B) ***Emergency surgery (S&F, pp. 703–704)*** ***V&A morbidity (S&F, p. 706)***

The choice of operation for bleeding duodenal ulcer depends on the surgeon. However, vagotomy plus antrectomy is associated with higher morbidity than vagotomy plus a drainage procedure in high-risk patients. Emergency surgery for bleeding duodenal ulcer increases perioperative mortality ten-fold when compared with the same surgery under elective conditions. Furthermore, postoperative complications, including wound infection and duodenal stump leakage, are much more frequent in patients undergoing emergency surgery. Proximal vagotomy with ulcer oversew is an option for patients with bleeding duodenal ulcer, depending on the experience of the individual surgeon.

(65–B, C)   *(S&F, pp. 704–705)*

Direct suture closure of the perforation alone without an omental patch has a high rate of failure. Perforations of more than 48 hours in duration and the presence of preoperative shock or severe coexisting medical illness are each associated with increased perioperative mortality. For gastric perforations, resection of the ulcer is desirable because "patched" perforations may recur. Although as many as 70% of highly selected patients can be managed medically alone with good results, age older than 70 years is associated with a higher mortality if surgery is delayed.

(66–A, B, C)   *(S&F, p. 582)*

Erythromycin, metoclopramide, and cisapride all may be useful in treating gastric stasis for the reasons stated, but the combination of erythromycin with cisapride MUST BE AVOIDED because of the risk of cardiac arrhythmias (torsades de pointes).

(67–A)   *(S&F, pp. 639–640)*

Malignant ulcers are usually caused when a tumor outgrows its blood supply, leading to necrosis. Because it is unlikely that the tumor would be present in both locations, the simultaneous coexistence of duodenal and gastric ulcers decreases the likelihood that gastric carcinoma is present.

(68–A, C, D)   *(S&F, pp. 733–737)*

The incidence of gastric cancer in the United States is 6 per 100,000 per year, with a 2:1 male-to-female ratio. *Helicobacter pylori* infection is associated with gastric cancer, reflecting the fact that it can progress to chronic atrophic gastritis, a premalignant lesion. Certain foods increase the risk of gastric cancer, including high starch diets, pickled vegetables, salted fish and meats, and smoked foods. Whole milk, citrus fruits, fresh vegetables, and refrigeration are not associated with gastric cancer.

(69–A)   *(S&F, pp. 623–624)*

Gastric metaplasia in the duodenum is thought to develop as a consequence of duodenal acid exposure, leading to epithelial damage with development of islands of gastric mucosa. Gastric metaplasia is rarely observed in patients with achlorhydria and hypochlorhydria and is more frequent in hypersecretory states such as Zollinger-Ellison syndrome. Gastric epithelium is a prerequisite attachment of *Helicobacter pylori* infection, which requires specific adhesin molecules not found in duodenal mucosa. Thus, duodenal *H. pylori* infection is always associated with metaplastic gastric epithelium. These two factors (gastric metaplasia and *H. pylori* infection) may compromise duodenal defenses sufficiently to cause duodenal ulceration. However, gastric metaplasia is also seen in some nonulcer subjects and in patients not infected with *H. pylori*.

(70–B)   *(S&F, p. 703)*

The mortality rate from in-hospital rebleeding from peptic ulcer is approximately 30%. Gastric ulcers are three times as likely to rebleed as duodenal ulcers. Each of the other factors is associated with an increased mortality from bleeding peptic ulcer.

(71–A, B)   *(S&F, pp. 681–682)*

Multiple endocrine neoplasia–1 (MEN-1) is an autosomal dominant genetic disorder characterized by tumors or hyperplasia of parathyroid, pancreatic islet, and pituitary glands. Gastrinoma is the most common type of islet cell tumor in MEN-1 patients, and half are malignant, not 10%. Unlike sporadic gastrinomas, gastrinomas associated with MEN-1 tend to be extrapancreatic, particularly in the wall of the duodenum. Hyperparathyroidism may unmask the presence of a gastrinoma by hypercalcemia stimulated gastrin release. Gastrinomas associated with MEN-1 are usually multiple.

(72–B)   *(S&F, p. 683)*

Steatorrhea in Zollinger-Ellison syndrome results from an abnormally low intraluminal pH in the duodenum. Pancreatic lipase has optimal activity between pH 6 and 8. For the lipase to function, colipase must first bind to triglycerides. Lipase then binds to colipase by electrostatic interactions. Colipase binding is not disrupted in Zollinger-Ellison syndrome. However, glycine conjugated bile salts precipitate out of solution below pH 5, preventing normal formation of mixed micelles. Also, fatty acids are protonated below a pH of 6.0, which further interferes with normal micelle formation. Ileal receptor function is normal.

(73–B)   *(S&F, p. 684)*

Postbulbar ulcers are often associated with gastrinomas. However, postbulbar duodenal or more distal small intestinal ulcers may also be seen in association with NSAID use, Crohn's disease, ischemia, radiation injury, and intra-arterial injection of 5-fluorouracil. Although patient B has a markedly elevated gastrin, he has hypochlorhydria rather than gastrinoma, as indicated by his high gastric pH after pentagastrin stimulation. Patients with hypochlorhydria may have hypergastrinemia and an exaggerated response to secretin. Such patients have a lower, rather than higher, risk of gastroduodenal ulcers.

(74–A, C)   *(S&F, pp. 689–690)*

Patients with lymph node involvement do not have improved survival with chemotherapy. Chemotherapy should not be used to reduce acid secretion. Omeprazole is superior to chemotherapy for decreasing acid secretion and its complications. Instead, the primary role of chemotherapy is improvement of symptoms owing to mass effect or invasive tumor. Decreases in both tumor mass and serum gastrin levels have been reported in more than half of patients treated by intra-arterial streptozotocin. Hepatic artery chemoembolization has been associated with high mortality (10%–14%) due to infection or hepatic abscess and has no proven advantage over conventional chemotherapy for the treatment of metastatic gastrinoma.

(75–1-E, 2-B, 3-C)   **(S&F, pp. 744–745)**

Endoscopic ultrasonography can differentiate extramural gastric compression from submucosal lesions. A pancreatic pseudocyst is a hypoechoic (dark) structure within the otherwise heterogeneous gray pancreatic parenchyma. An enlarged spleen may occasionally cause gastric indentations. The spleen has a relatively homogeneous echo pattern without distinct markings. A tortuous splenic artery typically appears as a tubular structure below the muscularis propria. None of these abnormalities alters the mucosal pattern.

(76–C)   **(S&F, pp. 737–742)**

In addition to carcinoma, polypoid submucosal lesions in the proximal stomach may represent gastric varices, extramural compression by an aberrant splenic artery, pancreatic pseudocyst, or leiomyoma. Snare cautery or needle aspiration could lead to untoward complications if a vascular lesion is present. Abdominal computed tomography scan is of little help in defining gastric wall lesions because it does not resolve the individual layers of the gastric wall. Transabdominal ultrasonography may help define certain gastric lesions.

(77–C)   **(S&F, pp. 740–742)**

Adenoma is an epithelial lesion, and therefore histopathology should indicate adenomatous changes of the mucosa. All the other lesions listed are submucosal, and thus endoscopic biopsy specimens usually show normal mucosa.

(78–D)   **(S&F, pp. 596–597)**

All of the conditions listed above except for the acquired immunodeficiency syndrome (AIDS) are associated with increased gastric acid secretion. Hypochlorhydria in patients with AIDS is clinically important because it may result in reduced absorption of acid-soluble drugs such as ketoconazole.

(79–B)   **(S&F, p. 669)**

The stomach and duodenum have anatomic proximity to the biliary tree and colon. Thus, most fistulous complications from penetrating gastric and duodenal ulcer disease involve these surrounding structures. The esophagus is not a site of fistulous complications in penetrating ulcer disease.

(80–A)   **(S&F, pp. 700–703)**

Antrectomy is contraindicated when severe inflammation surrounds the duodenal bulb because of the difficulty of resection and risk of leakage. Truncal vagotomy with antrectomy has a lower ulcer recurrence rate than truncal

vagotomy with a pyloroplasty (2.6% vs. 9.5%) and produces similar rates of dumping syndrome and postoperative diarrhea. Truncal vagotomy with antrectomy is indicated in patients with duodenal ulcer disease due to antral G-cell hyperplasia because most of the abnormal cells are removed by the procedure. Although most experienced surgeons report comparable mortality rates for truncal vagotomy with antrectomy versus truncal vagotomy with drainage procedure, the latter procedure is more appropriate for high-risk and elderly patients. Rates of rebleeding after each procedure are comparable (10%–15%).

(81–A)   **(S&F, pp. 706–707)**

Frank anemia may develop years after gastric surgery. Iron deficiency is the most common cause of anemia, but mixed deficiencies of iron, vitamin B_{12}, and folate may also occur. Pure megaloblastic anemia is rare unless the patient has undergone a major subtotal or total gastrectomy or has bacterial overgrowth. Multiple mechanisms may contribute to the development of anemia: (1) reduced food intake causes inadequate ingestion of iron, vitamin B_{12}, and folate; (2) reduced gastric acid secretion limits the solubility of iron in food and its conversion to the more soluble and absorbable ferrous form; (3) delivery of large, poorly digestible food particles into the proximal small intestine reduces the ability of pancreatic proteases to liberate heme iron from ingested meat; (4) alkaline reflux gastritis or stomal ulcers may increase intestinal blood loss; (5) reduced gastric acid secretion or the presence of a blind loop may lead to bacterial overgrowth, thereby reducing nutrient availability and absorption; and (6) gastric resection reduces intrinsic factor production and impairs vitamin B_{12} absorption.

(82–C)   **(S&F, pp. 700–701)**

Duodenal stump leakage occurs in the early postoperative period, often presents with catastrophic complications, and has a high mortality. Leakage of pancreaticobiliary contents into the peritoneal cavity usually leads to significant peritonitis. A marginal ulcer may occur in the presence of an incomplete vagotomy, retained antrum, continued use of exogenous noxious substances, or undiagnosed Zollinger-Ellison syndrome. Complications such as kinking of the jejunal loop or small bowel adhesions may also result in symptoms of postprandial abdominal pain, nausea, and vomiting in the early postoperative period.

(83–A)   **(S&F, p. 669)**

Sealing of the perforation with an omental patch and a parietal cell vagotomy (if stability of the patient allows) has a low rate of morbidity and ulcer recurrence. Partial or subtotal gastrectomy has a greater associated morbidity and is generally not warranted in what is probably an NSAID-related ulcer complication. Medical therapy has a role in treating perforated ulcers, but the peritoneal signs and the absence of comorbid conditions precluding surgery favor more definitive treatment.

(84–C)   **(S&F, p. 719)**

Biopsy specimens of the antrum would not reveal the existence of oxyntic gland gastritis. The lesser curve of the gastric body is often a transition zone and thus could be falsely interpreted as atrophic. The best location to sample is the mid body, greater curve.

(85–C)   **(S&F, pp. 665–668)**

Approximately 2% of ulcer patients develop obstruction. In contrast, perforation occurs in up to 5% of ulcer patients and hemorrhage in 15% to 25%. A positive saline load test consists of recovery of more than 400 mL of the instilled 750 mL of normal saline at 30 minutes after instillation. Recovery of 300 to 400 mL is highly suggestive. Gastric outlet obstruction is also suggested by intractable emesis or gastric retention, particularly if emesis contains food particles ingested more than 12 hours previously. Despite the availability of endoscopic balloon dilation for treatment of pyloric channel stenosis, surgical therapy is eventually required in the majority of patients with this disorder. Most patients presenting with gastric outlet obstruction have electrolyte abnormalities and dehydration due to vomiting. Volume repletion and correction of electrolyte abnormalities should be the initial step in management. Nasogastric suction may also help facilitate recovery of gastric tone.

(86–C)   **(S&F, pp. 653–654)**

Epidemiologic studies have shown that smoking is associated with both gastric and duodenal ulcers and the risk of ulceration is proportional to the amount smoked. Death rates from peptic ulcer disease are also greater in smokers. Follow-up studies of duodenal ulcer patients in whom *Helicobacter pylori* infection has been successfully treated indicate that patients who continue to smoke have an ulcer recurrence rate ranging from 0% to 13% at one year. This suggests that continued smoking may not be as important a risk factor for ulcer recurrence after eradication of *H. pylori* as when this organism is present.

References

Borody, T. J., George, L. L., Brandl, S., et al. Smoking does not contribute to duodenal ulcer relapse after *Helicobacter pylori* eradication. Am. J. Gastroenterol. *87*:1390, 1992.

Graham, D. Y., Lew, G. M., Klein, P. D., et al. Effect of treatment of *Helicobacter pylori* infection on the long-term recurrence of gastric or duodenal ulcer: A randomized controlled study. Ann. Intern. Med. *116*:705, 1992.

(87–A)   **(S&F, pp. 713–714)**

So-called alcoholic gastritis (a misnomer because there is little, if any, inflammation) may be seen after an alcoholic binge. It is diagnosed endoscopically by the finding of erosions and subepithelial hemorrhages and does not require biopsy confirmation in the appropriate clinical setting. Its appearance cannot be differentiated from other forms of hemorrhagic and erosive gastritis such as NSAID, stress, or ischemic gastritis.

(88–C, E)   **(S&F, pp. 680–681)**

Gastrinomas are endodermal in origin and arise from gastrin-producing tissue in the pancreas, as evidenced by the discovery of biologically active and inactive forms of progastrin and gastrin in adult pancreatic tissue. They are most commonly found in the head of the pancreas, whereas the most common site of extrapancreatic gastrinomas is the first or second portion of the duodenum. The majority of duodenal wall gastrinomas are located submucosally, and thus are easily missed on endoscopy. Other extrapancreatic sites include stomach, liver, and hilum of the spleen. The "gastrinoma triangle" is defined by the junction of the cystic and common bile ducts superiorly, the junction of the second and third portions of the duodenum inferiorly, and the junction of the neck and body of the pancreas medially. The vast majority of gastrinomas are found to reside within this anatomic triangle.

(89–E)   **(S&F, pp. 631–632)**

Prophylaxis against stress ulceration is not indicated for patients in whom serious illness will not be prolonged. For patients with more severe illness in whom prophylaxis is indicated, there is no clear advantage of one therapy over another.

(90–B)   **(S&F, p. 682)**

MEN-1 syndrome is composed of hyperparathyroidism (due to adenomas), pituitary adenomas, and islet cell tumors of the pancreas. Gastrinoma is the most common islet cell tumor complicating MEN-1 syndrome, affecting more than 60% of the patients.

(91–B)   **(S&F, p. 706)**

Iron deficiency is the most common cause of anemia in postgastrectomy patients. The cause is multifactorial and includes decreased oral intake, decreased absorption, and low-grade bleeding due to marginal ulceration. Vitamin B_{12} deficiency is also seen, but much less frequently.

(92–C)   **(S&F, p. 689)**

The goal of medical treatment in gastrinoma is to reduce hypersecretion sufficiently to allow healing of peptic disease. Healing of reflux esophagitis usually requires a greater reduction of acid secretion than duodenal or gastric ulcerations. Gastroesophageal reflux disease (GERD) occurs in approximately 25% of patients with Zollinger-Ellison syndrome and may be severe (15% of patients), resulting in peptic stricture. Some patients with severe GERD may require suppression of acid output to less than 1 mEq/hr. Also, patients with Zollinger-Ellison syndrome who have undergone a partial gastric resection (not recommended) need profound acid suppression.

(93–1-C, 2-D, 3-A, 4-B, 5-E)   **(S&F, pp. 659–669)**

Penetrating gastric or duodenal ulcers may produce fistulas connecting anatomically adjacent structures. When the colon is involved, seeding of the small intestine with bacteria may occur. Perforated ulcer, with resultant spillage of gastric contents, results in marked peritoneal inflammation and clinical signs and symptoms of peritonitis. Use of NSAIDs can contribute to intractable ulcer disease. Succussion splash can be demonstrated in up to 25% of patients with gastric outlet obstruction. Hypovolemic shock may be the initial presentation of bleeding peptic ulcer.

(94–A) **(S&F, pp. 645–652)**

Dissolution of some drugs, particularly weak bases, is decreased at neutral or high gastric pH. Ketoconazole, a weak base, has decreased dissolution and absorption when taken during acid suppressive therapy. Omeprazole, to be effective, must be concentrated and activated in the acidic compartments of actively secreting parietal cells. Omeprazole action is markedly compromised if it is administered during a period of acid inhibition by coadministration of an H_2 receptor antagonist. Cimetidine is metabolized by the hepatic cytochrome P-450 system. Thus, other drugs that are also metabolized via this mechanism, such as theophylline, phenytoin, and warfarin, may develop increased or even toxic serum levels in patients taking cimetidine at the usual recommended dosage. Although cimetidine interferes with metabolism of theophylline and phenytoin, their efficacy is unaffected by concurrent cimetidine administration. Ranitidine has less propensity to alter metabolism of these drugs, although there have been case reports of ranitidine-induced theophylline and phenytoin toxicity.

(95–E) **(S&F, p. 593)**

Omeprazole blocks transport of hydrogen ions (i.e., acid) out of parietal cells by irreversibly binding hydrogen–potassium adenosine triphosphatase, the enzyme responsible for active exchange of intracellular hydrogen ions for extracellular potassium ions. This enzyme is also known as the "proton pump."

(96–D) **(S&F, pp. 724–725)**

Ménétrier's disease is characterized by giant gastric folds in the fundus and body, hypochlorhydria, and hypoalbuminemia. The prominent histologic abnormality is foveolar hyperplasia. This disease is more common in men, has its usual onset in middle age, and rarely has a familial component. There have been reports of an increased risk of gastric carcinoma. Despite the similar radiographic appearance, there is no increased risk of gastric lymphoma.

(97–1-B, 2-A, 3-B, 4-A, 5-A) **(S&F, pp. 733–734)**

Gastric cancer may be divided into two histologic types: intestinal and diffuse. The intestinal type is commonly found in countries with a high incidence of gastric cancer and is typically associated with antecedent chronic atrophic gastritis and metaplasia. The diffuse type is more common in women and younger patients without prior metaplasia. The diffuse type extends widely with no distinct margins

and often contains cells with large mucous inclusions ("signet ring" cells). Intestinal type gastric cancer generally has a better prognosis than the diffuse type.

(98–A) **(S&F, pp. 697–700)**

The actions of gastrin and acetylcholine on the gastric parietal cell are synergistic. Vagotomy markedly reduces the responsiveness of partial cells to circulating gastrin.

(99–E) **(S&F, pp. 684–687)**

In Zollinger-Ellison syndrome, an upper gastrointestinal series may demonstrate prominent rugal folds, peptic and small bowel ulcerations, and large amounts of gastric fluid. Upper endoscopy often demonstrates the presence of thickened rugal folds and peptic ulceration, which may include giant or postbulbar ulcers. A fasting serum gastrin level of more than 1000 pg/mL is diagnostic of Zollinger-Ellison syndrome. Intravenous calcium infusion causes the serum gastrin level to increase markedly in patients with Zollinger-Ellison syndrome but not in patients with elevated gastrin levels due to other causes.

(100–A, C) **(S&F, p. 707)**

Postprandial nausea and vomiting followed by vasomotor symptoms is characteristic of a dumping syndrome. The latter symptoms are due to rapid filling of the small intestine with a high osmotic load and resulting fluid shifts into the lumen and reactive hypoglycemia. Simple sugars aggravate the vasomotor symptoms, whereas complex carbohydrates are recommended. Solid meals taken without liquid slow gastric emptying and ameliorate the symptoms.

(101–A, B, C) **(S&F, p. 697)**

Truncal vagotomy eliminates all innervation to the stomach, including the nerves responsible for normal antropyloric function. Gastric retention may result unless a drainage procedure is done. The loss of regulated gastric emptying caused by the drainage procedure contributes to dumping syndrome and postvagotomy diarrhea.

(102–D) **(S&F, pp. 706–708)**

Secretion of gastrin by antral G cells is regulated by extracellular pH. Retained distal antrum after ulcer surgery may result in hypergastrinemia if the antral tissue is bathed in neutral or alkaline secretions such as occur in the duodenum. Retained proximal antrum is not a reported cause of recurrent ulcers.

(103–E) **(S&F, pp. 654–655)**

Although certain foods, beverages, and spices cause dyspepsia, there is no convincing evidence that these foods cause, delay healing of, or reactivate peptic ulcers. In particular, ethanol is not a risk factor for peptic ulcer. In experimental settings, alcohol in high concentrations can damage the gastric mucosa. However, alcohol in the more moderate concentrations found in beverages does not appear to cause peptic ulceration. In this case, the reason to advise dietary modification would be to eliminate those foods that cause dyspepsia, not to reduce ulcer risk.

(104–A, B, C, D)   (S&F, p. 683)

Although a high rate of acid secretion is the main cause of diarrhea or steatorrhea in Zollinger-Ellison syndrome, high circulating levels of gastrin independent of acid secretion cause secretion (or impair absorption) of fluid in the small intestine. The optimum pH for most pancreatic enzymes is neutral to alkaline, whereas the duodenal and proximal ileal contents in Zollinger-Ellison syndrome are often quite acid. Bile salts precipitate at acid pH because of protonation of the carboxyl group, inhibiting formation of mixed micelles required for fat absorption. The osmotic effect of proton hypersecretion causes a significant increase in luminal flow rates, limiting the time available for digestion.

(105–B)   (S&F, pp. 699, 706)

Sham feeding is the preferred diagnostic test for determining the completeness of vagotomy. For postoperative patients, acid output after sham feeding should be less than 10% of maximal acid output. Congo red staining of the gastric mucosa may be used to detect areas that are still innervated by the vagus nerve. If more than 20% of the gastric surface area stains positive for acid production, the incidence of recurrent ulcers is increased. Insulin-induced hypoglycemia stimulates gastric acid secretion by means of the vagus nerve but has fallen out of favor owing to its associated risk. Secretin stimulation is useful in the diagnostic evaluation of gastrinoma but has no role in testing for incomplete vagotomy.

(106–B)   (S&F, pp. 742–746)

T2 lesions are defined by invasion into the muscularis propria but not through the serosa. In gastric cancers, any number of lymph nodes more than 2 cm removed from the primary lesion are classified as N2, independent of their size.

(107–B)   (S&F, p. 561)

Enteroendocrine cells, previously called basal granular cells, are characterized by secretory granules distributed in the cytoplasm between the nucleus and the cell base. These are true endocrine cells that release secretory granules into the lamina propria containing a variety of gastrointestinal hormones and peptides, including gastrin, secretin, somatostatin, motilin, serotonin, gastric inhibitory peptide, neurotensin, and enteroglucagon. They do not produce digestive enzymes or mucus in any appreciable amount.

(108–E)   (S&F, p. 659)

Exogenous factors such as tobacco use or NSAID use have been implicated in persistence of ulcer disease. Untreated *Helicobacter pylori* infection can contribute to intractable ulcer disease as well as the presence of a gastrinoma, as evidenced by a fasting gastrin level greater than 1000 pg/mL.

(109–B, C)   (S&F, pp. 742–743)

Middle-aged patients have a better prognosis than younger or older patients. The best predictor of survival appears to be the local depth of invasion. Lymph node involvement and metastases correlate with depth of invasion. Most studies show no difference in outcome between men and women. Serum carcinoembryonic antigen (CEA) levels are less frequently elevated in gastric cancer than in colon cancer. Fifty percent of patients have a serum level above 2.5 ng/mL, as do 10% of the normal population. Up to 50% of patients with unresectable disease have CEA levels greater than 5 ng/mL; however, only 15% with resectable disease have a CEA level greater than 5 ng/mL.

(110–A)   (S&F, pp. 668–669)

Sixty percent of perforations occur in the duodenal bulb, most commonly through the anterior wall. Twenty percent involve the antrum and 20% the body of the stomach. NSAID use is often associated.

(111–A)   (S&F, pp. 632–634)

Prevalence is defined as the proportion of the population with a given disease at a single point in time, over a period of time, or over a lifetime. *Incidence* is defined as the occurrence of new cases per population base in a given period of time. Yearly incidence of peptic ulcer is 1.5% to 3% whereas lifetime prevalence is 5% to 10% and is higher for males than for females. These data suggest that a small proportion of the population is responsible for most of the ulcer disease. For both gastric and duodenal ulcers, familial aggregation has been observed. First-degree relatives of patients with ulcers have an increased prevalence of ulcers. Familial forms of hyperpepsinogenemic and hypergastrinemic duodenal ulcers have been recognized. However, since *Helicobacter pylori* infection causes an increase in both pepsinogen and gastrin, these observations are likely related to familial clustering of *H. pylori*. Peptic ulcer prevalence increases with advancing age for both males and females. Age-related trends in peptic ulcer are probably, in part, related to trends of age-related differences in NSAID use, *H. pylori* infection, and smoking.

(112–A)   (S&F, pp. 687–688)

The primary goal for treatment of gastrinoma is complete surgical removal of tumor. A small, easily accessible solitary hepatic metastasis is amenable to resection and may result in cure. Enucleation is recommended for tumors in the body or head of the pancreas; however, tumors in the tail are treated by resection of the distal pancreas. If no tumor is localized during surgery, complete acid-reducing surgery, such as a total gastrectomy, should not be performed because medical therapy with proton pump inhibitors can usually manage the effects of acid hypersecretion and the greatest threat to life is no longer ulcer disease but rather tumor invasion.

(113–1-D, 2-C, 3-B, 4-E,   *(S&F, pp. 559–561)*
5-A, 6-A)

Gastrin is secreted by G cells found in the gastric antrum. Somatostatin is secreted by enteroendocrine cells (D cells) found in the oxyntic and antral glands. Histamine is secreted by enterochromaffin-like (ECL) cells found in fundic gastric glands. Glucagon is produced by A cells. Parietal cells contain a proton pump in the apical and canalicular microvilli that is responsible for acid secretion. Parietal cells also secrete intrinsic factor.

(114–A, C, E, F)   *(S&F, pp. 744–746)*

Diagnosis of abnormal gastric folds can be difficult. Even large punch biopsies are often normal, and diagnosis may require laparotomy with full-thickness biopsy. Endoscopic ultrasonography has emerged as an important adjunct for the evaluation of abnormal folds. The individual layers of the gastric wall are readily identified. Layers 1 (interface, superficial mucosa) and 2 (hypoechoic deep mucosa) represent the mucosa; layer 3, the submucosa; layer 4, the muscularis propria; and layer 5, the serosa. Primary gastric malignancies can spread predominantly within the submucosa. Metastatic cancers often mimic lymphoma by spreading as diffusely infiltrative processes within the submucosa (layer 3). Ménétrier's disease and gastritis produce a characteristic thickening of the hypoechoic second layer (deep mucosa).

(115–C)   *(S&F, pp. 624–628)*

Between 20% and 50% of patients with duodenal ulcers have elevated maximal acid output (MAO). Although some normal subjects have MAOs that fall into the higher range, the mean MAO of patients with duodenal ulcer is greater than that of controls. Proximal duodenal bicarbonate secretion is depressed in about 70% of patients with duodenal ulcer. However, duodenal pH, which reflects the net effect of duodenal delivery of gastric acid and the acid-neutralizing capacity of duodenal bicarbonate, does not consistently differ between duodenal ulcer patients and normal subjects. In duodenal ulcer patients, *Helicobacter pylori* infection is not clearly related to changes in gastric acid secretion.

(116–D)   *(S&F, p. 596)*

Proteins are the major food constituent that stimulates gastric acid secretion. Amino acids and peptides stimulate acid secretion by releasing gastrin. Carbohydrates and fats decrease gastric acid secretion when given alone, but when given mixed with proteins, gastric acid is stimulated. Ethanol causes a modest decrease in gastric secretion. Saline increases gastric acid secretion by causing gastric distention but is not as potent a stimulator as protein.

(117–E)   *(S&F, pp. 724, 726–727)*

When evaluating thickened gastric folds, the primary concern is to exclude an infiltrating neoplasm such as a lymphoma or carcinoma. Thick gastric folds are also seen in Ménétrier's disease and Zollinger-Ellison syndrome. Large gastric folds are not a prominent feature of any of the common causes of granulomatous gastritis, such as tuberculosis, syphilis, histoplasmosis, Crohn's disease, or sarcoidosis. Moreover, granulomatous gastritis generally involves the antrum.

(118–C)   *(S&F, pp. 753–754)*

Patients with familial polyposis coli can have associated gastric polyps. These are usually hyperplastic or occasionally adenomatous. Gardner's syndrome is an autosomal dominant disease with associated adenomatous polyps and polypoid hamartomas. Adenomas of the stomach should be completely removed in these patients.

(119–B, C, D)   *(S&F, pp. 684–685)*

The normal fasting gastrin level in serum is less than 100 pg/mL. The fasting gastrin level must be more than 1000 pg/mL to be diagnostic of Zollinger-Ellison syndrome. An increase in serum gastrin to more than 300 pg/mL after a protein meal may be used to diagnose antral G-cell hyperplasia. Modest hypergastrinemia is common after vagotomy, owing to the higher antral pH. However, basal gastrin levels are usually not elevated after antrectomy because most of the gastrin-producing cells have been removed.

Colon and Small Intestine

S&F Section X

---

120. Each of the following is a true statement regarding surveillance colonoscopy after complete resection of a colonic adenoma EXCEPT:

A. For sporadic adenomas, repeat colonoscopy should be performed at three years.

B. For malignant polyps, repeat colonoscopy should be performed at six months and yearly thereafter.

C. Colonoscopy will miss at least 30% of colon cancers when performed biennially for ulcerative colitis.

D. Colonoscopy will decrease colon cancer incidence by at least 75%.

E. The surveillance interval is independent of adenoma size.

---

121. Each of the following predicts poorer survival in colon cancer EXCEPT:

A. *p53* mutation

B. 18q deletion

C. K-*ras* mutation

D. Replication error–negative phenotype

E. Aneuploidy

---

122. A 62-year-old man with a 30-year history of ulcerative colitis underwent surveillance colonoscopy and was found to have low-grade dysplasia. Which of the following is the MOST appropriate next step?

A. Repeat colonoscopy with biopsy in two years.

B. Repeat colonoscopy with biopsy within eight weeks.

C. Perform abdominal computed tomography.

D. Discontinue sulfasalazine.

---

123. Each of the following is a true statement regarding the impact of NSAIDs on colon cancer EXCEPT:

A. Long-term sulindac therapy is an effective alternative to a total colectomy for treatment of familial adenomatous polyposis.

B. Aspirin effects on colon cancer have not been shown to be dose dependent.

C. NSAIDs may help prevent ulcerative colitis–associated colon cancers.

D. The effects of aspirin on colon cancer appear to be duration dependent.

E. All are true.

---

124. A 55-year-old man presents to the emergency department with a two-week history of intermittent nausea and vomiting accompanied by severe abdominal pain. The pain is located in the midabdomen. He is admitted and undergoes esophagogastroduodenoscopy and colonoscopy, both of which are normal. Over the next several days, his abdominal pain waxes and wanes. An obstructive series during an episode of pain demonstrates ileus consistent with obstruction in the distal small bowel. Enteroclysis demonstrates bowel loop thickening and the appearance of a mass in the midileum. The MOST appropriate next step in the management of this patient would be:

A. Angiography

B. Hypotonic duodenography

C. Exploratory laparotomy

D. Bone marrow aspiration and biopsy

E. Serum protein electrophoresis

---

125. A 22-year-old sexually active woman presents with the sudden onset of right upper quadrant pain radiating to her right shoulder. On further questioning, she reports a one- to two-week history of bilateral lower abdominal pain associated with a vaginal discharge. The physical examination revealed a temperature of 38.0° C, moderate right upper quadrant tenderness with guarding, and a white cervical discharge with cervical motion tenderness. Laboratory shows a leukocytosis with left shift and normal results of liver function tests. Which diagnosis is MOST compatible with this constellation of signs and symptoms?

A. Syphilitic hepatitis

B. Chlamydial pelvic inflammatory disease

C. Gonococcal perihepatitis

D. Appendicitis

E. Amebic abscess

---

126. Each of the following is a true statement about the risk of colon cancer in patients with inflammatory bowel disease EXCEPT:

A. Treatment with sulfasalazine reduces the risk.

B. Low-grade dysplasia on biopsy predicts less than 5% chance of having coexisting colon cancer.

C. Risk is associated with degree of bowel involvement.

D. Risk increases with time since diagnosis.

E. Carcinomas often arise without an adenomatous stage.

127. A surveillance colonoscopy in three years is indicated as part of a surveillance program in all of the following EXCEPT:
A. A 71-year-old man who had a single 5-mm tubular adenoma removed from his cecum
B. A 20-year-old patient who is part of a familial adenomatous polyposis kindred
C. A 50-year-old patient with three adenomas
D. A patient with a history of a malignant polyp
E. A patient with resected Dukes' B1 carcinoma

128. A 50-year-old woman requests a colonoscopy because her 75-year-old mother recently died of colon cancer. No other family member has had colon cancer, although her maternal aunt died of stomach cancer at age 40 and her father has ulcerative colitis well controlled on sulfasalazine. No medical history is available on her maternal grandparents, and her paternal grandparents died of coronary artery disease and diabetes. Colonoscopy would be clearly indicated for this woman IF (choose the best answer):
A. Flexible sigmoidoscopy showed a single 5-mm tubular adenoma at the rectosigmoid junction.
B. She had a 9-mm polyp with high-grade dysplasia removed last year.
C. The patient's 40-year-old sister has had ulcerative colitis requiring colectomy.
D. She had a hysterectomy six years ago for endometrial cancer.
E. Her older brother died of hepatoma at age 52.

129. A 25-year-old woman presents with three months of crampy abdominal pain, alternating diarrhea and constipation, and postprandial urgency. The pain always occurs either before or during a bowel movement, which gives relief. She has seen no blood or pus in the stool. She takes no medications. Family history is negative for inflammatory bowel disease or colon cancer. Physical examination is completely normal with the exception of borborygmi. Which of the following studies are warranted in this case? (one or more answers may be correct)
A. Sigmoidoscopy
B. Complete blood cell count, sedimentation rate
C. Stool examination for occult blood
D. Stool culture for routine bacterial pathogens
E. Empirical trial of a lactose-free diet

130. Each of the following statements about flat adenomas is true EXCEPT:
A. Macroscopically, flat adenomas are usually small (<10 mm) and flat or flat with a central depression.
B. Flat adenomas have a higher incidence of high-grade dysplasia than size-matched polypoid adenomas.
C. Compared with polypoid adenomas, flat lesions

are rare and account for less than 1% of all adenomas.
D. Flat adenomas are precursors of *de novo* carcinomas arising in nonpolypoid epithelium.
E. Multiple, flat adenomas clustering in the proximal colon suggest the patient has an attenuated form of familial adenomatous polyposis.

131. A 68-year-old patient is referred for persistently heme-positive stools. His hemoglobin level was initially in the low-normal range, and oral iron supplementation has raised it to mid-normal levels. His primary care physician has performed a single-contrast barium enema and rigid sigmoidoscopy, both of which were unrevealing. The patient is not on NSAIDs and has no upper gastrointestinal symptoms. The MOST appropriate next step would be to:
A. Observe the patient
B. Repeat the occult blood tests
C. Perform flexible sigmoidoscopy
D. Perform an air-contrast barium enema
E. Perform colonoscopy

132. A 50-year-old man presents with a three-month history of anorexia, epigastric pain, and weight loss with progressive nausea and vomiting over the past two weeks. At endoscopy, he has a large triangular ulcer in the fourth portion of the duodenum with apparent extraluminal compression. He denies taking NSAIDs, smoking, or recent alcohol ingestion. No history of peptic ulcer disease is present. Which of the following tests is LEAST indicated in the further management of this patient?
A. Computed tomography of the chest and abdomen
B. Bone marrow biopsy and aspiration
C. Serum and urine protein electrophoresis
D. Gastric emptying study
E. Fasting serum gastrin level

133. Measures of the malignant potential of an adenoma include all of the following EXCEPT:
A. Degree of dysplasia
B. Size
C. Histologic type
D. Patient's age
E. Number of adenomas

134. Specify whether the following statements are TRUE and, if true, whether they are related.
1. Mucosal cell mutations accumulate rapidly in patients with hereditary nonpolyposis colorectal cancer (HNPCC).
2. Annual screening by colonoscopy *or* flexible sigmoidoscopy plus air-contrast barium enema is recommended for HNPCC patients. Which of the following choices is correct?

Statement 1	Statement 2
A. T	T related

B. T   T unrelated
C. F   T
D. T   F
E. F   F

---

135. Considering the data supplied, which one or more of the following patients should have colonoscopic screening?
  A. A 60-year-old patient whose 67-year-old brother has a sigmoid colon cancer
  B. A 50-year-old patient in a familial adenomatous polyposis kindred
  C. A 55-year-old patient with a 5-mm tubular adenoma on flexible sigmoidoscopy
  D. A 44-year-old patient whose 50-year-old brother had a replication error–negative sigmoid cancer
  E. A 60-year-old patient who is part of a kindred of hereditary nonpolyposis colorectal cancer

---

136. Each of the following statements regarding screening for colon cancer is true EXCEPT:
  A. Screening sigmoidoscopy decreases mortality.
  B. Colonoscopy every three years is as effective as yearly colonoscopy in following sporadic adenoma patients.
  C. Fecal occult blood tests must be performed annually if they are to be effective.
  D. The protective effects of sigmoidoscopy extend for ten years.
  E. Carcinoembryonic antigen determination is an effective screening test in selected populations.

---

137. A 44-year-old woman with a six-year history of ulcerative colitis develops two months of vague right upper quadrant pain and generalized pruritus. A moderately elevated alkaline phosphatase level, minimal elevations of the serum aminotransferase levels, and a normal serum bilirubin level are present. Her symptoms and abnormal liver test results persist for six weeks. Hepatitis B surface antigen, anti-hepatitis C virus, and anti-hepatitis A virus IgM tests are all nonreactive. Serum ceruloplasmin, antimitochondrial antibody, antismooth muscle antibody, antinuclear antibody, and α_1-antitrypsin levels are unremarkable. A liver biopsy is performed and reveals a chronic inflammatory infiltrate in the portal tracts with concentric fibrosis around the bile ductules. Which one of the following statements regarding this patient is FALSE?
  A. Endoscopic retrograde cholangiopancreatography is necessary to confirm the diagnosis.
  B. This patient is most likely HLA-DR3, B8-positive.
  C. The liver disease is unlikely to progress.
  D. This patient has an increased risk of developing a bile duct carcinoma.

---

138. Which of the following infectious agents is NOT thought to be a cause of gastric ulcers?
  A. *Cryptosporidium*
  B. *Helicobacter pylori*
  C. Cytomegalovirus
  D. *Treponema pallidum*

---

139. A case-control study of screening sigmoidoscopy showed reduced mortality from distal colorectal cancer. However, a study comparing patients undergoing sigmoidoscopy with polypectomy did not show a lower subsequent risk of developing colon cancer compared with persons not undergoing sigmoidoscopy. Which of the following statements BEST explains these results?
  A. Polypectomy is not effective as a means of preventing subsequent colon cancer.
  B. Factors other than sigmoidoscopy were responsible for the decrease in mortality in the first study.
  C. Case-control studies are inherently less biased than retrospective studies.
  D. Both studies may be correct because the colonic distribution of cancers is moving distally.
  E. Both studies may be correct because the latter study did not control for colorectal cancer above the polypectomy site.

---

140. Match the following:
  1. Inflammatory pseudopolyps
  2. Colitis cystica profunda
  3. Pneumatosis cystoides intestinalis
  4. Benign lymphoid polyps
  5. Lipomas

  A. Found mainly in children
  B. Treated with oxygen therapy
  C. Often mistaken for colloid carcinoma
  D. Found mainly in the right colon
  E. Often seen in colons at increased risk of developing colon cancer

---

141. Which of the following statements about regulation of ion transport in the small intestine are TRUE?
  A. Ion transport is independent of intestinal blood flow.
  B. Metabolic acidosis is a potent stimulator of absorption.
  C. Metabolic alkalosis is a potent stimulator of absorption.
  D. Increased sympathetic input increases absorption and decreases secretion.

---

142. Each of the following luminal factors can cause diarrhea EXCEPT:
  A. Ursodeoxycholic acid
  B. Disaccharides
  C. Long-chain fatty acids
  D. Chenodeoxycholic acid
  E. Magnesium

143. Each of the following is a true statement about melanosis coli EXCEPT:
  A. It is a benign condition found in persons who chronically abuse anthracene cathartics.
  B. It usually disappears within 9 to 12 months after the offending cathartic is stopped.
  C. It has been associated with carcinoma of the colon, but the mechanism is unknown.
  D. The mucosal pigment is lipofuscin.
  E. The finding of melanosis coli on flexible sigmoidoscopy in a patient with a history of cathartic use should prompt a full colonoscopy.

144. Which one of the following statements regarding *Campylobacter jejuni* is FALSE?
  A. Contaminated or improperly cooked chicken is the most common mode of infection.
  B. Infection is found in many animals besides humans.
  C. Stool examination in affected patients is notable for the paucity of fecal leukocytes.
  D. The clinical course is characterized by a prodrome of coryza, headache, and malaise followed by waxing and waning diarrhea for several weeks.

145. Which of the following are TRUE statements about Hirschsprung's disease?
  A. It occurs in approximately 1 in each 5000 live births.
  B. Subsequent offspring of the same parents are not at increased risk.
  C. It is associated with Down's syndrome.
  D. The aganglionic segment invariably involves the rectosigmoid junction.

146. Each of the following has been identified as a risk factor for development of colonic adenoma EXCEPT:
  A. Sibling with colonic adenoma
  B. Smoking
  C. Consumption of a high-fat diet
  D. Chronic NSAID use
  E. Increasing age

147. A 40-year-old otherwise healthy patient is found to have an incidental 1.0-cm appendiceal carcinoid tumor. Which of the following is the MOST appropriate management?
  A. Simple appendectomy
  B. Simple appendectomy with yearly 24-hour urine collections for 5-hydroxyindoleacetic acid (5-HIAA)
  C. Simple appendectomy with yearly abdominal computed tomography
  D. Right hemicolectomy
  E. Right hemicolectomy with yearly 24-hour urine collections for 5-HIAA

148. A 40-year-old otherwise healthy patient is found to have an incidental 2.5-cm appendiceal carcinoid tumor. Which of the following is the MOST appropriate management?
  A. Simple appendectomy
  B. Simple appendectomy with yearly 24-hour urine collections for 5-hydroxyindoleacetic acid (5-HIAA)
  C. Simple appendectomy with yearly abdominal computed tomography
  D. Right hemicolectomy
  E. Right hemicolectomy with yearly 24-hour urine collections for 5-HIAA

149. Pathways between the central nervous system and the enteric nervous system include each of the following EXCEPT:
  A. Hormann's complex
  B. Cranial parasympathetics
  D. Thoracolumbar sympathetics
  D. Prevertebral ganglia
  E. Sacral parasympathetics

150. Which one of the following statements is TRUE with respect to the treatment of pseudo-obstruction of the colon (Ogilvie's syndrome):
  A. It is often exacerbated by treatment with cisapride.
  B. It should be treated with correction of metabolic, electrolyte, and fluid abnormalities.
  C. It often responds to oral laxatives such as lactulose.
  D. It rarely requires nasogastric or rectal suction.
  E. It responds to colonoscopic decompression in less than 50% of patients.

151. Each of the following is a true statement about irritable bowel syndrome (IBS) in childhood and adolescence EXCEPT:
  A. There is a high familial incidence.
  B. There is a female predominance.
  C. Children with IBS have normal growth and development.
  D. A majority of patients have a history of stress-induced onset.
  E. It is a common cause of referral to pediatric gastroenterologists.

152. A 40-year-old man, who had received extensive abdominal radiation ten years earlier for Hodgkin's disease, has chronic symptoms of postprandial bloating and periumbilical discomfort. Over the past several weeks he has noted persistent diarrhea. Routine stool studies for infectious agents are negative. Treatment with which of the following would MOST likely result in sustained improvement in his diarrhea?
  A. An oral mesalamine preparation

B. Bile acid–binding resins
C. A course of tetracycline
D. An H₂ receptor antagonist
E. A low-fat diet

---

153. Each of the following measures is useful in the management of acquired megacolon EXCEPT:
    A. Disimpaction of a fecal mass in the rectal vault
    B. Use of stimulant laxatives
    C. Use of bulking agents
    D. Trying to pass stool at the same time every day
    E. Surgical treatment

---

154. Which of the following statements are TRUE regarding ulcerative colitis in children?
    A. Prolonged corticosteroid treatment may suppress growth.
    B. A child with ulcerative colitis is less likely than an adult to have pancolitis.
    C. Ulcerative colitis does not present in infancy.
    D. Immunosuppressive therapy is contraindicated in children.

---

155. Each of the following statements about primary gastrointestinal lymphomas is true EXCEPT:
    A. Abdominal pain is a common presenting complaint.
    B. Abdominal mass is found in approximately one third of patients at presentation.
    C. The colorectal region is commonly involved.
    D. Massive hemorrhage is unusual.
    E. It often leads to gastric outlet obstruction or intussusception.

---

156. Each of the following malignancies has been reported with increased frequency in patients with Crohn's disease EXCEPT:
    A. Hodgkin's disease
    B. Colon cancer
    C. Squamous cell carcinoma of the anal canal
    D. Basal cell carcinoma
    E. Squamous cell carcinoma of the vulva

---

157. Which one of the following diseases is LEAST likely to be caused by a fiber-deficient diet?
    A. Diverticulosis
    B. Irritable bowel syndrome
    C. Appendicitis
    D. Constipation

---

158. Regarding the natural history of untreated colon polyps, which of the following statements are TRUE?
    A. Starting with a 10-mm polypoid mass, histology unknown, the probability of having colon cancer in five years is about 15%.

B. Starting with a 10-mm polypoid mass, histology unknown, the probability of having colon cancer in 20 years is about 25%.
    C. Starting with a 4-mm polypoid mass, histology unknown, the probability of having colon cancer in five years is less than 1%.
    D. Starting with a 4-mm polypoid mass, histology unknown, the probability of the lesion either staying the same size or shrinking in five years is greater than 90%.

---

159. Acute complications of schistosomiasis include each of the following EXCEPT:
    A. Biliary obstruction
    B. Cough and daily fevers to 39° C
    C. Appendicitis
    D. Pruritic, papular rash
    E. Dysentery

---

160. A patient with an ileal resection is placed on a bile acid–binding resin for treatment of chronic diarrhea. However, the diarrhea worsens. What is the MOST likely explanation?
    A. Patients with ileal resections frequently develop bacterial overgrowth.
    B. Bile acid–binding resins cause diarrhea.
    C. The bile acid binder has further depleted the bile acid pool.
    D. Bile acid binders may cause vitamin deficiencies.
    E. The patient most likely increased the consumption of poorly digestible carbohydrates.

---

161. Which of the following statements regarding diverticular bleeding are TRUE?
    I. Massive bleeding usually originates in the right colon.
    II. Bleeding may be aggravated by concurrent angiodysplasia.
    III. The lifetime risk of rebleeding after an initial diverticular hemorrhage is approximately 25%.
    IV. The lifetime risk of rebleeding after a second diverticular hemorrhage is approximately 10%.

    A. I and III
    B. II and IV
    C. I, II, and III
    D. All of the above

---

162. Each of the following is a true statement regarding surgical management of colorectal cancer EXCEPT:
    A. Prophylactic total colectomy is absolutely indicated in familial adenomatous polyposis once adenomas have developed.
    B. Surgery is indicated for curative therapy once the cancer has invaded the submucosa.
    C. Subtotal or total colectomy is indicated for colorectal cancers in hereditary nonpolyposis colorectal cancer.

D. A five-year survival of 20% can be obtained by resection of solitary hepatic metastases.
E. All are true.

---

163. Typical findings in Whipple's disease include all of the following EXCEPT:
A. Hepatosplenomegaly
B. Chronic cough
C. Cranial nerve deficits
D. Pericarditis
E. Peripheral adenopathy

---

164. Each of the following is a disadvantage of barium enema when compared with colonoscopy for colonic visualization EXCEPT:
A. Training for administering barium enemas is not as rigorous as in the past.
B. Barium enema cannot be used for ulcerative colitis surveillance.
C. Abnormal barium enemas often require diagnostic or therapeutic colonoscopy.
D. Barium enema lacks sensitivity for small polyps.
E. Barium enema lacks sensitivity in the sigmoid colon and at flexures.
F. All are true.

---

165. Which of the following is LEAST likely to present as megacolon?
A. *Blastocystis hominis* infection
B. Hirschsprung's disease
C. Inflammatory bowel disease
D. *Trypanosoma cruzi* infection
E. Colonic inertia

---

166. Adult *Schistosoma* worms traverse the portal vein but then migrate to tissues by preferred routes that help to determine the clinical presentation. Which of the following statements regarding the *Schistosoma* life cycle are TRUE?
A. *S. japonicum* preferentially migrates along the superior mesenteric vein.
B. *S. mansoni* tends to involve the descending colon and bladder because of its proclivity to follow the inferior mesenteric vein.
C. *S. haematobium* prefers the vesicle plexus, causing it to involve the pelvic organs and bladder.

---

167. Regarding the pathogenesis of traveler's diarrhea, which one of the following statements is FALSE?
A. The most common cause is enteroadherent *Escherichia coli.*
B. No pathogen can be identified in up to 40% of cases.
C. The major determinant of risk is the destination of the traveler.
D. Younger travelers have the highest risk.

---

168. At which point in the cell cycle is a proliferating cell MOST sensitive to X-irradiation?
A. G1
B. Early S phase
C. G2/M phase
D. The cell is equally sensitive throughout the cell cycle.
E. Late S phase

---

169. Each of the following statements regarding potassium transport in the intestine is true EXCEPT:
A. Small bowel potassium secretion is passive.
B. The colon secretes potassium into the lumen in exchange for sodium.
C. Potassium concentrations in the colonic lumen are greater than in serum.
D. Potassium exits the cell by means of a potassium channel.

---

170. The MOST common clinical presentation of small bowel carcinoid is:
A. Intermittent abdominal pain
B. Gastrointestinal bleeding
C. Intussusception
D. Carcinoid syndrome
E. Small bowel infarction

---

171. Match the following bacterial infectious agents with the corresponding clinical feature or fact.
1. *Salmonella typhi*
2. *Salmonella enteritidis*
3. *Shigella dysenteriae*
4. *Vibrio cholerae*

A. "Rose spot" rash
B. Signs of sepsis are rare
C. As few as 200 organisms can produce disease
D. Domestic animal zoonosis

---

172. Which of the following statements regarding Hirschsprung's disease are TRUE?
I. Stainable ganglion cells are generally absent in the dilated segment of bowel.
II. Rectal biopsy is usually diagnostic.
III. The aganglionic segment is always spastic but may be short.
IV. The rectoanal inhibitory reflex is preserved.

A. I and III
B. II and IV
C. I, II, and III
D. All of the above

---

173. Chronic intestinal radiation injury is primarily caused by:
A. Permanent damage to the mucosal crypt cell populations
B. Damage to the intestinal vascular epithelium
C. Disruption of brush border enzyme production

D. Loss of the normal villous structure
E. Formation of permanent fibrous bands

---

174. Each of the following statements regarding genetic predisposition in Crohn's disease is true EXCEPT:
A. Siblings of patients with Crohn's disease are 17 to 35 times more likely to develop Crohn's disease than the general population.
B. Data from monozygotic twins suggest an autosomal dominant pattern of inheritance.
C. Men and women are equally affected.
D. Ashkenazi Jews are more likely to develop Crohn's disease than are Jews of Russian or Polish origin.
E. The risk to offspring of a patient with Crohn's disease is similar to that of their siblings.

---

175. Of the following, the MOST sensitive and specific test for diagnosing small intestinal bacterial overgrowth is:
A. ^{14}C-bile acid breath test
B. Hydrogen breath test
C. Quantitative bacterial culture
D. ^{14}C-xylose breath test
E. Quantitation of urinary indican

---

176. Which of the following statements about sexual transmission of hepatitis are TRUE?
I. Sexual transmission of hepatitis A is primarily by oral-anal contact.
II. Hepatitis C can be detected by the polymerase chain reaction in semen and vaginal secretions.
III. Hepatitis B can be acquired transurethrally.
IV. Hepatitis B is associated with oral-anal sexual contact.

A. I and III
B. II and IV
C. I, II, and III
D. All of the above

---

177. True statements about Whipple's disease include all of the following EXCEPT:
A. It is fatal if not treated.
B. Response to antibiotics is slow.
C. It is caused by a gram-positive rod.
D. Pathologic specimens of the small bowel reveal prominent periodic acid–Schiff (PAS)-positive macrophages.
E. Lymphatic dilatation and fat accumulation are common pathologic features.

---

178. Each of the following statements regarding carcinoid crisis is true EXCEPT:
A. It usually occurs in foregut carcinoids.
B. It may be precipitated by stress, chemotherapy, or the induction of anesthesia.

C. The characteristic flushing of carcinoid syndrome is often absent.
D. It is usually associated with markedly elevated 5-hydroxyindoleacetic acid levels.

---

179. A 52-year-old man with ulcerative colitis who had been well in recent months reports lower abdominal cramping, subjective fever, arthralgias, and passage of six to eight bloody stools daily for the past two weeks. Stool studies are negative for bacterial or parasitic infection. A colonoscopy done six months ago revealed pancolitis. Which of the following is MOST likely to control the patient's acute symptoms?
A. Oral corticosteroids
B. Mesalamine suppositories
C. Azathioprine
D. 6-Mercaptopurine
E. Sulfasalazine

---

180. Rehydrating Hemoccult cards has been shown to approximately double the yield of colon cancers, while increasing the number of positive tests approximately four-fold. Each of the following statements about rehydration is true EXCEPT:
A. It increases the number of colon cancers discovered in earlier stages.
B. It decreases the mortality of colorectal cancer.
C. Rehydration of the slide increases the positive predictive value of the test.
D. Delayed development of the slide for one week decreases the sensitivity of the test.
E. Rehydration of the slide increases the sensitivity of the test.

---

181. Which of the following statements are TRUE regarding balantidiasis?
I. In the United States, balantidiasis is most common among institutionalized patients.
II. Three negative stool examinations for ova and parasites effectively exclude this condition.
III. The range of symptoms ranges from none to clinical dysentery.
IV. The only treatment is removal from the environment where the infection was acquired.

A. I and III
B. II and IV
C. I, II, and III
D. All of the above

---

182. Which one of the following statements about *Vibrio cholerae* infectious diarrhea is FALSE?
A. Fecal outputs of 15 to 20 L/day are common.
B. The organism is not invasive.
C. Bloody diarrhea is common.

D. Bacteremia is rare.

E. Patients often present with profound dehydration and hypovolemic shock.

---

183. The MOST common finding on abdominal examination of patients with clinically important malabsorption is:

A. Hyperactive bowel sounds

B. Epigastric tenderness

C. Positive heme test on the stool

D. Mild to moderate distention

E. Normal examination

---

184. A 55-year-old Vietnamese man has had progressive worsening of diarrhea for the last four months. His stool studies are remarkable for a quantitative fecal fat of 14 g/day. The LEAST likely diagnosis is:

A. Tropical sprue

B. Celiac sprue

C. Whipple's disease

D. Small bowel lymphoma

E. Pancreatic insufficiency

---

185. Each of the following statements about chronic intestinal pseudo-obstruction is true EXCEPT:

A. It is characterized by symptoms and signs of intestinal obstruction.

B. It may be caused by disorders of smooth muscle.

C. It may be associated with an occluding lesion of the intestinal lumen.

D. It can involve the esophagus and stomach.

E. It is caused by ineffective intestinal propulsion.

---

186. With respect to complications after ileoanal pouch anastomosis, which of the following statements is FALSE?

A. Impotence occurs in 1% to 2% of men after ileoanal pouch anastomosis.

B. Dyspareunia occurs in less than 10% of women after ileoanal pouch anastomosis.

C. Nocturnal fecal incontinence is common early on but usually diminishes after a year.

D. Pouchitis reflects vascular insufficiency and does not respond well to medical treatment.

E. Ileoanal pouch anastomosis has a complication rate of about 30%, with pelvic infections, small bowel obstruction, and pouch leakage being the most common.

---

187. Effective therapy for eosinophilic gastroenteritis includes which of the following?

I. Dietary manipulation

II. Sodium cromoglycate

III. Hydroxyurea

IV. Corticosteroids

A. I and III

B. II and IV

C. I, II, and III

D. IV only

E. All of the above

---

188. Which one of the following statements regarding carcinoembryonic antigen (CEA) is TRUE?

A. CEA is normal in most Dukes' A and B colon cancers.

B. CEA levels are useful in predicting disease outcome in colorectal cancer.

C. A rising CEA level and computed tomography have comparable sensitivity for detecting colorectal cancer recurrence.

D. All are true.

E. None is true.

---

189. Which one of the following syndromes is NOT associated with extracolonic malignancies?

A. Cowden's syndrome

B. Cronkhite-Canada syndrome

C. Muir-Torre syndrome

D. Turcot's syndrome

E. Lynch II syndrome

---

190. Which of the following is MOST commonly seen after total proctocolectomy?

A. Fat malabsorption

B. Vitamin B_{12} deficiency

C. Vitamin K deficiency

D. Salt depletion

E. Weight loss

---

191. TRUE statements about *Salmonella typhi,* the causative agent of typhoid fever, include:

A. Humans are the only natural reservoir of *S. typhi.*

B. The incubation period of typhoid fever is one to two days.

C. Patients with pre-existing gallbladder disease have a greater likelihood of becoming carriers.

D. Most strains are susceptible to ampicillin and chloramphenicol.

E. *S. typhi* can be isolated from the blood in about half of patients if cultured during the first week of illness.

---

192. A patient undergoes an extensive bowel resection and postoperatively is left with a jejunostomy and only the first 125 cm of jejunum. Which statement BEST describes future nutritional concerns?

A. The patient will likely require lifelong total parenteral nutrition.

B. The patient may eat but will require parenteral caloric supplements.

C. The patient will almost certainly be able to maintain normal hydration.

D. The patient should be able to maintain nutritional balance with oral feeding.

E. Normal oral nutrition is possible, but only if iron and folate supplements are given.

---

193. Which of the following colon cancer characteristics is associated with the BEST prognosis?

A. Mucinous histology

B. Scirrhous histology

C. Bulky tumor

D. Aneuploidy

E. Local inflammation

---

194. Which of the following statements regarding the epidemiology of intestinal parasitic infections are TRUE?

A. Sexual promiscuity increases viral and bacteria infections but not parasitic infections of the intestine.

B. Historically, parasitic infections were limited mainly to tropical and underdeveloped countries.

C. Crowding of children in day care centers has increased the prevalence of parasitic diseases.

D. Migration from third world countries to United States urban areas has had little impact on the prevalence of parasitic infections.

---

195. Which of the following is LEAST likely to mimic Crohn's disease of the terminal ileum?

A. Tuberculosis

B. Amebiasis

C. *Yersinia* infection

D. *Campylobacter jejuni* infection

E. Behçet's disease

---

196. Treatment of pseudomembranous colitis may include all of the following EXCEPT:

A. Use of antiperistaltic agents

B. Supportive measures such as intravenous fluids and correction of electrolyte abnormalities

C. Discontinuation of the offending antibiotic

D. Treatment with oral vancomycin, metronidazole, or bacitracin

---

197. Each of the following organisms may be associated with bloody diarrhea EXCEPT:

A. *Entamoeba histolytica*

B. *Shigella boydii*

C. *Campylobacter jejuni*

D. *Escherichia coli*

E. *Giardia lamblia*

---

198. In selecting a patient for an ileorectal anastomosis, all of the following are favorable selection factors EXCEPT:

A. Willing to undergo rectal surveillance

B. Age younger than 70

C. Minimal rectal inflammation

D. Good anal sphincter function

E. Low rectal compliance

---

199. Each of the following statements about staging is true EXCEPT:

A. Dukes' A malignancies and malignant polyps have the same prognosis.

B. Dukes' B lesions differ from Dukes' C lesions in presence of involved lymph nodes.

C. Increasing stage (A–C) is determined by the depth of penetration into and through the bowel wall.

D. Dukes' C1 lesions have a five-year survival greater than 50%.

E. Surgery in Dukes' D colon cancer is usually indicated even if metastatic disease cannot be resected for cure.

---

200. The major indirect cost of a mass screening program for colorectal cancer is:

A. Lost time from work

B. Public education costs

C. More frequent surveillance resulting from positive workups

D. Follow-up of false-positive screening tests

E. Complications during false-positive workups

---

201. Which one of the following statements about the Kock pouch (continent ileostomy) is TRUE?

A. It is the most common type of ileostomy after colectomy for ulcerative colitis.

B. Incontinence is seen in up to one third of pouches.

C. The pouch self-empties after sufficient pressure develops in the pouch to open the one-way valve.

D. Young women tend to have the worst outcome with this operation.

E. As opposed to ileoanal pouch anastomosis, pouchitis rarely develops.

---

202. An operation to remove a right ovarian cyst is being planned. Which of the following statements BEST addresses the role of incidental appendectomy at operation?

A. All patients in this circumstance should have an incidental appendectomy.

B. Incidental appendectomy should never be performed.

C. Patients between 30 and 50 years old are the most likely to benefit.

D. If the appendix is easily exposed it is worthwhile to remove it in patients older than 50 years old.

E. It is worthwhile in patients younger than 30 years old.

203. Each of the following statements regarding rectal carcinoids is true EXCEPT:
  A. They are usually detected incidentally in middle-aged adults.
  B. They are usually single lesions located 4 to 13 cm proximal to the dentate line.
  C. Although primary tumors are typically asymptomatic, metastatic rectal carcinoid usually causes carcinoid syndrome.
  D. Because rectal carcinoids over 2 cm frequently metastasize, treatment is surgical resection as for other rectal carcinomas.

204. Which of the following statements about pepsins are TRUE?
  A. They are released as a precursor that autoactivates in acidic pH.
  B. Pepsinogen is produced by chief cells in the gastric mucosa.
  C. Pepsinogen release is stimulated by gastrin, histamine, and cholinergic excitation.
  D. Pepsin activity is essential for normal protein absorption.

205. Fecal leukocytes are likely to be found in infections caused by all of the following EXCEPT:
  A. *Bacillus cereus*
  B. *Shigella flexneri*
  C. *Salmonella typhi*
  D. *Yersinia enterocolitica*
  E. *Clostridium difficile*

206. Which of the following conditions is LEAST likely to precipitate toxic megacolon?
  A. Ulcerative colitis
  B. Crohn's colitis
  C. Pseudomembranous colitis
  D. Collagenous colitis
  E. Amebic colitis

207. Which one of the following does NOT improve the specificity of fecal occult blood testing (FOBT)?
  A. Immunologic testing for human hemoglobin
  B. Avoiding antioxidant vitamins
  C. Avoiding peroxidase-containing vegetables
  D. Testing for porphyrin fluorescence
  E. All of the above improve the specificity of FOBT.

208. Which helminthic infection is associated with sexual transmission?
  A. *Ascaris lumbricoides*
  B. *Trichuris trichiura* (whipworm)
  C. *Ancylostoma duodenale* (hookworm)
  D. *Strongyloides stercoralis*

209. The major structural component of the cytoskeleton of plants is:
  A. Cellulose
  B. Lignin
  C. Pectin
  D. Starch

210. Secondary abnormalities caused by fat malabsorption include each of the following EXCEPT:
  A. Severe weight loss
  B. Proximal muscle weakness
  C. Depressed serum carotene
  D. Depressed serum albumin
  E. Prolonged prothrombin time

211. Which of the following is MOST commonly involved in eosinophilic gastroenteritis?
  A. Mucosal layer
  B. Submucosal layer
  C. Muscle layer
  D. Serosal layer

212. A 65-year-old woman who had received pelvic radiation for cervical cancer ten years earlier presents with persistent rectal bleeding. Colonoscopy reveals numerous mucosal telangiectases in the rectum. What would be the MOST appropriate next step in management?
  A. A diverting colostomy
  B. Proctectomy with colostomy
  C. Intensive topical therapy with glucocorticoid and mesalamine preparations
  D. Endoscopic cauterization
  E. Formalin enemas

213. Which of the following statements describing the effects of cholera are TRUE?
  I. Cholera produces a cytotoxin that impairs absorption and damages the mucosa.
  II. Cholera produces an enterotoxin that increases cyclic adenosine monophosphate and thus secretion.
  III. Sodium-coupled nutrient pathways (i.e., sodium-glucose) are damaged by the toxin.
  IV. Cholera toxin blocks electroneutral sodium chloride absorption.

  A. I and III
  B. II and IV
  C. I, II, and III
  D. All of the above

214. Which of the following are TRUE statements regarding the epidemiology of ulcerative colitis?
  A. The incidence of ulcerative colitis has remained stable over the past 30 years.

B. Ulcerative colitis is more common in Northern Europe than in Israel.

C. Twin studies have shown that a greater genetic influence exists for ulcerative colitis than for Crohn's disease.

D. Ten to 20 percent of patients with ulcerative colitis will have at least one other family member affected.

E. Ulcerative colitis may present from within the first year of life until the ninth decade.

---

215. Each of the following statements regarding nonrehydrated Hemoccult cards is true EXCEPT:

A. They are more sensitive for right colon lesions than left colon lesions.

B. Their sensitivity is reduced by consumption of fruits and vegetables.

C. False-positive results may occur due to consumption of animal hemoglobin.

D. They may be positive after upper gastrointestinal tract bleeding.

E. They are less sensitive than hydrated Hemoccult cards.

---

216. A 55-year-old man with a known metastatic carcinoid complains of a gradual increase in both the frequency and duration of flushing episodes to the point that he is no longer able to work. Which of the following drugs would be MOST likely to relieve his symptom of flushing?

A. Cimetidine

B. Cyproheptadine

C. Clonidine

D. Octreotide

E. Propranolol

---

217. The patient described in the previous question was treated with octreotide and experienced a significant reduction in the frequency and intensity of the flushing episodes. Which of the following statements regarding the continued use of octreotide are TRUE?

I. With continued daily use, his chances of developing cholelithiasis are 1 in 3.

II. Urinary 5-hydroxyindoleacetic acid levels are largely unaffected by octreotide treatment.

III. With continued daily use, tolerance to octreotide will ultimately limit its usefulness.

IV. Although useful for control of flushing, octreotide is not helpful in relief of carcinoid crisis.

A. I and III

B. II and IV

C. I, II, and III

D. All of the above

---

218. Match the following terms with their meanings.

1. Sensitivity
2. Specificity
3. Positive predictive value
4. Negative predictive value
5. Incidence
6. Prevalence

A. New cases appearing in the population over a given time period

B. The probability that a patient with a negative test will not have the disease

C. The cases existing in a population at a given time

D. The probability of a test's being positive in patients with the disease

E. The probability that a patient with a positive test will have the disease

F. The probability of a test's being negative in patients without the disease

---

219. Each of the following statements about intestinal adaptation after partial intestinal resection is true EXCEPT:

A. Initiating postoperative oral feeding enhances the crypt cell production rate.

B. The remaining small bowel frequently grows in length and diameter.

C. Adaptive changes are more prominent in the jejunum than the ileum.

D. Mean stool volume generally decreases over time.

E. Adaptive changes are thought to be mediated by growth factors.

---

220. The clinical finding that BEST differentiates distal bowel obstruction from paralytic ileus is:

A. Low-grade fever

B. Abdominal distention

C. Persistent vomiting

D. High-pitched bowel sounds

E. Poor skin turgor

---

221. Which of the following is MOST typical of antibiotic-associated pseudomembranous colitis?

A. Invasion of the bowel mucosa by *Clostridium difficile*

B. Presence of pseudomembranes with areas of normal intervening mucosa

C. Extension of pseudomembranes into the small bowel

D. The appearance of "volcanic eruptions" on mucosal histology

---

222. Which of the following statements about *Aeromonas* infection are TRUE?

A. It is associated with drinking untreated well or spring water.

B. Beta-lactam antibiotics are effective therapy.

C. Diarrhea may be chronic.

D. The disease is almost always benign and self-limited.

---

223. Which of the following measures is LEAST likely to be helpful in the management of acute colonic pseudo-obstruction (Ogilvie's syndrome)?

    A. Stopping oral feedings

    B. Nasogastric tube suction

    C. Rectal tube decompression

    D. Barium enema to exclude obstruction or volvulus

    E. Correction of associated electrolyte disturbances

---

224. Which one of the following statements about *Bacillus cereus* infection is FALSE?

    A. It can cause either an emetic or diarrheal illness.

    B. It is an aerobic gram-positive rod.

    C. It is not invasive.

    D. It typically produces fever.

---

225. Each of the following is a true statement regarding the anatomy of the duodenum EXCEPT:

    A. The duodenum is directly anterior to the descending aorta, and erosion through the aorta may cause catastrophic gastrointestinal bleeding.

    B. The liver is in immediate contact with the antero-superior aspect of the first portion of the duodenum.

    C. All of the duodenum is located intraperitoneally.

    D. The superior mesenteric artery and vein cross the third portion of the duodenum anteriorly.

    E. The pancreas is located immediately medial to the duodenum.

---

226. Nongranulomatous ulcerative jejunoileitis (also termed *idiopathic chronic ulcerative enteritis*) is BEST characterized by which one of the following?

    A. Gluten withdrawal benefits most patients.

    B. Treatment with prednisone induces remission in most patients.

    C. The clinical course is usually severe and often fatal.

    D. Malabsorption is rarely seen.

    E. It is usually seen complicating the course of celiac disease.

---

227. Bacterial overgrowth is a treatable but easily overlooked cause of malabsorption. Each of the following is associated with bacterial overgrowth EXCEPT:

    A. Addison's disease

    B. Diabetes mellitus

    C. Progressive systemic sclerosis

    D. Upper gastrointestinal tract surgery

    E. Vitamin B_{12} deficiency

---

228. Which one or more of the following are common pathologic features of small bowel mucosa from patients with celiac sprue?

    A. The intestinal crypts are elongated and villi are shortened.

    B. The total thickness of the mucosa is markedly reduced.

    C. Degenerative changes, including cytoplasmic vacuolization, are uncommon.

    D. There is a decrease in the number of absorptive cells.

---

229. In establishing the cause of pruritus ani, which of the following is LEAST appropriate?

    A. Skin biopsy

    B. Examination of a transparent adhesive tape that has been applied to the anal skin

    C. Inquiring about the recent use of oral antibiotics

    D. Inquiring about the recent topical applications of ointments, deodorants, powders, or soap

    E. Therapeutic trial of sclerotherapy for first-degree external hemorrhoids

---

230. Clinical manifestations of the carcinoid syndrome include which of the following?

    I. Flushing and diarrhea

    II. Asthma

    III. Pellagra

    IV. Aortic stenosis

    A. I and III

    B. II and IV

    C. I, II, and III

    D. All of the above

---

231. In a case of suspected celiac sprue, which one of the following tests would be MOST valuable in confirming the diagnosis?

    A. D-Xylose absorption test

    B. Abdominal computed tomography

    C. Endoscopic ultrasonography with examination of the pancreas

    D. Endoscopy with small bowel biopsy

    E. Hydrogen breath test

---

232. Which one of the following statements BEST describes the histologic findings in Crohn's disease?

    A. Chronic inflammation is limited to the mucosa.

    B. Granulomas are rarely seen on endoscopic mucosal biopsy, but they are almost always seen on resected surgical specimens.

    C. Resected specimens reveal chronic transmural inflammation, with granulomas being seen approximately one half of the time.

D. An acute inflammatory infiltrate is present with preservation of crypt architecture.

E. Apoptosis of glandular epithelium is commonly seen.

---

233. Which of the following statements regarding chloride movement in the intestine are TRUE?
  I. Most chloride absorption occurs by simple diffusion.
  II. Most cellular transport of chloride is linked to sodium.
  III. The chloride flux provides the principal driving force for fluid secretion.
  IV. Chloride accounts for the majority of luminal anions in the colon.

  A. I and III
  B. II and IV
  C. I, II, and III
  D. All of the above

---

234. Hamartomas are associated with all of the following EXCEPT:
  A. Juvenile polyposis
  B. Cowden's syndrome
  C. Turcot's syndrome
  D. Basal cell nevus syndrome
  E. All are associated with hamartomas.

---

235. Each of the following is a common cause of infectious diarrhea in adults EXCEPT:
  A. Rotavirus
  B. *Salmonella*
  C. *Shigella*
  D. *Campylobacter*
  E. Norwalk virus

---

236. Each of the following physiologic abnormalities is present in Hirschsprung's disease EXCEPT:
  A. Failure of the internal anal sphincter to relax after rectal distention
  B. Failure of the contracted segment to relax after administration of parasympathomimetic agents
  C. Increased resistance to stretch of the rectal wall
  D. Very high resting pressure in the internal anal sphincter
  E. Extension of the aganglionic segment from the internal anal sphincter

---

237. Specify whether flexible sigmoidoscopy or colonoscopy is more appropriate for evaluating each of the following conditions.
  1. Surveillance for neoplasms in inflammatory bowel disease
  2. Complicated sigmoid diverticular disease

  A. Flexible sigmoidoscopy
  B. Total colonoscopy

  3. Surveillance for neoplasms in Lynch's syndrome
  4. Acute severe hemorrhage

---

238. The MOST common cause of short bowel syndrome in children is:
  A. Necrotizing enterocolitis
  B. Mesenteric infarction
  C. Trauma
  D. Crohn's disease
  E. Congenital

---

239. Each of the following statements about *Yersinia enterocolitica* infection is true EXCEPT:
  A. Children older than the age of 5 with *Y. enterocolitica* infection often present with symptoms and signs indistinguishable from those of appendicitis.
  B. Infection in the terminal ileum often involves mesenteric lymph nodes and ulceration of Peyer's patches.
  C. *Y. enterocolitica* infection is most common in warm climates where the organism can proliferate in warm foods before ingestion.
  D. Culture in the bacteriology laboratory requires special techniques.
  E. The organism is resistant to beta-lactam antibiotics.

---

240. Each of the following conditions has a hereditary component EXCEPT:
  A. Sporadic colorectal cancer
  B. Sporadic adenomas
  C. Lynch I syndrome
  D. Cowden's disease
  E. Cronkhite-Canada syndrome

---

241. Match the maximum frequency of smooth muscle contractions to the appropriate intestinal tract site.
  1. Antrum   A. 3 per minute
  2. Duodenum   B. 8 per minute
  3. Ileum   C. 11 per minute

---

242. Manifestations of acute intestinal radiation injury include all of the following EXCEPT:
  A. Mucosal ulceration
  B. Gastrointestinal bleeding
  C. Villous blunting
  D. Stricture formation
  E. Nausea and vomiting

---

243. Each of the following statements regarding hookworm infection is true EXCEPT:
  A. Hookworm infestation typically presents as iron-deficiency anemia.

B. Infected patients should be treated with mebendazole and encouraged to wear shoes.
C. Unlike other helminthic infections, hookworm rarely causes eosinophilia.
D. With moderate to severe infestations the skin is noted to be dry (decreased sweating) and to have a yellow pallor.

---

244. Which of the following is LEAST likely to be a presenting symptom of irritable bowel syndrome?
A. Painless diarrhea
B. Constipation
C. Mucus in stool
D. Abdominal distention
E. Abdominal pain

---

245. Conditions associated with bacterial overgrowth of the small intestine include all of the following EXCEPT:
A. Billroth II partial gastrectomy and anastomosis
B. Scleroderma
C. Sustained hyperchlorhydria induced by the Zollinger-Ellison syndrome
D. Disordered migrating motor complex
E. Resection of the ileocecal valve

---

246. Each of the following is associated with pneumatosis cystoides intestinalis EXCEPT:
A. Jejunal ileal bypass for obesity
B. Peptic ulcer disease
C. Whipple's disease
D. Inflammatory bowel disease
E. Endometriosis

---

247. Which one of the following statements regarding the rectal anal region is TRUE?
A. The anatomic anal canal is 6 to 7 cm long.
B. The valves of Houston form an important component of the external anal sphincter.
C. Palpation of the lateral aspect of the rectum is important to rule out abscess formation in the ischiorectal space.
D. The internal and external hemorrhoidal plexus are located near the rectal sigmoid junction.
E. The lining of the rectum is composed of squamous epithelium.

---

248. Which of the following is the simplest and most effective test to confirm suspected bacterial overgrowth?
A. Glucose breath hydrogen test
B. Culture of the intestinal aspirate
C. Endoscopic biopsy of the small intestine
D. Gram stain of duodenal brushings
E. Stool for ova and parasites

---

249. Which of the following radiographic findings are consistent with a diagnosis of eosinophilic gastroenteritis?
  I. Achalasia-like esophagram with "bird's beak" lower esophageal sphincter
 II. Enlarged gastric folds
III. Pyloric stenosis
IV. Small bowel obstruction

A. I and III
B. II and IV
C. I, II, and III
D. IV only
E. All of the above

---

250. Important complications of diverticulitis include all the following EXCEPT:
A. Generalized peritonitis
B. Subphrenic abscess
C. Inflammatory diarrhea
D. Obstruction of the colon
E. Colovesical fistula

---

251. Food allergy syndromes associated with IgE-mediated disease include all of the following EXCEPT:
A. Allergic eosinophilic gastroenteritis
B. Gastrointestinal anaphylaxis
C. Food-induced colitis
D. Oral allergy syndrome
E. Infantile colic

---

252. Which of the following statements about patients with traveler's diarrhea are TRUE?
A. Treatment with antimotility drugs is often useful.
B. Prophylactic treatment with antibiotics can effectively prevent more than 80% of cases of traveler's diarrhea.
C. Enterotoxigenic *Escherichia coli* accounts for the majority of cases but *Entamoeba histolytica* is common enough (20%) to warrant metronidazole for empirical therapy.
D. Among different types of travelers, the risk of acquiring traveler's diarrhea is as follows: students more than business travelers more than persons visiting relatives.

---

253. The following factors are all necessary for the clinical expression of *Clostridium difficile* colitis EXCEPT:
A. An altered normal flora
B. Production of toxin
C. Presence of an underlying debilitating condition
D. Growth of the vegetative form of *C. difficile*

254. Which of the following statements are TRUE regarding amebic liver abscesses?
A. Ultrasonography and serologic testing have largely replaced abscess aspiration as diagnostic tools of choice.
B. Three negative stool examinations effectively rule out amebic liver abscess.
C. Amebic liver abscesses are three times more common in men than in women.
D. Amebic liver abscesses are easily curable and rarely life-threatening.
E. Patients usually have leukocytosis and eosinophilia.

255. Which of the following are TRUE statements regarding fecal impaction?
A. Patients with impaction have normal anal sphincter function but impaired rectal sensation of distention.
B. Medications that predispose to impaction include narcotics, anticholinergics, aluminum antacids, and bulk laxatives (fiber) without adequate hydration.
C. It often resolves after barium examination of the upper digestive tract.
D. Soapsuds enemas and oral lactulose may be used to facilitate disimpaction.

256. A 33-year-old woman presents with bloody diarrhea of one to two days' duration. She recently returned from a camping trip in Yosemite National Park where she drank water from a mountain stream. The LEAST likely diagnosis is:
A. Campylobacteriosis
B. Amebiasis
C. Shigellosis
D. Giardiasis

257. Which one of the following extraintestinal manifestations of ulcerative colitis does NOT correlate with the activity of the colitis?
A. Ankylosing spondylitis
B. Peripheral arthropathy
C. Episcleritis
D. Aphthous ulceration of the mouth
E. Erythema nodosum

258. The three most common locations of gastrointestinal carcinoids are:
A. Stomach, small bowel, appendix
B. Stomach, small bowel, ascending colon
C. Stomach, ascending colon, rectum
D. Small bowel, appendix, rectum
E. Appendix, ascending colon, rectum

259. Each of the following is a true statement about hereditary nonpolyposis colorectal cancer (HNPCC) EXCEPT:
A. Most lesions are proximal to the splenic flexure.
B. Most of the cancers do not arise from adenomas.
C. The average age for diagnosis of colon cancer is younger than 45 years.
D. The male-to-female ratio is approximately equal.
E. A replication error phenotype is associated with these tumors.

260. Each of the following is an important prognostic feature of gastrointestinal lymphoma EXCEPT:
A. Stage of the disease at the time of diagnosis
B. Cell type
C. Constitutional symptoms such as fever, night sweats, and weight loss
D. Patient age
E. White blood cell count

261. Of the following, which is the MOST common cause of small bowel obstruction?
A. Hernia
B. Volvulus
C. Adhesion
D. Intussusception
E. Tumor

262. Each of the following statements about the pathogenesis of acute appendicitis is true EXCEPT:
A. When intraluminal pressure in the appendix reaches 85 cm H_2O, the appendix becomes hypoxic.
B. Infections by viruses, bacteria, or parasites may initiate appendicitis.
C. Fecaliths are found obstructing the appendiceal lumen in the majority of cases.
D. Colonoscopic trauma may precipitate appendicitis.
E. Gangrene and perforation usually develop in 24 to 36 hours.

263. Match each syndrome with an associated characteristic.
1. Occurs mostly at night; aggravated by anxiety
2. Recent pelvic or spinal surgery
3. Levator muscle spasm
4. Straining at stool

A. Proctalgia fugax
B. Coccygodynia
C. Descending perineum syndrome
D. Chronic idiopathic anal pain

264. Match each statement with the corresponding phase of the migrating myoelectric complex (MMC). Each selection may be used once, more than once, or not at all.
1. Sphincter of Oddi exhibits maximal motor activity

A. Phase II
B. Phase III

2. Gallbladder fills with bile
3. Sphincter of Oddi exhibits decreased baseline pressure
4. Maximum emptying of bile into the duodenum

265. A patient with a proctocolectomy and extensive ileal resection is at risk for all of the following EXCEPT:
A. Vitamin B$_{12}$ malabsorption
B. Oxalate kidney stones
C. Vitamin K malabsorption
D. Gallstones
E. Calcium malabsorption

266. Of the following measures that have been proposed for primary prevention of colon cancer, which appears to have the LEAST effect in modulating colorectal cancer risk?
A. Dietary fiber supplements
B. Antioxidant vitamins (A, C, and E)
C. Calcium supplements
D. Dietary fat restriction
E. NSAID use

267. Of the following tests that may be useful in demonstrating gastrointestinal involvement with endometriosis, which is the LEAST likely to demonstrate the lesion:
A. Endovaginal sonography
B. Laparoscopy
C. Sigmoidoscopy
D. Esophagogastroduodenoscopy
E. Pelvic computed tomography

268. Although steatorrhea occurs in a variety of disease states, severe fat malabsorption usually indicates that the patient has:
A. Had previous gastric surgery that has impaired cholecystokinin release, mixing, and timing of emptying of gastric contents
B. Lymphatic obstruction from metastatic disease blocking chylomicron delivery to the circulation
C. Deficiency of exocrine pancreatic secretion of lipase and colipase impairing hydrolysis of triglyceride
D. Disruption of the enterohepatic circulation of bile salts by ileal or biliary disease impairing micelle formation and absorption

269. Which one or more of the following tissues may contain periodic acid–Schiff (PAS)-positive macrophages in patients with Whipple's disease?
A. Brain
B. Kidney
C. Skin
D. Eye
E. Heart

270. Match each malignant anal tumor with its distinguishing feature.
1. Epidermoid carcinoma
2. Bowen's disease
3. Extramammary Paget's disease
4. Malignant melanoma
5. Anorectal carcinoid tumor

A. Malignant lesions are uniformly fatal
B. Mucinous adenocarcinoma arising from apocrine glands
C. Pruritus ani
D. May resemble thrombosed hemorrhoid
E. Human papillomavirus types 16 and 18

271. A 41-year-old man who lives in a migrant labor camp complains of six weeks of frequent bloody diarrhea, tenesmus, and lower abdominal cramping. A stool sample is negative for ova and parasites, and the stool culture is negative for pathogens. His physician performs a flexible sigmoidoscopy and finds scattered colonic ulcers. The patient is started on prednisone, 40 mg/day. One week later, he presents to the emergency department with severe abdominal pain and vomiting. On examination he has a fever of 39° C and a moderately tender and slightly distended abdomen. Which of the following are TRUE statements regarding this patient?
A. A serum amebic titer would be of little use given the high prevalence of amebic dysentery in migrant labor camps.
B. An upright abdominal film should be performed as soon as possible to exclude megacolon.
C. Given the vomiting, he should be switched to intravenous corticosteroids at stress doses.
D. Colonoscopy should be performed after an overnight bowel preparation to establish a definitive diagnosis and stage the extent of colonic involvement.

272. Multiple concentric circumferential diaphragmatic strictures in the small intestine are MOST likely to be a complication of which of the following?
A. NSAIDs
B. Crohn's disease
C. Radiation
D. Tuberculosis
E. Lymphoma

273. Each of the following is a true statement about lipomas of the gastrointestinal tract EXCEPT:
A. On probing with a biopsy forceps, an indentation is seen—the "cushion" sign.
B. They should be removed because of their malignant potential.
C. They are most commonly seen in the distal ileum, cecum, or ileocecal valve area.
D. They may cause symptoms due to intussusception, obstruction, or bleeding.
E. They can grow up to 5 cm in diameter.

274. Examples of bacterial metabolism of drugs within the intestinal lumen include:
   A. Conversion of sulfasalazine to sulfapyridine plus mesalamine
   B. Deconjugation of biliary-secreted conjugates of chloramphenicol
   C. Degradation of digoxin to inactive metabolites
   D. Metabolism of L-dopa to dopamine
   E. All of the above

275. In patients with Crohn's disease, adenocarcinoma of the small intestine:
   A. Occurs usually in an uninvolved segment
   B. Occurs no more frequently than in an age-matched population
   C. Occurs with a 100-fold greater frequency than in an age-matched population
   D. Should be screened for annually
   E. Is usually detected at an early stage owing to obstructive symptoms

276. Each of the following has been associated with ano-rectal fistulas EXCEPT:
   A. Crohn's disease
   B. Carcinoma
   C. Radiation therapy
   D. External hemorrhoids
   E. Chlamydial infections

277. Which of the following statements are TRUE regarding ulcerative colitis and pregnancy?
   A. Maintenance therapy should be stopped.
   B. Women with ulcerative colitis have more difficulty conceiving a child.
   C. Women with ulcerative colitis are at increased risk of spontaneous abortion.
   D. Pregnancy does not increase the risk of relapse in ulcerative colitis.

278. An anal fissure:
   A. Is most likely to arise in the anterior midline
   B. Is usually painless
   C. When chronic, is usually accompanied by a sentinel pile
   D. Often requires antibiotics to aid healing
   E. Is treated by strengthening the internal sphincter to retard anal stretching during defecation

279. A 55-year-old man presents to the emergency department complaining of progressive abdominal pain and distention with intermittent vomiting over the past 24 hours. He denies prior medical problems except for an appendectomy 20 years earlier. On physical examination he has a low-grade fever, a distended abdomen with high-pitched bowel sounds, and diffuse abdominal tenderness without rebound or guarding.

Which of the following is the LEAST likely diagnosis?
   A. Incarcerated internal hernia
   B. Obstruction due to adhesions
   C. Adynamic paralytic ileus
   D. Sigmoid volvulus
   E. Obstructing carcinoma

280. Referring to the case in question 279, which of the following is LEAST indicated in the initial evaluation of this patient?
   A. Supine and upright radiographs of the abdomen
   B. Serum electrolytes
   C. Complete blood cell count
   D. Peritoneal lavage
   E. Upright chest radiograph

281. Referring to the case in question 279, the patient was found to have a leukocytosis, a serum Na level of 133 mEq/L, K level of 3.4 mEq/L, Cl level of 96 mEq/L, and HCO_3 of 16 mEq/L. An abdominal film showed dilated loops of small bowel with air-fluid levels and a paucity of colonic gas. After two hours of resuscitation and nasogastric suction, he developed localized tenderness in the right lower quadrant but was otherwise unchanged. Which of the following is warranted?
   A. Broad-spectrum antibiotics and continued close monitoring for evidence of perforation
   B. Colonoscopic decompression and attempted reduction of a cecal volvulus
   C. Immediate laparotomy
   D. Gentle Hypaque enema to exclude colonic obstruction and possibly reduce a sigmoid volvulus
   E. Mesenteric arteriography to exclude intestinal ischemia

282. Match the following colonic polyps with their histologic appearance:
   1. Adenoma
   2. Hyperplastic polyp
   3. Juvenile polyps
   4. Peutz-Jeghers polyps
   5. Pneumatosis cystoides intestinalis

   A. Excessive lamina propria and dilated cystic glands
   B. Basophilic, elongated nuclei in a picket fence pattern
   C. Normal mucosa
   D. "Starfish" appearance on cross section
   E. Branching bands of smooth muscle

283. Which of the following statements about tuberculosis of the gastrointestinal tract are TRUE?
   A. It may be caused by either *Mycobacterium tuberculosis* or *Mycobacterium bovis*.
   B. It may be clinically indistinguishable from Crohn's disease.
   C. It commonly involves the ileocecal region.
   D. It is often diagnosed by identification of acid-fast organisms in the stool.
   E. It frequently requires surgical intervention.

284. A patient with Crohn's disease limited to the colon is being evaluated for a flare of disease activity. Extraintestinal manifestations that might be noted on physical examination include all of the following EXCEPT:
A. Iritis
B. Aphthous stomatitis
C. Erythema nodosum
D. Clubbing
E. Granulomatous skin ulcers

285. The diagnosis of intestinal worms is best made by stool examinations for all of the following EXCEPT:
A. *Ascaris*
B. Whipworm
C. *Strongyloides*
D. Hookworm

286. Which of the following statements regarding the diagnosis of *Clostridium difficile* colitis are TRUE?
A. The absence of pseudomembranes on endoscopic examination excludes the diagnosis.
B. The most commonly available diagnostic test involves detection of toxin in stool.
C. Toxin titers correlate directly with severity of disease.
D. Stool cultures for *C. difficile* are the "gold standard" for diagnosis.

287. Which one of the following statements about primary benign tumors of the small intestine is FALSE?
A. Adenomas and leiomyomas are more common than angiomas and neurogenic tumors.
B. They are usually asymptomatic and are often found incidentally.
C. They may produce intermittent intestinal obstruction.
D. They have their peak incidence in the second and third decades.

288. Each of the following statements regarding small bowel carcinoids is true EXCEPT:
A. Approximately half are located within 2 feet of the ileocecal valve.
B. They are often multicentric in origin.
C. The tendency to metastasize is directly related to the size of the primary tumor.
D. After liver metastases occur, the disease progresses rapidly, with a median survival of less than one year.

289. In which of the following disorders does biopsy of the small intestine NOT show periodic acid–Schiff (PAS)-positive macrophages?
A. Whipple's disease

B. *Mycobacterium avium-intracellulare* infection
C. Tropical sprue
D. Disseminated histoplasmosis
E. Macroglobulinemia

290. A previously healthy 27-year-old woman reports six months of recurrent diarrhea, bilateral lower abdominal cramps, rectal urgency, and tenesmus in association with a 4-kg weight loss. Stool examined three times for ova and parasites is negative, and stool culture reveals no pathogens. A flexible sigmoidoscopy reveals mild proctitis with normal-appearing mucosa proximal to the rectum. Biopsies of the rectum reveal chronic inflammation with crypt distortion. Which of the following tests would be MOST helpful?
A. Stool sample to test for *Mycobacterium avium-intracellulare*
B. Lumbosacral radiographs
C. Small bowel radiographs after oral barium contrast
D. An upper endoscopy with small bowel biopsy

291. Each of the following is a true statement concerning hereditary nonpolyposis colorectal cancer (HNPCC) and sporadic colorectal cancer EXCEPT:
A. The interval from normal mucosa to development of cancer is the same in both.
B. The mechanisms by which genetic abnormalities occur are different.
C. HNPCC malignancies are more often diploid than sporadic malignancies.
D. The frequency of metachronous malignancies is greater in HNPCC than in sporadic colorectal cancers.
E. HNPCC malignancies arise from adenomas.

292. Which one or more of the following are associated with an increased risk of colonic adenomas?
A. Ureterosigmoidostomy
B. Acromegaly
C. *Streptococcus bovis* bacteremia
D. Increasing age
E. All of the above
F. None of the above

293. Match the preferred drug treatment with the appropriate disease. Answers may be used once, more than once, or not at all.
1. Rectal gonorrhea
2. Syphilitic hepatitis
3. *Chlamydia trachomatis* proctitis
4. Acute hepatitis B

A. Azithromycin, 1 g single dose, or doxycycline, 100 mg b.i.d. for 7 days
B. Ceftriaxone, 250 mg IM, plus doxycycline, 100 mg b.i.d. for 7 days
C. Interferon alfa, 5 million units IM Monday–Friday for six months

D. Benzathine penicillin G, 2.4 million units IM

E. Benzathine penicillin G, 2.4 million units IM every week for three weeks

F. No treatment

---

294. The MOST common cause of short bowel syndrome in adults is:
A. Severe necrotizing enteric infection
B. Mesenteric infarction
C. Radiation enteritis
D. Crohn's disease
E. Trauma

---

295. The diagnosis of eosinophilic gastroenteritis requires each of the following EXCEPT:
A. Gastrointestinal symptoms
B. Eosinophilic infiltration of one or more areas of the gastrointestinal tract
C. Absence of eosinophilic infiltration of organs outside the gastrointestinal tract
D. Peripheral blood eosinophilia
E. Absence of parasites

---

296. Each of the following conditions is associated with development of small intestinal lymphoma EXCEPT:
A. Celiac sprue
B. Dermatitis herpetiformis
C. Epstein-Barr virus infection
D. Chronic phenobarbital therapy
E. Human immunodeficiency virus infection

---

297. A patient with diarrhea and a history of ileal resection is being evaluated. The extent of resection is unknown. Which of the following would be the MOST appropriate test to guide therapy?
A. Colonoscopy with ileal biopsy
B. Schilling test
C. D-Xylose test
D. Quantitative fecal fat
E. Secretin test

---

298. The MOST reliable and practical therapy for food allergies is:
A. Dapsone
B. Elimination diet
C. Combination therapy with cromolyn and H_1 and H_2 receptor antagonists
D. Desensitization therapy

---

299. Which one of the following statements regarding *Shigella dysenteriae* is FALSE?
A. The major site of attack is the colon.
B. It is a common pathogen in livestock.

C. Multiple, small-volume, bloody, mucoid stools are characteristic.
D. Bacterial resistance to ampicillin and sulfa is common, but resistance to trimethoprim-sulfamethoxazole and ciprofloxacin in the United States remains uncommon.

---

300. Which of the following statements regarding *Clostridium difficile* are TRUE?
A. It is recovered frequently from the stools of healthy adults.
B. Toxin production is necessary for the expression of disease.
C. High carriage rates are seen in infants without evidence of disease.
D. It is a nosocomial pathogen in hospitals and nursing homes.
E. Certain strains cause more severe disease than others.

---

301. Each of the following is a defining characteristic of the irritable bowel syndrome EXCEPT:
A. Motor disorder of the intestine
B. Altered bowel habits
C. Abdominal pain
D. Lactose intolerance
E. Exclusion of organic diseases

---

302. Which of the following is NOT associated with the precipitation of toxic megacolon in patients with severe, acute ulcerative colitis?
A. Anticholinergics
B. Cyclosporine therapy
C. Barium enema
D. Hypokalemia
E. Colonoscopy

---

303. The features of colonic diverticula that correlate with increased risk of diverticulitis include each the following EXCEPT:
A. Wide anatomic distribution
B. Large size
C. Large number
D. Appearance early in life
E. Presence for more than ten years

---

304. Which one or more of the following are complications associated with celiac sprue?
A. Ulceration of the small bowel
B. Stricture of the small bowel
C. Lymphomatous transformation
D. Refractory sprue

---

305. A 47-year-old man with a 12-year history of celiac sprue who has recently been in good health with

normal weight presents with three months of worsening diarrhea and a 15-lb weight loss. He has continued the same diet over the past 12 years. Of the following, the MOST useful initial diagnostic test is:
A. Hydrogen breath test
B. Abdominal computed tomography
C. Right upper quadrant ultrasonography
D. Endoscopy with biopsy
E. Endoscopic retrograde cholangiopancreatography

306. Which of the following foods should be removed from the diet of patients with celiac sprue?
A. Rice
B. Corn
C. Rye
D. Soybeans

307. Which of the following side effects of sulfasalazine are due to the sulfapyridine moiety?
A. Male infertility
B. Hypersensitivity rash
C. Hemolytic anemia
D. Nausea
E. Headache

308. Which of the following statements about irritable bowel syndrome (IBS) are TRUE?
I. It is diagnosed more commonly in females than in males, but the prevalence is similar.
II. It is the most common cause for referral to a gastroenterologist.
III. More than one third of IBS patients experienced sexual abuse as children.
IV. Symptoms begin before age 35 in 90% of cases.

A. I and III
B. II and IV
C. I, II, and III
D. All of the above

309. A 50-year-old patient noted to have iron deficiency anemia by her primary care physician is referred to you. You note buccal pigmentation. In addition to evaluating possible gastrointestinal sources of blood loss, appropriate further studies would include:
A. Abdominal ultrasonography
B. Head computed tomography
C. α-Fetoprotein evaluation
D. Endoscopic retrograde cholangiopancreatography
E. Bone marrow biopsy

310. Which of the following are TRUE statements regarding the medical treatment of endometriosis?
A. Low-dose estrogen-progestin compounds are successful in treating severe disease.

B. Danazol inhibits release of follicle-stimulating hormone and luteinizing hormone and diminishes symptoms due to endometriosis.
C. Use of gonadotropin-releasing hormone agonists is associated with pronounced bone loss.
D. Surgical treatment is indicated for repeated intussusception.
E. Progesterone is contraindicated in the treatment of endometriosis.

311. *Entamoeba histolytica* can be transmitted sexually. Which of the following statements are TRUE regarding this disease in its sexually transmitted form?
I. It often causes nonspecific complaints, including flatulence, diarrhea, and cramping.
II. Isolates found in homosexual men are usually invasive strains.
III. It can be spread via the fecal-oral route or by direct rectal transplantation.
IV. Systemic complications such as liver abscesses are common.

A. I and III
B. II and IV
C. I, II, and III
D. All of the above

312. Which of the following is the MOST likely cause in a patient presenting with extensive jejunal ulceration?
A. B-cell lymphoma
B. T-cell lymphoma
C. Advanced adenocarcinoma
D. Caustic substance ingestion
E. *Yersinia* infection

313. Which of the following are TRUE statements regarding treatment of pseudomembranous colitis?
A. Oral vancomycin and metronidazole are equally effective.
B. Fewer relapses are seen when patients are treated with oral vancomycin.
C. Patients who are improving spontaneously need not be treated.
D. Relapses should always be treated with a different antibiotic.
E. Cholestyramine is useful in treating relapses.

314. Each of the following is an indication for abdominal-perineal resection with permanent sigmoid colostomy for rectal cancer EXCEPT:
A. Poorly differentiated morphology
B. Bulky tumor deep in the pelvis
C. Extensive local spread of the tumor
D. Tumor less than 5 cm from the anus
E. All of the above

315. Regarding developmental abnormalities of the small intestine, each of the following is true EXCEPT:
    A. Clinical manifestations of jejunoileal atresia include polyhydramnios, bilious emesis, abdominal distention, and failure to pass meconium.
    B. The presence of a meconium ileus is consistent with cystic fibrosis.
    C. Bleeding is an unusual complication of Meckel's diverticulum in children younger than 2 years old.
    D. Malrotation is an uncommon developmental anomaly presenting with bleeding, ileal obstruction, and volvulus.
    E. The presence of Meckel's diverticulum can be confirmed by an indium scan.

316. The total radiation dose below which chronic radiation bowel damage is rare:
    A. Is 4000 rads
    B. Is 6000 rads
    C. Is 8000 rads
    D. Cannot be predicted
    E. Is dependent on tumor characteristics

317. Each of the following factors delays gastric emptying EXCEPT:
    A. Acidic pH of duodenal contents
    B. Hypertonic duodenal contents
    C. Decreased duodenal bile acid concentration
    D. Fat present in the ileum
    E. Hypotonic duodenal contents

318. The single MOST useful method to distinguish acquired megacolon from congenital megacolon (Hirschsprung's disease) is:
    A. Anorectal manometry
    B. A superficial rectal mucosal biopsy
    C. A barium enema
    D. A colonic transit time study
    E. The physical examination

319. Each of the following is a true statement about cell proliferation in the small intestine EXCEPT:
    A. Undifferentiated crypt cells divide most actively.
    B. Cells begin to differentiate into absorptive cells in the upper crypt area.
    C. Crypt cells express surface proteins for digestion and absorption.
    D. Cell migration and maturation require four to six days.
    E. Because of rapid cell division, intestinal epithelium is sensitive to mitotic inhibitors.

320. Each of the following is a true statement about anorectal hemorrhoids EXCEPT:
    A. Small symptomatic hemorrhoids often can be treated easily with a high-fiber diet.
    B. Band ligation is the treatment of choice for fourth-degree prolapsed hemorrhoids.
    C. Infrared photocoagulation results in fibrosis and relief in symptoms in the majority of patients.
    D. Sclerotherapy is successful in the majority of patients with first-degree hemorrhoids.
    E. Recurrences are unusual after hemorrhoidectomy.

321. Which one of the following statements about nonspecific ulcerative proctitis is FALSE?
    A. It is the only manifestation in about one third of patients with ulcerative colitis.
    B. It is a chronic condition requiring long-term therapy.
    C. It can be mimicked by *Clostridium difficile*.
    D. The histologic appearance of nonspecific ulcerative proctitis cannot be distinguished from chronic ulcerative colitis.
    E. It can be treated effectively with mesalamine or corticosteroid enemas.

322. Each of the following statements is true EXCEPT:
    A. Pseudocarcinomatous invasion is a distinct entity from carcinoma in situ.
    B. Carcinoma in situ has no metastatic potential.
    C. The primary difference between carcinoma in situ and a malignant polyp is the size of the carcinomatous focus.
    D. Recurrence after endoscopic removal of a malignant polyp correlates with the degree of differentiation.
    E. All are true.

323. Each of the following is a useful test in diagnosing food allergies EXCEPT:
    A. Medical history
    B. Prick skin test
    C. Double-blind placebo-controlled oral food challenge
    D. Food-specific IgG antibody levels
    E. Two-week elimination diets

324. Cytomegalovirus (CMV) may be transmitted during sexual contact. Which statements are TRUE regarding sexually acquired CMV?
    I. It is transmitted by ingestion of virus particles.
    II. An acute infection may be asymptomatic.
    III. It can result in acute ulcerative proctocolitis.
    IV. Viral shedding typically occurs only during acute infection.

    A. I and III
    B. II and IV
    C. I, II, and III
    D. All of the above

325. A 24-year-old man presents complaining of a bloody mucopurulent anal discharge, tenesmus, and diarrhea. His symptoms have been present for more than four months without improvement. He is a sexually active homosexual. Stool cultures and three ova and parasite studies by the referring family physician were negative. Barium enema three weeks ago was read as consistent with ulcerative colitis. Rigid sigmoidoscopy revealed a granular, friable mucosa; nodules with erythema; and a cobblestone appearance with strands of mucus. Biopsy specimens revealed diffuse inflammation with crypt abscesses, granulomas, and a few giant cells. Which of the following are appropriate in the management of this patient?

   I. Trial of prednisone, 20 mg/day for four weeks, and reassess
   II. Drawing of blood for human immunodeficiency virus serologic test
   III. Trial of sulfasalazine, 3 g/day for four weeks, and reassess
   IV. Draw blood for lymphogranuloma venereum (LGV) titer

   A. I and III
   B. II and IV
   C. I, II, and III
   D. All of the above

326. Match the following syndromes with their associated feature.

   1. Peutz-Jeghers syndrome
   2. Muir-Torre syndrome
   3. Gardner's syndrome
   4. Cowden's syndrome
   5. von Recklinghausen's disease

   A. Desmoid tumors
   B. Café au lait spots
   C. Facial trichilemmomas
   D. Buccal pigmentation
   E. Sebaceous tumors

327. Each of the following is a true statement about sexual abuse and constipation EXCEPT:

   A. Severe irritable bowel syndrome in women necessitating hospitalization is commonly associated with a history of sexual abuse.
   B. Child victims of sexual abuse often develop severe abdominal pain or constipation.
   C. Somatic reactions to sexual abuse include constipation and anismus.
   D. Victims of childhood sexual abuse receive many unnecessary operations for constipation.
   E. All are true.

328. Each of the following is a true statement about mucosa-associated lymphoid tissue (MALT) lymphomas EXCEPT:

   A. Most lymphomas are of B-cell lineage.
   B. The hallmark of the MALT lymphoma is the lymphoepithelial lesion.
   C. A plasma cell infiltrate is found in approximately one third of cases.

   D. The most common site within the gastrointestinal tract is the rectum.
   E. They may be confused with pseudolymphoma.

329. Match the fat-soluble vitamin on the right with the statement that most accurately describes it on the left. Answers may be used once, more than once, or not at all.

   1. α-Tocopherol is the most potent form of this vitamin.
   2. Beta-carotene is a precursor of this vitamin.
   3. Active adults do not require any intake of this vitamin.

   A. Vitamin A
   B. Vitamin D
   C. Vitamin E
   D. Vitamin K

330. A 24-year-old man describes a three-day history of right lower quadrant pain associated with daily fevers. Physical examination is notable for a temperature of 39° C and right lower quadrant tenderness. Further questioning reveals a three-month history of intermittent diarrhea and weight loss. Which of the following would be the next MOST reasonable step in management of the patient?

   A. Intravenous corticosteroid therapy
   B. Barium small bowel series
   C. Colonoscopy
   D. Abdominal computed tomography
   E. Careful observation

331. Which of the following statements concerning irritable bowel syndrome (IBS) patients are TRUE?

   A. Patients are frequently awakened from sleep by symptoms.
   B. Food induces colonic hypermotility for hours after ingestion.
   C. Rectal distention produces an exaggerated colonic motor response.
   D. Cholinergic agents produce paradoxical colonic motor activity in IBS patients.

332. Which of the following statements are TRUE regarding tapeworm infections?

   I. *Hymenolepis nana* (dwarf tapeworm) is the most common tapeworm in the United States and is unique because it typically causes systemic symptoms.
   II. *Taenia solium* may exhibit hyperinfection that can lead to diffuse visceral cysticercosis.
   III. *Diphyllobothrium latum* may grow to ten meters long and cause vitamin B_{12} deficiency.
   IV. Cysticercosis requires the ingestion of inadequately cooked pork that is contaminated with viable larvae of *T. solium*.

   A. I and III
   B. II and IV
   C. I, II, and III
   D. All of the above

333. Which statements regarding pancreatic proteases are TRUE?
  I. All are secreted from the pancreas as proenzymes.
  II. Trypsinogen is converted to trypsin by chymotrypsin.
  III. Trypsin, chymotrypsin, and elastase are all endopeptidases.
  IV. Proteases cleave proteins to individual amino acids in order for them to be absorbed.

  A. I and III
  B. II and IV
  C. I, II, and III
  D. All of the above

334. Each of the following is true regarding hemorrhagic colitis caused by *Escherichia coli* serotype 0157:H7 EXCEPT:
  A. Patients initially have moderate to severe watery diarrhea followed by several days of bloody diarrhea.
  B. The right and transverse colon is most severely affected.
  C. Diagnosis can be established by microscopic examination of the stool.
  D. The disease process usually runs a self-limited course over five to ten days.
  E. Antibiotic treatment neither shortens nor attenuates the illness.

335. A patient is noted to have a 7-mm polyp. Rank the following conditions from the lowest to the highest risk of the polyp harboring a malignancy.
  A. Sporadic adenoma
  B. Hereditary nonpolyposis colorectal cancer
  C. Familial adenomatous polyposis
  D. Hyperplastic polyp
  E. Hamartoma

336. Regarding chronic appendicitis:
  A. It is a common consequence of incomplete appendectomy.
  B. It is a relatively common cause of abdominal pain in school-aged children.
  C. It is more common in children with cystic fibrosis.
  D. It is more common in the elderly.
  E. It is effectively treated with oral antibiotics.

337. Which of the following statements regarding infection with *Ascaris* are TRUE?
  A. The exceptional size of the worm and the large parasite burden often enable the careful examiner to palpate collections of worms.
  B. Although pyrantel pamoate is the drug of choice, the second best drug, mebendazole, also has a broad spectrum of activity against other common helminths.
  C. Symptoms are typically limited to abdominal discomfort and malnutrition.
  D. A common symptom of a large worm burden is diarrhea.

338. All of the following measures are useful for stopping a hospital epidemic of pseudomembranous colitis EXCEPT:
  A. Treatment of hospital personnel who are asymptomatic carriers
  B. Enteric precautions
  C. Assigning patients to private bathroom facilities
  D. Identification of environmental vehicles of transmission

339. The Schilling test may be abnormal in each of the following diseases EXCEPT:
  A. Ileal mucosal disease
  B. Gastric mucosal disease
  C. Disease of the exocrine pancreas
  D. Jejunal mucosal disease
  E. Bacterial overgrowth in the jejunum

340. Diverticulitis is similar to appendicitis in each of the following ways EXCEPT:
  A. It begins with acute suppuration in the lumen.
  B. The clinical syndrome may present with focal pain in the lower half of the abdomen.
  C. Microperforation is common.
  D. Peritonitis is a potential complication.

341. A 23-year-old male homosexual presents with complaints of malaise, high fever with chills, and diffuse muscle aches. The review of systems is otherwise negative, and he has no history of drug use. He denies prior sexually transmitted diseases, but his partner has been treated for urethral discharge in the past. His physical examination reveals a thin man with a temperature of 39.3° C and a pulse of 110 beats per minute. The rest of his examination is normal except for a holosystolic murmur at the apex with radiation to the axilla. Laboratory examination reveals leukocytosis with a left shift. The human immunodeficiency virus (HIV) test result is pending. What is the MOST likely diagnosis based on the available data?
  A. Primary HIV infection
  B. *Mycobacterium avium-intracellulare* infection
  C. Disseminated cytomegalovirus infection
  D. *Neisseria gonorrhoeae* endocarditis
  E. Disseminated *Chlamydia trachomatis* infection

342. Which of the following factors is MOST important in allowing the regrowth of normal intestinal epithelium from stem cells after radiation therapy?
A. Tumor size
B. Functional status of the patient
C. Nutritional supplementation during therapy
D. Rest period between radiation doses
E. Tumor type

343. Each of the following is a true statement about the irritable bowel syndrome EXCEPT:
A. It includes visible abdominal distention and relief of pain with bowel movements.
B. It is a motor disorder limited to the colon.
C. It does not predispose to cancer.
D. It may present with incapacitating abdominal pain.
E. Stools tend to be more frequent and looser with onset of pain.

344. Each of the following has been identified as a neurotransmitter in the enteric nervous system EXCEPT:
A. Cholecystokinin
B. Somatostatin
C. Gastrin
D. Nitric oxide
E. Vasoactive intestinal peptide

345. Chronic complications of schistosomiasis include each of the following EXCEPT:
A. Colon cancer
B. Intestinal obstruction
C. Hepatic encephalopathy
D. Protein-losing enteropathy
E. Intestinal fistulas

346. Each of the following statements about pouchitis after ileoanal pouch anastomosis is true EXCEPT:
A. Pouch biopsies reveal nonspecific inflammation.
B. The underlying disorder has no effect on future development of pouchitis.
C. Bacterial overgrowth may be an etiologic factor.
D. Patients may develop arthritis during episodes of pouchitis.
E. Some patients with pouchitis may have unrecognized Crohn's disease.

347. Each of the following statements about appendiceal perforation is true EXCEPT:
A. Perforation within 12 hours of the onset of pain is unusual.
B. Although perforation is common in children younger than 2 years old, it is unusual in older children.
C. Forty to 75 percent of adults older than 60 years old have appendiceal perforation by the time of operation.
D. Perforation is recognized preoperatively in the majority of patients.
E. High fever and duration of symptoms for more than 36 hours are suggestive of perforation.

348. Symptoms of carbohydrate malabsorption such as bloating, abdominal cramps, and diarrhea suggest which of the following?
A. Decreased levels of brush border enzymes
B. Decreased secretion of cholecystokinin in response to a meal
C. Excess acidity causing inactivation of pancreatic enzymes
D. Decreased output of pancreatic amylase due to pancreatitis

349. Which of the following statements are TRUE about Hirschsprung's disease?
I. The onset of significant symptoms can be late in life.
II. Clinical features overlap with those of idiopathic constipation.
III. Spontaneous remissions may occur.
IV. Distal narrowing is always seen on a barium enema.

A. I and III
B. II and IV
C. I, II, and III
D. All of the above

350. Which of the following statements regarding the relationships between ulcerative colitis, Crohn's disease, and smoking are TRUE?
A. Ulcerative colitis is less common in smokers.
B. Crohn's disease is less common in smokers.
C. Former heavy smokers are at an increased risk of developing ulcerative colitis.
D. Nicotine patches have an effect similar to that of smoking.

351. Which of the following statements about carbohydrate metabolism and absorption are TRUE?
A. Starch comprises about 50% of the digestible carbohydrates in a western diet.
B. Lactose, glucose, and galactose are the three major dietary monosaccharides.
C. Glucose and galactose are absorbed by the enterocyte by facilitated diffusion.
D. Dietary starch is composed of long chains of glucose molecules.

352. An otherwise healthy patient is successfully treated for an appendiceal abscess with intravenous antibiotics and computed tomographic–guided drainage of

the abscess. Of the following, what is the MOST reasonable future management?
A. Elective appendectomy in two months
B. Elective appendectomy before discharge
C. Repeated computed tomography at three-month intervals for one year
D. No further management
E. Long-term oral antibiotics

353. Vasoactive intestinal peptide released from islet cell tumors causes diarrhea by which mechanism?
A. Increased intracellular calcium, which inhibits sodium chloride absorption and stimulates chloride secretion
B. Increased intracellular cyclic adenosine monophosphate, which inhibits sodium chloride absorption and stimulates chloride secretion
C. Irreversible inhibition of the apical sodium channel
D. Disruption of intercellular tight junctions

354. Each of the following statements regarding strongyloidiasis is true EXCEPT:
A. Skin manifestations are common in both acute and chronic disease.
B. Like hookworm and *Ascaris*, *Strongyloides* infection is initiated by ingestion of eggs.
C. Cure rates with mebendazole are only about 50%, decreasing the drug's usefulness as a broad-spectrum anthelminthic.
D. *Strongyloides* infection is more likely to be fatal than *Ascaris*, hookworm, or whipworm infection.

355. Vitamin B_{12} is bound by several proteins during its absorption. Which of the following is the CORRECT sequence in which cobalamin is bound?
A. Intrinsic factor–R protein–ileal receptor–transcobalamin
B. Transcobalamin–intrinsic factor–ileal receptor–R protein
C. R protein–intrinsic factor–ileal receptor–transcobalamin
D. Intrinsic factor–R protein–ileal receptor–transcobalamin

356. Which of the following drugs is contraindicated in pregnant women with ulcerative colitis?
A. Sulfasalazine
B. Corticosteroids
C. 6-Mercaptopurine
D. Azathioprine
E. None of the above

357. All of the following statements regarding immunoproliferative small intestinal disease are true EXCEPT:
A. It is most often found in populations from the Mediterranean basin.

B. It has a natural course that includes a reversible premalignant stage followed by a frankly malignant lymphomatous transformation.
C. It usually involves the entire length of the small intestine microscopically.
D. It rarely leads to chronic diarrhea, malabsorption, or weight loss.

358. What is the MOST common anatomic distribution of involvement in Crohn's disease?
A. Small bowel and colon
B. Small bowel alone
C. Colon alone
D. Perianal disease alone
E. Equally distributed throughout the gastrointestinal tract

359. Each of the following statements about fat intake and absorption in the United States is true EXCEPT:
A. Approximately 40% of daily energy requirements are met by fats.
B. The most common dietary fatty acids are oleate (C18:1) and palmitate (C16:0).
C. Movement of digested dietary lipid across the brush border membrane is by active transport.
D. Linoleic acid (C18:2) and linolenic acid (C18:3) are essential fatty acids.

360. Which one or more of the following diseases have been implicated as predisposing factors for salmonellosis?
A. Sickle cell anemia
B. Acquired immunodeficiency syndrome (AIDS)
C. Schistosomiasis
D. Leukemia
E. Malaria

361. Each of the following statements about the onset of diffuse ulceration in patients with celiac sprue is true EXCEPT:
A. Associated symptoms include increased abdominal pain and weight loss.
B. An underlying lymphoma is frequently present.
C. Symptoms typically respond to reinstitution of a gluten-free diet.
D. Treatment with steroids frequently is complicated by intestinal perforation.
E. Some patients may require surgical resection.

362. Eosinophilic gastroenteritis may involve which of the following?
I. Esophagus
II. Stomach
III. Large intestine
IV. Small intestine

A. I and III

B. II and IV
C. I, II, and III
D. All of the above

363. Which of the following are TRUE statements about thrombosed external hemorrhoids?
A. They occur mainly in young adults as a result of heavy lifting, childbirth, or straining to defecate.
B. They are often painless and noted by the patient only after bleeding.
C. They can be forced into the anal canal to minimize discomfort.
D. They usually respond within three to seven days to analgesics, stool softeners, and topical emollients.

364. Hyperplastic polyps differ from adenomas in which of the following respects?
A. Endoscopic appearance
B. Malignant potential
C. Distribution within the colon
D. Histologic appearance
E. None of the above

365. Which one of the following radiographic findings are characteristic of chronic intestinal pseudo-obstruction?
I. Air-fluid levels on plain abdominal films
II. Megaduodenum on upper gastrointestinal series
III. Megacolon on barium enema
IV. Normal upper gastrointestinal series and barium enema

A. I and III
B. II and IV
C. I, II, and III
D. All of the above

366. Match the vitamin with the statement that most accurately describes it. Answers may be used once, more than once, or not at all.
1. Dietary recommendations are 0.2 mg/day in adults and 0.4 mg/day during pregnancy.
2. This vitamin is bound to transcobalamin II in the portal circulation.
3. The only important dietary sources of this vitamin are the seeds of plants.

A. Vitamin C
B. Vitamin B_{12}
C. Folic acid
D. Thiamine

367. An 18-year-old sexually active woman notes a 24-hour history of fever, anorexia, and poorly localized lower abdominal pain. She denies vaginal discharge. A serum pregnancy test is negative. Which of the following tests would be MOST useful in guiding therapy?
A. Abdominal radiography
B. Computed tomography
C. Culdocentesis
D. Ultrasonography
E. Barium enema

368. Evidence that type I (IgE-mediated) hypersensitivity reactions play a role in the pathogenesis of eosinophilic gastroenteritis includes each of the following EXCEPT:
A. Tissue and blood eosinophilia
B. Increased incidence of atopy
C. Elevated IgE levels
D. Response to corticosteroids
E. Response to H_2 blockers

369. Which one of the following statements regarding the prognosis of eosinophilic gastroenteritis is TRUE?
A. It is related to the degree of peripheral eosinophilia.
B. It is related to the type of tissue layer involvement.
C. It is generally poor given the increased risk of gastrointestinal malignancy.
D. It is generally good if obstruction and malnutrition can be avoided.

370. Which of the following is the MOST reliable test for diagnosing acute diverticulitis?
A. Plain supine and upright abdominal radiographs
B. Barium contrast studies
C. Ultrasonography
D. Computed tomography of the abdomen
E. Careful endoscopic examination with a flexible sigmoidoscope

371. Which of the following diagnostic tests is LEAST helpful in establishing the diagnosis of schistosomiasis?
A. Needle biopsy of the liver
B. Examination of concentrated stool specimens for ova and parasites
C. Rectal biopsy
D. Serologic complement fixation test

372. Which one of the following statements about chylomicron formation and transport is TRUE?
A. Chylomicrons are the major transport particle for triglycerides in the fasting state.
B. Chylomicrons have a fatty acid composition similar to very low density lipoprotein.
C. Chylomicrons require apoprotein B for synthesis and secretion.
D. The chylomicron core consists of cholesterol esters and phospholipids.

373. Each of the following statements regarding age and colon cancer is true EXCEPT:
- A. Age 45 is the average for diagnosis of cancer in hereditary nonpolyposis colorectal cancer.
- B. Age 67 is the average age for diagnosis of sporadic colon cancer.
- C. Age 39 is the average age for diagnosis of colon cancer in familial adenomatous polyposis.
- D. Age younger than 30 at diagnosis is associated with a poor prognosis.
- E. All are true.

374. Gastroscopic findings of eosinophilic gastroenteritis may include the presence of enlarged gastric folds. Which of the following disorders has the MOST similar gastroscopic appearance?
- A. Zollinger-Ellison syndrome
- B. *Helicobacter pylori* infection
- C. NSAID-associated gastropathy
- D. Portal hypertensive gastropathy
- E. Angiodysplasia

375. The differential diagnosis of eosinophilic gastroenteritis includes which of the following?
- I. Helminthic infestation
- II. Drug allergy
- III. Allergic granulomatosis (Churg-Strauss syndrome)
- IV. Crohn's disease

- A. I and III
- B. II and IV
- C. I, II, and III
- D. All of the above

376. Which of the following statements regarding amebiasis are TRUE?
- A. Stool examination is a much more reliable way to diagnose amebiasis than giardiasis.
- B. Colonic disease is three to ten times more common in men than in women.
- C. Antibiotics may help because amebae need bacteria to initiate and maintain colonic infection.
- D. Amebiasis must be distinguished from inflammatory bowel disease to avoid excess mortality caused by steroid therapy in infected patients.
- E. Metronidazole can be routinely expected to eradicate colonic amebae.

377. Each of the following antimicrobial agents commonly leads to *Clostridium difficile* colitis EXCEPT:
- A. Trimethoprim-sulfamethoxazole
- B. Metronidazole
- C. Cephalosporins
- D. Nafcillin

378. A 36-year-old woman seeks evaluation for chronic intermittent abdominal pain dating back several years that has become worse since the death of her mother six months ago. She states that the pain is diffuse over the lower abdomen, aggravated by meals, and relieved by defecation. She also reports more frequent and looser stools with the onset of pain. Which of the following clinical features would NOT support the diagnosis of irritable bowel syndrome in this patient?
- A. Small stools
- B. Weight loss
- C. Patient not awakened by pain
- D. Visible abdominal distention
- E. Severe intensity of pain

379. Referring to the case in question 378, which of the following diagnostic investigations is LEAST indicated?
- A. Stool Hemoccult test
- B. Complete blood cell count with differential
- C. Erythrocyte sedimentation rate
- D. Flexible sigmoidoscopy
- E. Esophagogastroduodenoscopy

380. Referring to the case in question 378, subsequent testing confirms the diagnosis of irritable bowel syndrome (IBS). Which of the following treatment modalities is likely to be the MOST beneficial?
- A. High-fiber diet
- B. Trial of metronidazole
- C. Reassurance and psychological support
- D. Trial of antispasmodics as needed for pain
- E. Lactose-free diet

381. The migrating motor complex refers to the:
- A. Cyclical pattern of electrical activity that occurs in the rectum as distention occurs
- B. Electrical activity in the small intestine caused by vasoactive intestinal peptide and cholecystokinin
- C. Cyclical electrical pattern migration along the length of the intestine
- D. Accentuated electrical pattern seen during ileus
- E. Electrical pattern that leads to defecation after a meal

382. Match the following causes of bacterial food poisoning with a characteristic feature.
- 1. *Bacillus cereus*
- 2. *Vibrio parahaemolyticus*
- 3. *Staphylococcus aureus*
- 4. *Listeria monocytogenes*
- 5. *Clostridium perfringens*

- A. Uncooked rice
- B. Incubation period approximately three hours
- C. Seafood
- D. Milk and milk products
- E. Roasted, boiled, stewed, or steamed meats

383. Regarding treatment of colorectal cancer, which of the following are TRUE?
  A. Treatment with levamisole plus 5-fluorouracil increases the time to tumor recurrence.
  B. Treatment with levamisole plus 5-fluorouracil does not affect overall five-year survival.
  C. Adjuvant therapy for stage B2 and C colon and rectal cancer includes both radiation and chemotherapy.
  D. Portal vein infusion of adjuvant chemotherapy reduces liver metastasis better than systemic therapy.
  E. Approximately 20% of hepatic metastases are potentially curable with surgery.

384. The only intestinal nematode large enough to produce a significant risk of mechanical obstruction of the small bowel, appendiceal orifice, ileocecal valve, and biliary tree is:
  A. *Ancylostoma duodenale* and *Necator americanus* (hookworm)
  B. *Strongyloides stercoralis*
  C. *Ascaris lumbricoides*
  D. *Trichuris trichiura* (whipworm)

385. Which of the following are TRUE statements regarding the joint involvement associated with ulcerative colitis?
  A. Most patients with sacroiliitis are HLA-B27 positive.
  B. Peripheral arthropathy usually involves the small joints of the extremities in a symmetric fashion.
  C. Proctocolectomy has no impact on the course of ankylosing spondylitis.
  D. Ankylosing spondylitis does not develop until after colonic symptoms have been present for some time.

386. Which of the following therapies is the LEAST helpful in maintaining long-term remission in patients with ulcerative colitis?
  A. Azathioprine
  B. Olsalazine
  C. Corticosteroids
  D. Sulfasalazine
  E. Mesalamine enemas

387. A 45-year-old woman with multiple previous ileal resections for Crohn's disease notes a three-week history of episodic upper abdominal pain but no change in bowel habits. A barium small bowel series reveals no active disease or strictures. Which of the following would have the HIGHEST diagnostic yield?
  A. Colonoscopy
  B. Abdominal computed tomography
  C. Upper endoscopy
  D. Stool for ova and parasites
  E. Abdominal sonogram

388. Which of the following statements regarding *Blastocystis hominis* are TRUE?
  I. It is a rare but important pathogen found in stool examined for ova and parasites.
  II. It is often present without symptoms.
  III. Immunosuppressed patients are less likely to have symptoms than are normal persons.
  IV. The decision to treat should be based on the organism burden.

  A. I and III
  B. II and IV
  C. I, II, and III
  D. All of the above

389. Symptoms of late-onset radiation proctitis:
  A. Usually respond to corticosteroid enemas
  B. Usually respond to mesalamine enemas
  C. Usually resolve spontaneously
  D. Are generally poorly responsive to standard medical therapies
  E. Are treated most effectively with sucralfate enemas

390. Which one of the following is NOT associated with abnormalities in the adenomatous polyposis coli (APC) gene?
  A. Muir-Torre syndrome
  B. Familial adenomatous polyposis
  C. Gardner's syndrome
  D. Hereditary flat adenoma syndrome
  E. All of the above are associated with APC gene abnormalities

391. Each of the following is a clinically important species of *Schistosoma* EXCEPT:
  A. *S. haematobium*
  B. *S. mekongi*
  C. *S. amazoni*
  D. *S. mansoni*
  E. *S. japonicum*

392. A 27-year-old woman has severe Crohn's colitis that is refractory to intensive medical therapy with steroids and immunosuppressive agents. A recent colonoscopy revealed disease extending from the sigmoid to cecum only. The ileum and rectum are normal. Which of the following would be the MOST reasonable surgical approach?
  A. Ileal pouch anal anastomosis
  B. Ileal pouch distal rectal anastomosis
  C. Ileoanal anastomosis

D. Ileorectal anastomosis
E. Brooke ileostomy

393. Allergic eosinophilic gastroenteritis is frequently associated with each of the following EXCEPT:
A. Intense intestinal mucosal infiltration with eosinophils
B. Prompt response to corticosteroid therapy
C. Postprandial vomiting
D. Prompt response to elimination diets
E. Peripheral eosinophilia

394. A 22-year-old female heterosexual presents complaining of a sore throat, odynophagia, dysphagia, and fever. Her physical examination revealed a temperature of 38.0° C and marked pharyngeal erythema with ulcers over tonsils and posterior pharynx. Laboratory analysis reveals a negative rapid streptococcal screen. She is sexually active and admits to all forms of sexual contact. Her sexual partner has had no symptoms suggestive of sexually transmitted diseases. What is the MOST likely diagnosis of those listed below?
A. Cytomegalovirus infection
B. *Neisseria gonorrhoeae* infection
C. Herpes simplex virus–2 infection
D. *Chlamydia trachomatis* infection

395. Pseudomembranous enterocolitis in the preantibiotic era was believed to be associated with which organism?
A. *Escherichia coli*
B. *Staphylococcus aureus*
C. *Streptococcus faecalis*
D. *Staphylococcus epidermidis*

396. Each of the following statements regarding the symptoms of colorectal cancer is true EXCEPT:
A. Constitutional symptoms of shortness of breath, fatigue, and angina are more common at presentation in cancers proximal to the splenic flexure.
B. Obstruction is more common in colorectal cancers distal to the splenic flexure.
C. Palpable masses are more common in proximal colorectal cancers.
D. Hematochezia is more common in distal colorectal cancers.
E. Napkin ring lesions are more common in the proximal colon.

397. Which one of the following statements regarding vitamin B_{12} is TRUE?
A. It is found almost entirely in vegetable sources.
B. It binds intrinsic factor in the stomach when the pH is less than 3.

C. Intrinsic factor is secreted by parietal cells.
D. The intrinsic factor/cobalamin complex is absorbed in the duodenum.

398. Each of the following statements about the ^{14}C-xylose breath test is true EXCEPT:
A. It has a high specificity.
B. It is less sensitive than the ^{14}C-bile acid breath test.
C. It is simple to perform.
D. Xylose is catabolized by gram-negative aerobes, which are almost always part of the overgrowth flora.
E. The 30-minute breath sample is more reliable than the 60- or 90-minute samples.

399. Which of the following statements pertaining to sodium transport in the small intestine are TRUE?
I. All sodium transport is coupled to chloride or glucose.
II. Nutrient absorption is generally linked to sodium transport.
III. Sodium-glucose cotransport requires the hydrolysis of adenosine triphosphate.
IV. Sodium is removed from the cell by the sodium/potassium pump.

A. I and III
B. II and IV
C. I, II, and III
D. All of the above

400. Each of the following regarding whipworm infection is true EXCEPT:
A. Whipworm is common in the United States, afflicting millions of persons.
B. Whipworm primarily colonizes the lumen of the colon.
C. Microscopic examination of the stool is required to diagnose whipworm.
D. Mebendazole is the drug of choice, but two courses may be required for eradication.

401. Each of the following statements regarding the anatomy of the anorectum is true EXCEPT:
A. The lower 2 cm of the anal canal is lined by stratified squamous epithelium.
B. The upper portions of the anal canal and rectum are supplied by autonomic nerves and hence are relatively insensitive to pain.
C. The valves of Houston provide an important sphincter preventing incontinence.
D. Lymph from the lower anal canal drains through the inguinal lymph nodes.

402. Which of the following are TRUE statements regarding *Coccidioides* infections?
I. Endoscopic biopsy of small intestine is usually required to diagnose *Isospora* infection.
II. Trimethoprim-sulfamethoxazole is the treatment of choice for *Isospora*.
III. Cryptosporidiosis causes a self-limited diarrheal illness in patients with a normal immune system.
IV. Eradication of *Cryptosporidium* using paromomycin should be attempted in patients with acquired immunodeficiency syndrome because infection is often fatal.

A. I and III
B. II and IV
C. I, II, and III
D. All of the above

403. Match the symptom(s) with the most likely site of bowel obstruction.

1. Proximal small bowel
2. Distal small bowel
3. Colon

A. Intermittent feculent emesis, moderate distention
B. Progressive pain and tenderness, marked distention
C. Frequent emesis that relieves pain, minimal distention

404. A 35-year-old man develops the onset of lower abdominal pain, hematochezia, and increased bowel frequency. Two years earlier the patient underwent a total colectomy with ileoanal pouch anastomosis. Endoscopy reveals erythema and friability in the pouch. Stool culture and examination for ova and parasites are negative for pathogens. What would the MOST appropriate treatment at this point be?
A. Oral prednisone
B. Hydrocortisone enemas
C. Mesalamine enemas
D. Metronidazole
E. 6-Mercaptopurine

405. Which one of the following statements regarding iron metabolism is TRUE?
A. In nonvegetarian adults, the majority of ingested iron is absorbed.
B. Most absorption occurs in the proximal small intestine.
C. The ferric form is better absorbed than the ferrous form.
D. Iron is absorbed by simple diffusion only.

406. Solitary rectal ulcer syndrome is:
A. Usually due to an infectious cause
B. More common in older men
C. Located 1 to 2 cm above the anal verge.
D. Treated effectively by sucralfate retention enemas
E. Often confused with inflammatory bowel disease

407. Each of the following is a true statement about tropical sprue EXCEPT:
A. The risk of developing tropical sprue during brief visits to endemic areas is high.
B. It occurs most commonly in expatriates after two or more years in the tropics.
C. The disease is most prevalent in India, Southeast Asia, and the Caribbean, with tropical Africa and South America being much less affected.
D. It represents much less of a health hazard to children living in endemic areas than adults.

408. Patients who have undergone a total proctocolectomy have an increased incidence of:
A. Cholelithiasis
B. Adenocarcinoma of the terminal ileum
C. Urolithiasis
D. Gout
E. Hypocalcemia

409. The incidence of acute appendicitis appears to be declining in western countries. What is the MOST likely explanation?
A. Development of improved antibiotics
B. Increased use of more refined grains
C. Increased dietary fiber and improved hygiene
D. An increase in the size of the appendiceal orifice
E. Methodologic flaws in epidemiologic studies

410. Mucosal defects causing maldigestion include each of the following EXCEPT:
A. Whipple's disease
B. Lactase deficiency
C. Intestinal resection
D. Zollinger-Ellison syndrome

411. Infectious diarrhea due to which of the following organisms has been associated with the hemolytic-uremic syndrome?
A. *Bacillus cereus*
B. *Escherichia coli*
C. *Staphylococcus aureus*
D. *Listeria monocytogenes*
E. *Clostridium perfringens*

412. Each of the following statements regarding syphilitic gastritis is true EXCEPT:
A. It may produce epigastric pain and weight loss without nausea and vomiting.
B. Serologic tests for syphilis are typically negative at this stage.
C. Barium studies show loss of normal gastric mucosal pattern.

D. Endoscopy reveals diffuse gastric mucosal ulceration.

D. Endoscopy reveals diffuse gastric mucosal ulceration.

413. Each of the following statements regarding iron absorption is true EXCEPT:
A. Although vegetarian diets contain less total iron than meat diets, the bioavailability of the iron is similar in meats and vegetables.
B. Daily iron absorption is approximately 1.0 mg/day in healthy adults.
C. The proportion of dietary iron absorbed decreases with increasing dietary loads.
D. Most iron absorption occurs in the proximal small intestine.

414. TRUE statements regarding infectious diarrhea due to *Salmonella* include:
A. Humans represent the only known reservoir of infection.
B. Typical presentation is with nausea and emesis followed by diarrhea lasting four days.
C. Antibiotics usually improve the rate of clinical recovery.
D. The quinolones are highly active against *Salmonella* species *in vitro*.
E. Multiple drug resistance is common.

415. Which of the following statements regarding the D-xylose test are TRUE?
A. D-Xylose is absorbed by passive diffusion proportional to mucosal surface area.
B. D-Xylose is metabolized to glucose plus galactose by the small intestine.
C. The test does not require a timed urine collection.
D. D-Xylose absorption is reduced by bacterial overgrowth.
E. The test is often abnormal even in patients with mild or distal small bowel disease.

416. Celiac sprue is associated with all of the following EXCEPT:
A. Dermatitis herpetiformis
B. Secondary hyperparathyroidism
C. Demyelinating central nervous system lesions
D. Anemia
E. Large joint arthritis

417. Which of the following are associated with increased risk of colon cancer in patients with ulcerative colitis?
I. Duration of disease
II. Severity of disease
III. Extent of disease
IV. History of toxic megacolon

A. I and III

B. II and IV
C. I, II, and III
D. All of the above

418. Which of the following statements MOST accurately reflects the relationship between pregnancy and Crohn's disease?
A. Active disease at the time of conception has no effect on the outcome of the pregnancy.
B. The majority of patients in remission at conception will experience flare of the disorder at some point during the pregnancy.
C. Only about one third of patients with active disease at the time of conception will achieve remission during pregnancy.
D. Patients in remission have higher rates of spontaneous abortions and stillbirths when compared with age-matched controls.
E. Patients with Crohn's disease should be counseled against becoming pregnant.

419. A patient undergoes proctocolectomy with ileostomy for Crohn's colitis. All of the following statements regarding prestomal ileitis are true EXCEPT:
A. Symptoms of mechanical obstruction are often present.
B. There is an increased output from the ileostomy.
C. Endoscopy reveals punched-out ulcerations.
D. Fever is frequently present.
E. It typically occurs in patients who had "backwash ileitis" at the time of colectomy.

420. An essential amino acid is defined as:
A. An amino acid that cannot be synthesized endogenously
B. An amino acid that cannot be synthesized in quantities necessary for metabolic processes
C. An amino acid that cannot be synthesized unless the corresponding keto acid is available exogenously
D. An amino acid that cannot be synthesized unless the corresponding keto acid is available from carbohydrate metabolism

421. Laboratory findings typical of celiac sprue include all of the following EXCEPT:
A. Iron-deficiency anemia
B. Prolonged prothrombin time
C. Megaloblastic anemia
D. Thrombocytopenia

422. Which of the following statements are TRUE about Hirschsprung's disease?
A. A barium enema may miss the diagnosis if the aganglionic segment is short.
B. The characteristic finding on barium enema is distal rectal narrowing with proximal dilation.

C. A normal deep rectal biopsy excludes the diagnosis.

D. Absence of the rectoanal inhibitory reflex confirms the diagnosis.

E. Excess acetylcholinesterase on routine rectal biopsy together with appropriate anorectal manometry precludes the need for a deep rectal biopsy.

---

423. Each of the following is a true statement about Ogilvie's syndrome EXCEPT:

A. The characteristic time course is chronic.

B. It is a form of pseudo-obstruction localized to the colon.

C. Most patients have a coexisting primary medical problem.

D. Abdominal films show gaseous distention throughout the colon and rectum.

---

424. Which of the following blood tests BEST discriminates between anorexia nervosa and diffuse small bowel disease such as celiac sprue?

A. Hematocrit

B. Red blood cell folate

C. Vitamin B_{12}

D. Serum folate

E. Mean corpuscular volume

---

425. Which infectious form of proctitis is MOST likely to lead to abscesses, fistulas, and rectal strictures?

A. *Chlamydia* (lymphogranuloma venereum type)

B. *Neisseria gonorrhoeae*

C. *Treponema pallidum*

D. *Entamoeba histolytica*

E. Cytomegalovirus

---

426. All of the following are typical features of acute appendicitis. Arrange them in the chronological sequence in which they typically occur.

A. Fever

B. Anorexia, nausea or vomiting

C. Pain at some site in the abdomen

D. Pain over the appendix

---

427. Which of the following statements regarding the clinical course of pseudomembranous colitis are TRUE?

A. Bloody diarrhea is common.

B. It can appear more than four weeks after stopping antibiotics.

C. The severity correlates with the dose of the antibiotic.

D. The absence of stool leukocytes excludes the diagnosis.

E. It can present as a toxic megacolon.

---

428. A 32-year-old Irish man with no previous medical illness presents with progressive diarrhea and weight loss over the previous three months. There is no history of ethanol consumption. Stools are foul smelling and occasionally float. Based on the history, the MOST likely diagnosis is:

A. Celiac sprue

B. Bacterial overgrowth

C. Pancreatic insufficiency

D. Whipple's disease

E. Intestinal tuberculosis

---

429. Match the disease process with the associated biopsy findings:

1. *Schistosoma mansoni*
2. Hirschsprung's disease
3. Cystic fibrosis
4. Rectal amyloidosis

A. Absence of ganglion cells

B. Ova in squash preparation in mucosal specimen

C. Prominent goblet cells and crypts packed with mucus

D. Green birefringence with Congo red stain

---

430. Each of the following is a true statement regarding motility of the small intestinal wall EXCEPT:

A. Ring contractions tend to sweep caudad.

B. The fundamental frequency of ring contractions is highest at the duodenum and decreases caudad.

C. Sleeve contractions tend to produce cephalad movement of luminal contents and decrease mixing.

D. Ring and sleeve contractions often occur simultaneously, maximizing the mixing of intestinal contents.

E. The density of the submucosal and myenteric plexuses is highest in the duodenum and lowest in the rectum.

---

431. Each of the following is a cause of chronic intestinal pseudo-obstruction EXCEPT:

A. Familial visceral myopathies

B. Myxedema

C. Progressive systemic sclerosis

D. *Helicobacter pylori* infection

E. Parkinson's disease

---

432. Which one of the following statements concerning infectious diarrhea due to *Escherichia coli* is FALSE?

A. Enteropathogenic *E. coli* (EPEC) lead to invasion with bloody diarrhea.

B. Enteroinvasive *E. coli* (EIEC) produce a shiga-like toxin.

C. Enterohemorrhagic *E. coli* (EHEC) are most often of the serotype 0157:H7.

D. Enterotoxigenic *E. coli* (ETEC) produce an enterotoxin similar to that produced by *Vibrio cholerae*.

433. Which of the following hormones causes net sodium absorption in the intestine?
I. Aldosterone
II. Glucocorticoids
III. Epinephrine
IV. Somatostatin

A. I and III
B. II and IV
C. I, II, and III
D. All of the above

434. A 55-year-old patient is referred to you by his local physician for heme-positive stools. On colonoscopy, a 0.7-cm tubular adenoma is found and removed. Which one or more of the following follow-up regimens are acceptable?
A. Repeat colonoscopy in three years
B. Flexible sigmoidoscopy in five years
C. Occult blood testing yearly with flexible sigmoidoscopy in three years
D. Flexible sigmoidoscopy and barium enema in three years
E. All of the above are currently acceptable.
F. None of the above is currently acceptable.

435. Regarding giardiasis, each the following statements is true EXCEPT:
A. *Giardia* require passage through nonhuman hosts to maintain their life cycle.
B. The pathophysiology of diarrhea in this infection is unknown.
C. Both quinacrine and metronidazole are excellent treatment options.
D. Duodenal aspiration is a reliable means of diagnosis, but stool studies are less reliable.
E. *Giardia* infections often occur after drinking pristine stream water in the Rocky Mountains.

436. Which of the following statements regarding eosinophilia in helminthic infections are TRUE?
I. Because the whipworm life cycle involves little tissue invasion, eosinophilia is uncommon.
II. A brisk eosinophil response is common in strongyloidiasis and may lead to Charcot-Leyden crystals in the stool.
III. Hookworm causes a consistent but mild eosinophilia.
IV. Eosinophilia is generally mild in ascariasis.

A. I and III
B. II and IV
C. I, II, and III
D. All of the above

437. A 65-year-old woman who presents with the sudden onset of abdominal pain is found to have a perforated jejunal ulcer at laparotomy. Which of the following drugs is MOST likely to be associated with this clinical scenario?
A. Alcohol
B. Antibiotics
C. Enteric-coated potassium tablets
D. Prednisone
E. NSAIDs

438. Which of the following pathologic features are specific for ulcerative colitis?
A. Crypt abscesses
B. Mucosal infiltration with neutrophils and plasma cells
C. Epithelial flattening and ulceration
D. Pseudopolyps
E. None of the above

439. Which of the following provides the strongest evidence for an environmental role in colorectal cancer?
A. The change in colorectal cancer rates in migrant populations
B. The redistribution of colorectal cancer toward the right colon
C. The fact that industrialized countries tend to have higher rates of colorectal cancer than developing nations
D. The fact that bile acids (noncarcinogenic) are converted to secondary bile acids (co-carcinogenic) by colonic bacteria
E. The fact that colorectal cancers have accumulated more genetic abnormalities than adenomas

440. Which of the following are TRUE statements about constipation?
I. Stercoraceous perforation is a complication of prolonged constipation.
II. Patients with prolonged constipation have an increased risk of colon cancer.
III. Patients with anterior mucosal prolapse (rectal prolapse) often have no history of constipation or straining.
IV. Hemorrhoids are commonly caused by constipation.

A. I and III
B. II and IV
C. I, II, and III
D. All of the above

441. The clinical features of eosinophilic gastroenteritis are determined by the predominant mucosal layer involved. Serosal layer involvement MOST typically presents with which of the following?
A. Colicky abdominal pain, weight loss, and diarrhea
B. Protein-losing enteropathy, malabsorption

C. Crampy abdominal pain, intestinal obstruction
D. Eosinophilic ascites
E. Nausea and vomiting

---

442. A 35-year-old man with Crohn's disease of the small bowel was successfully brought into remission with high-dose prednisone. Two attempts at tapering the corticosteroids over the previous six months have resulted in recurrent flares when the prednisone was lowered below 20 mg/day. Which of the following is the MOST appropriate next step in management?
A. Total parenteral nutrition
B. Metronidazole
C. Methotrexate
D. Maintain prednisone at 20 mg/day
E. 6-Mercaptopurine

---

443. Which of the following are TRUE statements about Hirschsprung's disease?
A. It usually manifests shortly after birth by failure to pass meconium.
B. Twenty percent of affected infants develop diarrhea due to pseudomembranous enterocolitis.
C. Inheritance is autosomal recessive.
D. A short aganglionic segment usually presents in the neonatal period whereas a long aganglionic segment presents later in life.

---

444. Each the following statements about diverticular pathology is true EXCEPT:
A. Most are actually pseudodiverticula.
B. Right colonic diverticula are more likely to cause massive bleeding.
C. Myochosis predisposes to diverticula.
D. The diverticula protrude through the taenia coli.
E. Diverticula are most common in the sigmoid colon.

---

445. Infectious agents that cause diarrhea and primarily affect the small intestine include all of the following EXCEPT:
A. *Vibrio cholerae*
B. Enterotoxigenic *Escherichia coli*
C. Norwalk virus
D. *Campylobacter jejuni*
E. *Giardia lamblia*

---

446. Which of the following contribute to shock in acute intestinal obstruction?
  I. Intestinal wall edema
 II. Decreased gut absorption
III. Increased gut secretion
IV. Translocation of bacteria from the gut lumen to mesenteric lymph

A. I and III

B. II and IV
C. I, II, and III
D. All of the above

---

447. Each of the following is a true statement about the treatment of fecal impaction EXCEPT:
A. Initial therapy is partial removal of the fecal mass by digital disimpaction.
B. Proximal sigmoid masses can be broken up using a sigmoidoscope with gentle irrigation.
C. Complications of disimpaction include sepsis, hypotension, and perforation.
D. Tap water enemas are hazardous because of the risk of hyponatremia.
E. Oral doses of osmotic laxatives may be used to prevent recurrence.

---

448. Vitamin B_{12} is malabsorbed in bacterial overgrowth of the small bowel because:
A. Bacterial enzymes cleave vitamin B_{12} from intrinsic factor.
B. Bacteria take up vitamin B_{12} and vitamin B_{12}–intrinsic factor complexes.
C. Vitamin B_{12} is a fat-soluble vitamin that is malabsorbed by patients with steatorrhea.
D. Rapid transit does not allow enough contact time in the terminal ileum.

---

449. Each of the following is a true statement regarding idiopathic small intestinal ulcers EXCEPT:
A. They are more common in the ileum than in the jejunum.
B. Intermittent small bowel obstruction is common at presentation.
C. Perforation is a common complication.
D. Biopsy shows chronic inflammation with a prominent granulomatous component.
E. Diagnosis is frequently made at laparotomy.

---

450. A 60-year-old man receives 55 Gy (5500 rads) of radiation to the pelvis for the treatment of prostate cancer. Which of the following BEST describes his chances for developing symptoms of chronic radiation proctitis?
A. 5%
B. 40%
C. 90%
D. Future risk is unpredictable.
E. Patients with prostate cancer rarely sustain chronic radiation bowel injury.

---

451. A 35-year-old woman with ulcerative colitis for five years calls angrily complaining that the life insurance company has more than doubled her premiums after obtaining your office records. She has been asymptomatic on sulfasalazine for one year. Which one of the following statements regarding this situation is TRUE?

A. The higher rate is justified because of the increased risk of colon cancer.

B. The higher rate is justified because of the risk of death from fulminant colitis.

C. The insurance company is overestimating her risk of premature death and should be challenged.

D. The patient is being unreasonable.

Colon and Small Intestine

■■■■*Answers*

(120–B)   *(S&F, pp. 1876–1881)*

Unfavorable prognostic factors at the time of polypectomy include poorly differentiated morphology, invasion of veins or lymphatics, malignancy at the tumor margin, or invasion into the submucosa. If one or more of these is present, the risk of tumor recurrence is substantially increased and surgical resection of the polyp site should be performed. If none is present, then repeat colonoscopy should be performed at three to six months to examine the polypectomy site and surveillance performed every three years thereafter. Yearly colonoscopy is not required. The National Polyp Study found that colonoscopy every three years is as effective as yearly examination and will decrease the incidence of colon cancer by 76% to 90%. Adenoma size per se is not a determinant of the surveillance interval.

■■■■**References**

Winawer, S. J., Zauber, A. G., Ho, M. N., et al. Prevention of colorectal cancer by colonoscopic polypectomy: The National Polyp Study Workgroup. N. Engl. J. Med. *329*:1977, 1993.
Winawer, S. J., Zauber, A. G., O'Brien, M. J., et al. Randomized comparison of surveillance intervals after colonoscopic removal of newly diagnosed adenomatous polyps: The National Polyp Study Workgroup. N. Engl. J. Med. *328*:901, 1993.

(121–C)   *(S&F, pp. 1923–1924)*

K-*ras* mutations are believed to occur earlier in the adenoma-carcinoma stage than 18q or *p53* mutations. However, there does not seem to be any prognostic significance to this independent stage of the cancer. Most other DNA abnormalities have been associated with poorer survival.

■■■■**References**

Ahlquist, D. A., and Thibodeau, S. N. Will molecular genetic markers help predict the clinical behavior of colorectal neoplasia? [Editorial; comment]. Gastroenterology *102*:1419, 1992.
Brentnall, T. A., Crispin, D. A., Rabinovitch, P. S., et al. Mutations in the *p53* gene: An early marker of neoplastic progression in ulcerative colitis. Gastroenterology *107*:369, 1994.
Kinzler, K. W., and Vogelstein, B. Cancer therapy meets *p53*. N. Engl. J. Med. *331*:49, 1994.
Thibodeau, S. N., Bren, G., and Schaid, D. Microsatellite instability in cancer of the proximal colon. Science *260*:816, 1993.

(122–B)   *(S&F, p. 1756)*

If low-grade dysplasia is found, a repeat examination should be performed within a few weeks to confirm the diagnosis. If confirmed, most experts would recommend colectomy. Deferring colectomy until high-grade dysplasia appears is associated with an increased risk of metastatic malignancy and is no longer recommended.

(123–A)   *(S&F, p. 1894)*

Sulindac has been shown to be effective in decreasing adenoma formation and even causing regression of some existing polyps. However, the response is not complete and sulindac cannot be used in place of subtotal colectomy in affected persons. Whether sulindac is effective as an adjunct after subtotal colectomy has not yet been determined. The epidemiologic evidence thus far suggests that frequency and duration may be factors in the aspirin effects; however, the minimal effective dosage has not been established. Treatment of ulcerative colitis with sulfasalazine (which liberates 5-aminosalicylic acid in the colon) may also be associated with a lower risk of developing cancer. The prevailing theory is that the antiproliferative effects of aspirin, 5-aminosalicylic acid, and other NSAIDs are due to inhibition of prostaglandin synthesis.

■■■■**References**

Bond, J. H. Polyp guideline: Diagnosis, treatment, and surveillance for patients with nonfamilial colorectal polyps: The Practice Parameters Committee of the American College of Gastroenterology. Ann. Intern. Med. *119*:836, 1993.
Giardiello, F. M., Hamilton, S. R., Krush, A. J., et al. Treatment of colonic and rectal adenomas with sulindac in familial adenomatous polyposis. N. Engl. J. Med. *328*:1313, 1993.

(124–C)   *(S&F, pp. 1861–1862)*

Given the demonstration of bowel loop thickening as well as detection of a potential tumor in the midileum, exploratory laparotomy is indicated. The patient's abdominal pain is most likely the result of intermittent intussusception caused by the tumor. If the enteroclysis had not shown abnormal findings, other appropriate diagnostic tests would have included computed tomography of the abdomen as well as small bowel enteroscopy.

(125–C)   *(S&F, p. 1951)*

Subphrenic gonococcal infection (Fitz-Hugh–Curtis syndrome) involving the surface of the liver may have signs and symptoms similar to those of acute cholelithiasis. Such symptoms usually occur in young, sexually active women who may have evidence of pelvic inflammatory disease. Gonococci are presumed to reach the liver by direct spread from infected fallopian tubes through the peritoneal cavity. Patients usually present with sudden onset of upper abdominal pain with tenderness in the right subcostal area. Leukocytosis and an elevated erythrocyte sedimentation rate are usually present. Hepatic enzyme levels may be mildly elevated. Cervical cultures are usually positive for *Neisseria gonorrhoeae* even when cervical discharge is absent. Antibiotic treatment causes rapid resolution of symptoms.

Syphilitic hepatitis is usually asymptomatic with a disproportionate increase in the alkaline phosphatase and/or bilirubin value.

(126–B) **(S&F, pp. 1755–1758)**

Current data suggest that treatment of ulcerative colitis with sulfasalazine is associated with a decreased risk of developing colorectal cancer. Approximately 40% of patients having high-grade dysplasia and 20% of patients having low-grade dysplasia on endoscopic surveillance biopsy specimens will have coexisting carcinoma somewhere within their colon. The finding of definitive dysplasia of any grade on biopsy thus argues for colectomy.

Reference

Pinczowski, D., Ekbom, A., Baron, J., et al. Risk factors for colorectal cancer in patients with ulcerative colitis: A case-control study. Gastroenterology *107*:117, 1994.

(127–A) **(S&F, p. 1877)**

Single small (<10 mm) tubular adenomas are not really associated with any higher risk of colon cancer than the background population in whom the status of colon adenomas is unknown; therefore, solitary, diminutive tubular adenomas need not necessarily be followed with surveillance colonoscopy. Familial adenomatous polyposis kindred members who are at risk but have not yet developed adenomas should be screened by flexible sigmoidoscopy annually and by colonoscopy every three years. These persons are at risk because they may belong to the newly recognized attenuated forms of adenomatous polyposis coli or may exhibit incomplete penetrance of the genetic defect. Commercial availability of tests for adenomatous polyposis coli may obviate the need for endoscopic screening in many of these kindreds. Hereditary nonpolyposis colorectal cancer is characterized by patients having an average or slightly above average number of adenomas. However, the lack of DNA proofreading function predisposes these adenomas to develop mutations rapidly. Therefore, cancer may arise in the adenomas in these patients at an accelerated rate. The predilection of these lesions for the right colon necessitates colonoscopy. All of the other patients can be colonoscoped at three-year intervals. In cases D and E, the patients should also have one colonoscopy three to six months after resection to re-examine the polypectomy or anastomosis site.

References

Bronner, C. E., Baker, S. M., Morrison, P. T., et al. Mutation in the DNA mismatch repair gene homologue hMLH1 is associated with hereditary nonpolyposis colon cancer. Nature *368*:258, 1994.

Giardiello, F. M., Krush, A. J., Petersen, G. M., et al. Phenotypic variability of familial adenomatous polyposis in 11 unrelated families with identical APC gene mutation. Gastroenterology *106*:1542, 1994.

Leach, F. S., Nicolaides, N. C., Papadopoulos, N., et al. Mutations of a mutS homolog in hereditary nonpolyposis colorectal cancer. Cell *75*:1215, 1993.

Lynch, H. T., Smyrk, T. C., Watson, P., et al. Genetics, natural history, tumor spectrum, and pathology of hereditary nonpolyposis colorectal cancer: An updated review. Gastroenterology *104*:1535, 1993.

Nicolaides, N. C., Papadoulos, N., Liu, B., et al. Mutations of two PMS homologues in hereditary nonpolyposis colon cancer. Nature *371*:75, 1994.

Spirio, L., Olschwang, S., Groden, J., et al. Alleles of the APC gene: An attenuated form of familial polyposis. Cell *75*:951, 1993.

(128–D) **(S&F, pp. 1876–1877)**

Studies have shown that a single small tubular adenoma does not predict risk of synchronous adenomas in the proximal colon. The National Polyp Study has shown that surveillance colonoscopy need not be done more frequently than every three years. Ulcerative colitis of duration or more than eight years is associated with increased risk for developing colon cancer. However, ulcerative colitis in a parent or sibling does not warrant colonoscopy in an asymptomatic patient. Primary hepatoma is not associated with an increased risk of colon cancer.

The patient may be at increased risk for developing colon cancer if she belongs to a Lynch II kindred, which predisposes to a spectrum of malignancies including stomach, endometrial, ovarian, small bowel, kidney, and bladder cancer. Because she has already had endometrial cancer at age younger than 45 years and has a family history of Lynch II syndrome–associated cancers, she should be screened for colorectal cancer with colonoscopy.

References

Bond, J. H. Polyp guideline: Diagnosis, treatment, and surveillance for patients with nonfamilial colorectal polyps: The Practice Parameters Committee of the American College of Gastroenterology. Ann. Intern. Med. *119*:836, 1993.

Lynch, H. T., Smyrk, T. C., Watson, P., et al. Genetics, natural history, tumor spectrum, and pathology of hereditary nonpolyposis colorectal cancer: An updated review. Gastroenterology *104*:1535, 1993.

(129–A, B, C, E) ***Rome criteria (S&F, p. 1537)***
Minimal test (S&F, p. 1542)

The patient fits the Rome criteria for the diagnosis of the irritable bowel syndrome, and a probable diagnosis can be made based on history. The presence of constipation argues against an acute bacterial colitis, so stool cultures would not be warranted. Minimal laboratory studies to exclude anemia and leukocytosis, and a sigmoidoscopy complete the evaluation in most patients.

(130–C) **(S&F, p. 1869)**

Although frequently missed by colonoscopy, flat adenomas actually account for about 10% of all adenomas and are clinically important because the risk of severe dysplasia and carcinoma is much higher in these lesions. The familial form of multiple, predominantly proximal flat adenomas has now been genetically proven to be an attenuated form of familial adenomatous polyposis.

(131–E) **(S&F, pp. 1926–1927)**

The patient was iron deficient, as evidenced by his response to iron. Visualization of the colon is indicated in all elderly patients who are truly iron deficient and have heme-positive stools. The fact that he is no longer iron deficient has no role in your decision. Repeating his fecal occult blood tests should also not affect your decision because malignancies are known to bleed intermittently. Flexible sigmoidoscopy would be a possible alternative if the patient had a high-quality air contrast barium enema already.

(132–D)   *(S&F, pp. 1848–1850)*

A large triangular ulcer with extrinsic compression of the duodenum is considered by some to be pathognomonic of duodenal lymphoma. The usual evaluation of suspected lymphoma includes options A, B, and C. The fasting gastrin level is indicated because a gastrin-secreting tumor can also produce large distal duodenal ulcers as part of the Zollinger-Ellison syndrome. A gastric emptying study would provide little diagnostic or therapeutic information about this patient.

(133–D)   *(S&F, pp. 1868, 1875–1877)*

Patient age per se is not a predictor of the presence of malignancy in a polyp, although age is associated with more and larger polyps. All of the other factors are associated with a greater risk of malignancy within an adenoma.

(134–D)   *(S&F, p. 1932)*

Mutations accumulate rapidly in hereditary nonpolyposis colorectal cancer (HNPCC) mucosal cells owing to defective repair of DNA base-pair mismatches. These mutations predispose adenomas to degenerate rapidly into frank malignancies. Thus, small adenomas (<1 cm) in HNPCC harbor dysplasia much more often than in sporadic adenomas. Flexible sigmoidoscopy plus air-contrast barium enema is not adequate for surveillance in these patients because many neoplasms form in the proximal colon in HNPCC where flexible sigmoidoscopy cannot detect them. In addition, barium enemas are relatively insensitive for smaller neoplasms that pose a greater risk in this population. Colonoscopy should be performed annually instead.

■■■**References**

Bronner, C. E., Baker, S. M., Morrison, P. T., et al. Mutation in the DNA mismatch repair gene homologue hMLH1 is associated with hereditary nonpolyposis colon cancer. Nature 368:258, 1994.
Leach, F. S., Nicolaides, N. C., Papadopoulos, N., et al. Mutations of a mutS homolog in hereditary nonpolyposis colorectal cancer. Cell 75:1215, 1993.
Lynch, H. T., Smyrk, T. C., Watson, P., et al. Genetics, natural history, tumor spectrum, and pathology of hereditary nonpolyposis colorectal cancer: An updated review. Gastroenterology 104:1535, 1993.
Nicolaides, N. C., Papadopoulos, N., Liu, B., et al. Mutations of two PMS homologues in hereditary nonpolyposis colon cancer. Nature 371:75, 1994.

(135–E)   *(S&F, pp. 1876–1877)*

Although the average age at diagnosis of hereditary nonpolyposis colorectal cancer (HNPCC) is younger than 45, 20% of the cancers occur in patients older than 50 and cases occurring in patients up to age 83 have been documented. A 60-year-old patient who has not previously been screened but is clearly part of an HNPCC family should be colonoscoped unless the gene abnormality for his or her kindred has been defined and he or she is negative. The patient in option A is at slightly increased risk statistically. However, the brother's age and location of the cancer are against this being due to a hereditary syndrome. A 50-year-old patient in a familial adenomatous polyposis (FAP) kindred can be screened with flexible sigmoidoscopy. The risk of gene carriage is 4% if no adenomas are present at age 30; and if this patient has no adenomas at age 50, his chances of having the FAP phenotype are virtually nil. A single adenoma less than 10 mm on flexible sigmoidoscopy does not predict more proximal adenomas. A single first-degree relative with colorectal cancer increases the patient's odds of developing colorectal cancer two- to three-fold. However, patient D's brother had his cancer in the left colon and it was replication error (RER) negative (90% of HNPCC cancers will be RER positive), making it unlikely that his colon cancer was due to HNPCC. This patient should be screened with a flexible sigmoidoscopy within the next year.

■■■**Reference**

Lynch, H. T., Smyrk, T. C., Watson, P., et al. Genetics, natural history, tumor spectrum, and pathology of hereditary nonpolyposis colorectal cancer: An updated review. Gastroenterology 104:1535, 1993.

(136–E)   *(S&F, pp. 1927–1931)*

Carcinoembryonic antigen (CEA) is not effective as a screening test in any population. Its clinical utility is limited to patients already diagnosed with colon cancer who are then found to have elevated CEA levels. CEA levels can then be used to monitor for recurrence after surgery.

■■■**References**

Nicolaides, N. C., Papadopoulos, N., Liu, B., et al. Mutations of two PMS homologues in hereditary nonpolyposis colon cancer. Nature 371:75, 1994.
Selby, J. V., Friedman, G. D., Quesenberry, C. P., Jr., and Weiss, N. S. A case-control study of screening sigmoidoscopy and mortality from colorectal cancer. N. Engl. J. Med. 326:653, 1992.
Winawer, S. J., Zauber, A. G., Ho, M. N., et al. Prevention of colorectal cancer by colonoscopic polypectomy: The National Polyp Study Workgroup. N. Engl. J. Med. 329:1977, 1993.

(137–C)   *(S&F, p. 1750)*

The patient most likely has primary sclerosing cholangitis (PSC), but endoscopic retrograde cholangiopancreatography is necessary to confirm the diagnosis and exclude other causes of bile duct obstruction. PSC is a progressive disease that is associated with increased risk of cholangiocarcinoma.

(138–A)   *(S&F, p. 1659)*

Cytomegalovirus (CMV) was first associated with ulcers in renal transplant patients; however, CMV has also been reported in association with peptic ulcers in nonimmunocompromised hosts. The proof that syphilis causes gastric ulcers comes from the demonstration of the organism in the gastric mucosa, appropriate serology, and evidence that lesions regress after antibiotic therapy. Gastric syphilis is usually observed during the secondary stage of the disease. *Treponema pallidum* spirochetes can be demonstrated in gastric biopsy specimens by silver staining and fluorescent antibody techniques.

(139–E)   **(S&F, pp. 1879–1881)**

Because we know that polypectomy decreases the subsequent risk of developing colon cancer from other studies, A and B are unlikely to account for these seemingly disparate results. Case-control studies are retrospective studies. Statement D is incorrect because the change in distribution of colon cancer cannot reconcile the two studies. Statement E is correct because the second study did not control for colorectal cancer above the site of the polypectomy, which is more likely after polypectomy than in controls.

(140–1-E, 2-C, 3-B, 4-A, 5-D)   **(S&F, pp. 1883–1887)**

Inflammatory pseudopolyps develop during healing after inflammation. They occur in inflammatory bowel disease and may occasionally be large and solitary, mimicking a neoplastic mass. Colitis cystica profunda is a benign, rare lesion consisting of dilated, mucus-filled glands in the submucosa and resulting in solitary (occasionally multiple) large polyps. Their primary clinical significance is that they may be confused with colloid carcinoma. Pneumatosis cystoides intestinalis is multiple air-filled cysts within the submucosa of the colon and small intestine and may produce a polypoid appearance. In its benign form, it is often associated with chronic obstructive pulmonary disease and scleroderma. In its more malignant form, it may be produced by invasion by gas-forming bacteria in the setting of severe inflammation or ischemia. It typically responds to inhaled oxygen therapy. Lymphoid tissue is present throughout the colon and hypertrophied follicles may be mistaken for polyps. Occasionally, they may grow large enough to produce symptoms (pain, bleeding) or may become pedunculated. Lymphoid polyps are more common in children. Lipomas tend to be solitary, asymptomatic, and detected incidentally. Colonic lipomas are most common on the right side and tend to occur near the ileocecal valve. Removal of these lesions is usually unnecessary.

(141–B, D)   **(S&F, pp. 1461–1462)**

Volume status and intestinal blood flow can alter ion transport. There is evidence to suggest that both active absorption and secretion are associated with increased intestinal blood flow. Metabolic acidosis is a potent stimulator of absorption, whereas metabolic alkalosis appears to inhibit absorption. These effects appear to be mediated by the sodium–hydrogen and chloride–bicarbonate exchangers. Increased sympathetic input, which occurs with hypovolemia, results in a decrease in secretion and probably increases absorption. Loss of sympathetic neural regulatory mechanisms in diabetic autonomic neuropathy is associated with the development of "diabetic diarrhea."

(142–A)   **(S&F, pp. 1462–1465)**

Unlike the kidney, the intestinal epithelium cannot sustain an osmotic gradient. Thus, any osmotically active compound will produce diarrhea if not absorbed. Cations such as magnesium or anions such as sulfate are poorly absorbed by the normal gut. Disaccharides are a frequent source of nonabsorbable solute because they must be converted to simple sugars before they can cross the apical membrane. The most frequent clinical example is lactose intolerance. Chenodeoxycholic acid but not ursodeoxycholic acid can cause diarrhea when given in therapeutic doses. The mechanism is believed to be stimulation of chloride secretion. Long-chain fatty acids that enter the colon may cause diarrhea by a similar mechanism.

(143–E)   **(S&F, pp. 1992–1993)**

Melanosis coli is a black pigment, lipofuscin, in the colonic mucosa. The pigment is often diffuse but is found mainly in the cecum and proximal colon. Melanosis coli has also been reported in patients with carcinoma of the colon, but the mechanism and significance are unknown. Melanosis coli is a benign condition and requires no further evaluation in a patient with an appropriate history of cathartic use.

(144–C)   **(S&F, pp. 1612–1613)**

The reservoir of *Campylobacter jejuni* is enormous, including primarily cattle, sheep, swine, and domesticated animals; and the disease is often transmitted to humans by improperly prepared meats, especially chicken. The disease, while causing significant colonic invasion and colitis as the dominating symptom, is characteristically preceded by a systemic prodrome. The stool is usually packed with leukocytes.

(145–A, C)   **(S&F, pp. 1811–1813)**

Hirschsprung's disease occurs in approximately 1 of each 5000 live births and is familial. There is an overall incidence of 3.6% among siblings of all index cases. Association of congenital megacolon with Down's syndrome is ten times more frequent than would be expected by chance. Approximately 2% of the patients with congenital megacolon have Down's syndrome. The aganglionic segment invariably involves the internal anal sphincter and extends proximally a variable length.

(146–D)   **(S&F, pp. 1872–1873)**

Any first-degree relative with a history of either colon cancer or colonic adenomas increases the risk of an individual having colonic adenomas. The risk is further increased if the age at diagnosis in the relative was younger than 60. The association between red meat (a high-fat diet) and smoking for development of adenomas has been strengthened by results from recent publications. Increasing age is the single most important risk factor for the development of adenomas. In retrospective studies, chronic NSAID use, especially of aspirin, has been negatively correlated with the incidence of adenomas; prospective studies looking at chemoprevention of adenomas by NSAIDs are in progress.

References

Giovannucci, E., Rimm, E. B., Stampfer, M. J., et al. A prospective study of cigarette smoking and risk of colorectal adenoma and colorectal cancer in United States men. J. Natl. Cancer Inst. *86*:183, 1994.
Sandler, R. S., Lyles, C. M., McAuliffe, C., et al. Cigarette smoking, alcohol, and the risk of colorectal adenomas. Gastroenterology *104*:1445, 1993.

(147–A)   **(S&F, p. 1832)**

Simple appendectomy is the standard treatment for appendiceal carcinoids 1 cm or less in diameter. For lesions 1 to 2 cm in diameter, a right hemicolectomy had been advocated to reduce risk of recurrence. This view was not supported by clinical trials, however. Current recommendations are for simple appendectomy for appendiceal carcinoids less than 2 cm in size with no additional follow-up required.

(148–D)   **(S&F, pp. 1832–1833)**

Appendiceal carcinoids larger than 2 cm have a definite risk of metastasis. A more aggressive operation is indicated in those patients who are otherwise healthy. The presence of vascular invasion and involvement of the mesoappendix are also factors that favor more aggressive surgery.

(149–A)   **(S&F, pp. 1439–1440)**

The central nervous system and enteric nervous system are intimately connected by multiple pathways. The craniosacral pathway involves the vagal and sacral (pelvic) segments. The thoracolumbar sympathetics provide adrenergic stimulus through prevertebral ganglia. Many of these pathways have motor as well as sensory components.

(150–B)   **(S&F, p. 1828)**

Initial treatment of Ogilvie's syndrome consists of correcting metabolic electrolyte and fluid abnormalities, discontinuing narcotic and anticholinergic drugs, and instituting decompression via a nasogastric or rectal tube. Laxatives are generally not helpful and should be avoided, especially nonabsorbable sugars such as lactulose that increase intraluminal gas. Multiple drugs have been tried to increase colonic motility. Recent reports suggest that cisapride may produce a clinical response in many patients and should be tried. Colonoscopic decompression, when necessary, is effective in up to 90% of patients. Endoscopically placed rectal decompression tubes may decrease early recurrence.

(151–B)   **(S&F, p. 1536)**

A high familial incidence of irritable bowel syndrome (IBS) has been reported. In three fourths of children with IBS, one or both parents or one or more siblings have a functional gastrointestinal disorder. The female predominance that exists in adults is not found in children. In many series, boys outnumber girls, suggesting that more boys outgrow the syndrome or that females have a later onset or both. Children with IBS have normal growth and development. Three fourths of school-aged children with IBS have a history of onset of symptoms with stressful school problems or parental marital problems. It is estimated that two thirds of referrals to pediatric gastroenterologists are because of functional disorders.

(152–C)   **(S&F, p. 1706)**

Chronic radiation injury to the small bowel may present as impaired motility or stricture, as suggested by the patient's chronic stable symptoms. Patients with impaired motility or stricture are at high risk for bacterial overgrowth due to stasis. Treatment with a course of tetracycline would be the therapy most likely to result in sustained improvement of the diarrhea.

(153–B)   **(S&F, pp. 1816–1817)**

The goal of medical management of megacolon or megarectum is to empty the bowel of stool and to keep it empty. Disimpaction is indicated if there is a large fecal mass in the rectal vault. Bulking agents and large volumes of water are dietary devices to assist in daily defecation. Preparations containing senna, cascara, bisacodyl, and other stimulant laxatives should be avoided. Patients are encouraged to pass stools at the same time every day, usually after meals to take advantage of the gastrocolic response. For patients failing medical management, surgery is an option.

(154–A)   **(S&F, pp. 1758–1759)**

Prolonged corticosteroid treatment may suppress the growth rate in children with ulcerative colitis; however, active colitis itself will also cause growth retardation, and careful attention must be paid to height and weight percentiles at each visit. Ulcerative colitis can present within the first few months of life. Pancolitis is more common in children with ulcerative colitis than in adult patients. Immunosuppressive drugs can be used as steroid-sparing agents in children with ulcerative colitis.

(155–C)   **(S&F, pp. 1848–1849)**

Primary gastrointestinal lymphomas in the United States most frequently affect the stomach and/or small bowel, with the colorectal region rarely involved. Abdominal pain is the most common presenting complaint, often with anorexia, weight loss, and malaise. Proximal lesions may cause nausea and vomiting, whereas distal lesions lead to abdominal distention. Malabsorption is a relatively rare occurrence in most lymphomas but has been associated with T-cell lymphomas of the gut.

(156–D) **(S&F, pp. 1728–1729)**

Except for basal cell carcinoma, all of the malignancies listed have been reported with increased frequency in patients with Crohn's disease.

(157–C) **(S&F, p. 1779)**

Appendicitis is commonly caused by obstruction of the appendiceal lumen, leading to accumulation of infected secretions. Most cases occur in children, and the obstruction is usually caused by hyperplasia of lymphoid tissue, suggesting the presence of an adjacent infection rather than fiber deficiency. Factors predisposing to constipation include a low intake of fiber, physical inactivity, lack of toilet facilities, pregnancy, and certain drugs. Most patients with mild to moderate constipation benefit from treatment with wheat bran or viscous polysaccharides. Patients with constipation and irritable bowel syndrome often respond to dietary fiber or fiber supplements, whereas those with diarrhea often report improvement even though stool weight increases. Dietary fiber may protect against the development of diverticulosis by making the colonic contents softer, bulkier, and easier to propel, thus reducing intraluminal pressures.

(158–B, C, D) **(S&F, pp. 1875–1876)**

What is known of the natural history of untreated polyps is based on small (usually retrospective) series of cases. Nonetheless, based on serial barium enema measurements, the risk of a 10-mm polypoid mass (histology unknown) developing into carcinoma at 5, 10, and 20 years is 2.5%, 8%, and 24%, respectively. The natural history of diminutive (<5 mm) polyps is even more benign, with 96% either staying the same size or regressing in size over five years and fewer than 1% turning into cancer.

(159–A) **(S&F, pp. 1672–1674)**

Most cercariae die after penetrating the skin in humans and are absorbed. Repeated exposure may cause a hypersensitivity response including a pruritic papular rash. With migration through the lungs, acute schistosomiasis can produce cough and daily spiking fevers to more than 39° C. The immune response to the flukes can produce an allergic reaction with urticaria and facial swelling similar to serum sickness. Patients often have painful adenopathy and an enlarged spleen and liver. Acute involvement in the intestine may produce a severe dysentery that is occasionally fatal (especially in children). Infestation of the appendix can even produce acute appendicitis. Biliary obstruction, however, is not seen in acute schistosomiasis.

(160–C) **(S&F, p. 1550)**

Diarrhea after an ileal resection is usually caused either by bile acid malabsorption and bile salt–induced colonic secretion (<100 cm resection) or by bile salt malabsorption with bile salt pool depletion and fatty acid–induced colonic secretion (>100 cm resection). The clinical finding of worsening diarrhea with treatment with binding resins suggests further bile salt depletion.

(161–C) **Anatomy (S&F, p. 1791)**
Rebleeding (S&F, p. 1793)

The two most common causes of serious colonic bleeding are diverticula and angiodysplasia. Recent data suggest that concurrent angiodysplasia and diverticula may predispose to more frequent bleeding. In instances where the site of massive diverticular bleeding can be identified, right colonic diverticula were the source in the majority of cases. The chances of a second hemorrhage in the months or years after an initial diverticular hemorrhage are 20% to 25%. Once bleeding recurs, the chance of another bleeding episode increases to 50% or more.

(162–A) **(S&F, p. 1893)**

Although prophylactic total colectomy is the most effective method of preventing colorectal cancer in very high risk patients, several groups have obtained reasonable success with rectum-sparing operations followed by three- to six-month sigmoidoscopies and adenoma fulguration, resulting in a risk of malignancy of approximately 10%. Trials of NSAIDs such as sulindac or indomethacin enemas in conjunction with rectum-sparing surgery may yield even better results. The high rate of synchronous and metachronous colorectal cancers in patients with hereditary nonpolyposis colorectal cancer (approximately one third) necessitates subtotal or total colectomy.

Reference

Lynch, H. T., Smyrk, T. C., Watson, P., et al. Genetics, natural history, tumor spectrum, and pathology of hereditary nonpolyposis colorectal cancer: An updated review. Gastroenterology *104*:1535, 1993.

(163–A) **(S&F, pp. 1589–1590)**

Whipple's disease is a systemic disease characterized by many extraintestinal manifestations. Choices B through E are classic manifestations; however, hepatosplenomegaly is uncommon.

(164–F) **(S&F, pp. 185, 1790–1794, 1813, 1875)**

All are true. However, air-contrast barium enema with flexible sigmoidoscopy enjoys a considerable cost advantage over colonoscopy such that many managed-care groups prefer the cost advantage despite the lower sensitivity. Unfortunately, training in barium procedures has become somewhat less rigorous, owing to the emphasis on the more "glamorous" radiologic procedures such as interventional radiology, computed tomography, and magnetic resonance imaging. As a result, national radiologic organizations are re-emphasizing the importance of adequate training in these procedures.

(165–A) **(S&F, pp. 1810–1811)**

Megacolon is a descriptive term rather than a disease. In adults, it is diagnosed when the diameter of the rectosigmoid or descending colon on a radiograph is more than 6.5 cm, the ascending colon more than 8 cm, or the cecal diameter more than 12 cm. *Congenital megacolon* is the term often applied to Hirschsprung's disease. Toxic megacolon is a feared complication of inflammatory bowel disease and severe infectious colitis. The most common background for acquired megacolon is colonic inertia, a condition afflicting children and the elderly. *Blastocystis hominis* is an intestinal parasite that, when abundant, may cause watery diarrhea but not megacolon.

(166–A, C)   **(S&F, pp. 1672–1673)**

Schistosoma japonicum prefers the superior mesenteric vein and is therefore the main schistosome to involve the small intestine. *Schistosoma mansoni* has a striking tendency to follow the inferior mesenteric vein and preferentially involves the descending colon; however, the bladder is spared. *Schistosoma haematobium* prefers the vesicle plexus, often involves the pelvic organs and bladder, and may also involve the rectum distally.

(167–A)   **(S&F, pp. 1616–1617)**

The most common cause of traveler's diarrhea is enterotoxigenic *Escherichia coli* (40% to 60% of cases) acquired by ingesting fecally contaminated food or beverages. The highest risk destinations include Latin America, Africa, the Middle East, and Asia, where 25% to 50% of travelers are affected. Despite careful study, no pathogen can be identified in up to 40% of cases. Younger travelers, particularly those from 20 to 29 years of age, have the highest risk. Risky foods include uncooked vegetables, meat, seafood, tap water, and unpeeled fruits.

(168–C)   **(S&F, p. 1697)**

A proliferating cell is most sensitive to the ionizing effects of radiation during G2 and mitosis, because normal repair mechanisms are unable to act before the radiation-induced mutations become fixed by DNA replication. Resistance to radiation builds during the G1 and S phases.

(169–B)   **(S&F, p. 1458)**

Small bowel potassium movement is passive and largely reflects the negative electrical potential difference developed across the epithelium. In contrast, the colon can actively secrete potassium using an adenosine triphosphate–dependent mechanism that is independent of sodium fluxes. Several secretory stimuli enhance both chloride and potassium secretion, suggesting the two processes may be linked. Potassium exits the cell across the basolateral membrane via a potassium channel.

(170–A)   **(S&F, p. 1834)**

The most common clinical presentation of small bowel carcinoid is periodic abdominal pain. Pain typically results from intermittent small bowel obstruction, usually due to "kinking" of the small bowel from an exuberant fibrotic reaction surrounding the tumor. Gastrointestinal bleeding and intussusception are distinctly uncommon. Carcinoid syndrome is a late manifestation of disease, generally occurring only after hepatic metastases are present. Small bowel infarction may be a manifestation of ischemia or obstruction due to carcinoid syndrome but is not as common as intermittent abdominal pain.

(171–1-A, 2-D, 3-C, 4-B)   **V. cholerae (S&F, p. 1596)**
                                S. typhi (S&F, p. 1610)
                              S. enteritidis (S&F, p. 1606)

A classic sign of typhoid fever is the "rose spot," an evanescent rash that is evident early in the course of the disease. Over 1700 serotypes of nontyphi *Salmonella* have been identified in a multitude of domestic animals. *S. enteritidis* is a prominent member of this group. *Shigella dysenteriae* can cause disease with ingestion of very few organisms. Ingestion of 100,000 organisms causes disease in more than 75% of persons, and clinical disease can be brought about by ingestion of as few as 200 organisms. This is in contrast to *Salmonella* and *Escherichia coli,* which generally require orders of magnitude of larger numbers of organisms to produce disease. *Vibrio cholerae* is not invasive and does not cause bacteremia or sepsis. The other organisms can all produce bacteremia and/or sepsis.

(172–C)   **(S&F, pp. 1811–1814)**

In Hirschsprung's disease, neurons are absent in the diseased segment, the affected bowel is spastic, and there is no rectoanal inhibitory reflex. The disease may involve only a very short aganglionic segment that can be missed on barium enema. The absence of the rectoanal inhibitory reflex is the best way to make the diagnosis in patients with ultra short-segment Hirschsprung's disease.

(173–B)   **(S&F, p. 1698)**

Chronic intestinal radiation injury is due to effects of radiation on the vascular epithelium leading to an obliterative endarteritis with subsequent mucosal ischemia. Fibrosis and stricturing may result.

(174–B)   **(S&F, pp. 1711–1712)**

The concordance rate for developing Crohn's disease in monozygotic twins is substantially less than 100%, suggesting that simple mendelian inheritance cannot account for the familial patterns.

(175–C)   **(S&F, pp. 1531–1533)**

The gold-standard test for detection of bacterial overgrowth is quantitative bacterial culture. Samples can be obtained through a nasojejunal tube or during endoscopy. Fluids must be kept under anaerobic conditions until plating and serially diluted to determine bacterial titers. Normal titers are less than 10,000 organisms/mL, whereas patients with clinically significant small bowel overgrowth typically have more than 100,000 organisms/mL. All of the other tests are of value in screening patients with suspected overgrowth but are less sensitive or specific.

(176–A)   *(S&F, pp. 1956–1957)*

The major mechanism of transmission of hepatitis A virus (HAV) is ingestion of virus shed in feces. Among patients at a clinic for sexually transmitted diseases, 30% of homosexual and 12% of heterosexual men showed evidence of anti-HAV. The annual incidence of hepatitis A in susceptible homosexual men was 22%, with acquisition of hepatitis A associated with a greater number of sexual partners and with oral-anal sexual exposure. In contrast, hepatitis B virus (HBV) is efficiently transmitted by heterosexual contact. High titers of HBV are found in semen, but not in urine or feces. HBV in males may be acquired transurethrally, because insertive anal intercourse in one study appeared to carry an even greater risk for infection than did receptive anal intercourse. Sexual transmission of hepatitis C virus (HCV) probably occurs, but at much lower rates than for HBV. HCV has not been detected in saliva, semen, urine, stool, or vaginal secretions of infected patients by polymerase chain reaction, reflecting the much lower viral titers commonly seen with HCV.

(177–B)   *(S&F, pp. 1585–1586)*

The response of Whipple's disease to antibiotics is usually rapid and dramatic.

(178–C)   *(S&F, p. 1837)*

Probably the most dramatic manifestation of the carcinoid syndrome is carcinoid crisis. It occurs most frequently in patients with foregut carcinoids who have greatly elevated 5-hydroxyindoleacetic acid levels. Stress, chemotherapy, and the induction of anesthesia may precipitate the crisis. Patients usually develop an intense, generalized flushing that may persist for hours or days. There may be exacerbation of diarrhea and abdominal pain, and central nervous system abnormalities, including coma, may occur. Although carcinoid crisis can be a terminal event, patients may by resuscitated through standard measures.

(179–A)   *(S&F, pp. 1753–1754)*

Systemic corticosteroid therapy is most likely to control an acute flare of pancolitis. Azathioprine and 6-mercaptopurine take at least several weeks to act and are not useful in this situation. Sulfasalazine alone is unlikely to control symptoms of this severity. Suppositories do not treat the entire colon.

(180–C)   *(S&F, pp. 1928–1931)*

Fecal occult blood testing has been shown to decrease the mortality of colorectal cancer in randomized, prospective studies that show an increase in the yield of cancers in earlier stages and a reduction in mortality by 15% to 43%. Rehydration of the slide doubles the sensitivity but quadruples the number of false-positive test results, thus decreasing the positive predictive value of the test.

Reference

Mandel, J. S., Bond, J. H., Church, T. R., et al. Reducing mortality from colorectal cancer by screening for fecal occult blood: Minnesota Colon Cancer Control Study. N. Engl. J. Med. *328*:1365, 1993.

(181–A)   *(S&F, pp. 1661–1662)*

Balantidiasis is generally a rare condition. However, serious outbreaks have occurred in the United States among institutionalized individuals. Three stool examinations are not sufficient to exclude this diagnosis. At least six to seven fresh specimens must be analyzed before this disease can be excluded. Fresh specimens are required because the examiner is looking for motile ciliates and not eggs. The spectrum of presentation for balantidiasis includes asymptomatic carriers and patients with mild diarrhea, dysentery, and even appendicitis. Early recognition is extremely difficult because there are many asymptomatic carriers. Balantidiasis is readily treated with tetracycline or alternates such as iodoquinol or metronidazole.

(182–C)   *(S&F, p. 1595)*

Vibrio cholerae is not invasive and therefore does not cause bacteremia or bloody diarrhea. It readily attaches to upper small intestinal mucosa, from where it elaborates a toxin that stimulates adenylate cyclase activity in enterocytes, leading to increased levels of cyclic adenosine monophosphate and massive fluid loss by intestinal epithelial cells. This leads to the clinical findings of profound dehydration and hypovolemic shock.

(183–E)   *(S&F, pp. 1514–1518)*

Each of the findings listed may be present in patients with malabsorption. However, none is common enough to be characteristic. The most common finding in malabsorption is a normal abdominal examination.

(184–C)   *(S&F, p. 1589)*

All of these processes can cause malabsorption and diarrhea. However, Whipple's disease is extremely uncommon (if it occurs at all) in persons from Southeast Asia. The overwhelming majority of patients with Whipple's disease are white men; only a small number of patients from India and one case from Japan have been reported.

(185–C)   *(S&F, pp. 1820–1822)*

Chronic intestinal pseudo-obstruction is a clinical syndrome caused by ineffective intestinal propulsion. It is characterized by symptoms and signs of intestinal obstruction in the absence of an occluding lesion of the intestinal lumen. Disorders of smooth muscle, the myenteric plexus, or extraintestinal nervous system may be associated with the syndrome. Chronic intestinal pseudo-obstruction can also involve the esophagus and stomach.

(186–D)   *(S&F, pp. 1764–1766)*

The etiology of pouchitis is unclear but seems to reflect the propensity of the individual to develop bowel inflammation. Patients undergoing ileoanal pouch anastomosis for Crohn's disease have a higher incidence of pouchitis than patients with polyposis. The small bowel mucosa in the pouch undergoes adaptation that includes variable degrees of villous atrophy and inflammation. For reasons that are unclear, most patients with pouchitis respond dramatically to metronidazole, although a few with severe symptoms who fail to respond ultimately must have the pouch resected.

(187–D)   **(S&F, pp. 1685–1686)**

Dietary manipulation, if beneficial, is generally only temporary. Scattered reports suggest a good response to sodium cromoglycate. However, this has not been confirmed in controlled trials. Hydroxyurea has been useful in the hypereosinophilic syndrome, but its role in eosinophilic gastroenteritis has not been defined. Corticosteroids are the mainstay of both acute therapy and maintenance.

(188–D)   **(S&F, pp. 1925, 1931, 1935)**

Carcinoembryonic antigen may be useful in preoperative staging and postoperative follow-up of patients with large bowel cancer but has a low predictive value for diagnosis in symptomatic patients. The test's low sensitivity and specificity combine to make it unsuitable for screening large populations. Its sensitivity is only 36% in patients with Dukes' A and B lesions, compared with 75% in Dukes' D disease when 2.5 mg/mL is used as the upper limit of normal.

(189–B)   **(S&F, pp. 1897–1900)**

Cronkhite-Canada syndrome is characterized by gastrointestinal hamartomas that are of the juvenile retention type. These have a slightly increased risk of developing malignancy secondary to adenomatous epithelium that sometimes develops within the hamartomas. However, no extracolonic malignancies have been associated with this syndrome.

▮▮▮▮Reference

Burt, R. W., and Groden, J. The genetic and molecular diagnosis of adenomatous polyposis coli. Gastroenterology *104*:1211, 1993.

(190–D)   **(S&F, pp. 1762–1763)**

The colon is capable of avid salt absorption, especially during conditions of low salt intake. Without the colon there is an obligate loss of 30 to 40 mEq of sodium per day.

(191–A, C, D)   **(S&F, pp. 1609–1611)**

Unlike nontyphoidal salmonellosis in which the infecting organisms are nearly ubiquitous in the environment, the only reservoir of *Salmonella typhi* is humans. The incubation period of this infection is usually 7 to 14 days. Blood cultures are positive in 90% of cases during the first week, and patients continue to be bacteremic for several weeks if untreated.

(192–D)   **(S&F, p. 1549)**

Digestion and absorption are nearly complete in the first 100 cm of jejunum in normal humans. Patients with more than 100 cm of jejunum are typically able to maintain a positive caloric and occasionally a positive water balance with oral feeding. Iron and folate are absorbed in the duodenum and very proximal jejunum, so supplements are usually unnecessary.

(193–E)   **(S&F, pp. 1923–1924)**

Primary tumors with extensive local inflammation are associated with fewer metastatic foci and a better prognosis. This suggests that immunologic recognition of abnormal cells may be an important defense mechanism against spread of malignancies.

(194–B, C)   **(S&F, p. 1648)**

Sexual promiscuity, migration from third world countries, and increased use of day care centers have all contributed to the observed increase in parasitic infections in the United States. Historically, these infections were primarily limited to tropical and underdeveloped countries, but this is clearly changing.

(195–D)   **(S&F, p. 1721)**

Campylobacter jejuni, though capable of causing a disease lasting weeks, typically involves the colon and not the ileum. Isolated amebiasis of the ileum is very rare, but amebic involvement of the ileum (and colon) can produce features indistinguishable from inflammatory bowel disease. The remaining entities can produce ileal disease that can be difficult to distinguish from Crohn's disease.

(196–A)   **(S&F, p. 1641)**

Antiperistaltic agents should be avoided when treating pseudomembranous colitis because of the risk of precipitating toxic megacolon.

(197–E)   **(S&F, pp. 1618–1619)**

Giardia rarely causes bloody diarrhea.

(198–E)   **(S&F, pp. 1767–1768)**

All of the factors listed are favorable except low rectal compliance. The more compliant the rectum is, the better it can function as a reservoir and the lower the number of stools per day.

(199–C)   **(S&F, pp. 1922–1923)**

The difference in stage B and stage C cancers is in the presence or absence of lymph nodes rather than depth of penetration. Malignant polyps are a particular subtype of Dukes' A lesions. Patients with Dukes' C1 lesions (i.e., less than four positive lymph nodes) have a 65% five-year survival. Palliative surgery to prevent bowel obstruction is indicated even if the disease is widely metastatic as long as the patient is able to withstand surgery.

(200–C) **(S&F, p. 1928)**
Surveillance is by far the most important contributor to the hidden costs (i.e., costs not directly resulting from screening). It is "the submerged part of the iceberg," even as surveillance regimens become increasingly less aggressive. Both D and E are direct costs incurred during screening.

Reference

Ransohoff, D. F., and Lang, C. A. Screening for colorectal cancer. N. Engl. J. Med. *325*:37, 1991.

(201–B) **(S&F, pp. 1764–1765)**
The Kock pouch operation is performed relatively rarely. Incontinence is seen in up to one third of patients and frequently requires reoperation for correction. Young women who have the pouch created at the time of initial operation tend to have the best results. Pouchitis develops with a frequency similar to that seen with ileoanal pouch anastomosis. The pouch is emptied voluntarily by inserting a catheter in the nipple valve.

(202–E) **(S&F, pp. 1784–1785)**
Given the declining incidence of appendicitis with advancing age, there is little justification for incidental appendectomy in patients older than 50 years old. Patients younger than 30 years old are the most likely to benefit if the primary operation is not compromised.

(203–C) **(S&F, p. 1833)**
The typical patient with rectal carcinoid is a middle-aged adult who is found to have the lesion incidentally at routine proctosigmoidoscopy. In contrast to small bowel carcinoids that are often multiple, rectal carcinoids are usually single tumors. They are generally located between 4 and 13 cm above the dentate line. Larger lesions (>2 cm) are more likely to metastasize and when detected should be treated by surgical resection as for other rectal carcinomas. Rectal carcinoids rarely produce serotonin. Thus, they rarely cause carcinoid syndrome even when metastatic.

(204–A, B, C) **(S&F, p. 1482)**
Digestion of protein begins in the stomach by the action of pepsins secreted by chief cells in the gastric mucosa. Pepsins are converted from their precursor pepsinogens by autohydrolysis and release of a small peptide fragment at an acidic pH. Pepsinogen is produced by chief cells. Regulation closely mirrors acid secretion and is stimulated by gastrin, histamine, and cholinergic excitation. Subjects who are achlorhydric or who have lost control of gastric emptying have no problem with assimilation of protein, suggesting that gastric proteolysis is not an essential component of digestion.

(205–A) **Bacillus cereus (S&F, p. 1627)**
Fecal leukocytes (S&F, p. 1619)
Bacillus cereus is an aerobic spore-forming gram-positive rod frequently present in uncooked rice. It causes an acute (usually epidemic) food poisoning syndrome characterized by either profound vomiting or watery diarrhea, depending on the toxin produced. It is not invasive so fecal leukocytes would not be expected. All the rest produce an acute colitis, and fecal leukocytes are shed to a varying degree.

(206–D) **(S&F, p. 1811)**
The large intestine is particularly susceptible to dilatation. Toxic megacolon is a feared complication of many conditions affecting the colon. Once thought to be restricted to ulcerative colitis, it is now clear that Crohn's colitis, amebic colitis, pseudomembranous colitis, and other infectious causes can lead to this life-threatening complication. Collagenous or microscopic colitis is a relatively benign disorder not associated with toxic megacolon.

(207–B) **(S&F, p. 1928)**
Specificity is defined as the true negative rate (i.e., the probability that a test will be negative in a patient without the disease). The formula for calculating this can be expressed as true-negatives ÷ (false-positives + true-negatives). Thus, a test that decreases the number of false-positive results will increase the specificity of a test. Immunologic testing for human hemoglobin, avoiding peroxidase-containing vegetables, and testing for porphyrin fluorescence will all decrease the false-positive results and hence increase the specificity of the test. Avoiding antioxidant vitamins, on the other hand, reduces false-negative results, a beneficial effect to be sure as the sensitivity of the test is increased, but false-negative results do not influence specificity.

(208–D) **(S&F, pp. 1947–1948)**
Direct person-to-person transmission is possible only for helminths that do not require a period of maturation outside the host. *Enterobius* (pinworm) and *Strongyloides* have been associated with sexual transmission. *Strongyloides stercoralis* infects the human host by penetration of the skin as filariform larvae that travel through capillaries to enter the lungs where they develop into adolescent worms. They are usually coughed up, swallowed, and invade the small bowel mucosa where they reside. The females release eggs that may develop into infective filariform larvae. During rectal intercourse, filariform larvae within the rectal lumen may penetrate the skin of the penis directly. Penetration of oral mucosa by infective larvae may also occur. *Ascaris lumbricoides* is a large roundworm with worldwide distribution. Infection is through the ingestion of embryonated eggs from contaminated food or drink. *Trichuris*

trichiura has a worldwide distribution but is most commonly found in the tropics and in areas with poor sanitation. Infection occurs through the ingestion of stale fecal material. The embryo requires a period of three to five weeks outside the body to reach the infective stage. *Ancylostoma duodenale* is not transmitted sexually. Eggs in feces are deposited in the soil and hatch in one to two days. They develop into filariform larvae that penetrate the skin and are then carried to the lung.

(209–A)   **(S&F, p. 1479)**

The trend has been away from the use of the term *dietary fiber* and toward more precise chemical definitions of each of the components. Instead of dietary fiber, some advocate the use of the term *complex carbohydrate* to define a group that not only would comprise cellulose, lignin, and food gums such as pectin and guar but would also include starch. Dietary fiber is essentially composed of plant cell wall material. The major structural component of the cytoskeleton of plants is cellulose.

(210–D)   **(S&F, pp. 1514–1516)**

Malabsorption of fat may cause marked weight loss due to calorie deprivation. Proximal muscle weakness, prolonged prothrombin time, and depressed serum carotene are all caused by malabsorption of fat-soluble vitamins. Depressed serum albumin is not a feature of fat malabsorption but commonly reflects protein malnutrition or loss of albumin into the stool.

(211–A)   **(S&F, pp. 1681–1682)**

The most prevalent type of eosinophilic gastroenteritis is the mucosal layer subtype. Patients present with colicky abdominal pain, nausea, vomiting, diarrhea, and weight loss. Evidence of malabsorption, protein-losing enteropathy, or iron-deficiency anemia may be present. Muscle layer disease is less common; serosal layer disease is rare. Submucosal disease is not recognized as a separate subtype.

(212–D)   **(S&F, p. 1705)**

Endoscopic cauterization with a thermal device or neodymium:yttrium-aluminum-garnet (Nd:YAG) laser would be the most reasonable next step. Topical therapy would be unlikely to have any effect on vascular lesions. Surgical treatment should be reserved for patients unresponsive to endoscopic treatment. There is as yet limited experience with formalin enemas.

(213–B)   **(S&F, pp. 1464–1465)**

Bacterial toxins produce diarrhea by different mechanisms. Cytotoxins, like those produced by *Shigella,* kill mammalian cells, usually by inhibition of protein synthesis. This leads to impaired absorption and damage to the mucosa. However, cholera produces an enterotoxin that binds the basolateral brush border membrane, where it produces

an unregulated increase in cyclic adenosine monophosphate. The result is blockage of electroneutral sodium chloride absorption and massive stimulation of chloride secretion. Sodium-coupled nutrient pathways are unaltered by the toxin. This allows for oral rehydration therapy in which sodium absorption is driven by nutrients (e.g., glucose), permitting water absorption to continue in the presence of massive diarrhea.

(214–A, B, D, E)   **(S&F, pp. 1735–1737)**

Twin studies show a much greater genetic influence for Crohn's disease than for ulcerative colitis. The other statements are true.

(215–B)   **(S&F, pp. 1928–1931)**

Vegetables such as broccoli, turnips, cantaloupe, cauliflower, and radish contain peroxidases that can give false-positive results. Although vitamin C consumption can give false-negative results, it is virtually impossible to consume enough vitamin C from fruits and vegetables to prevent the test from becoming positive in the presence of hemoglobin.

(216–D)   **(S&F, pp. 1838–1840)**

Occasional success has been reported in the treatment of metastatic carcinoid with cimetidine, propranolol, and clonidine, although more commonly they fail to significantly reduce symptoms. Cyproheptadine has both antihistaminic and antiserotonergic effects, but it works more effectively at reducing diarrhea than flushing. The most effective medical therapy is octreotide (150 mg subcutaneously every eight hours), and it is the treatment of choice for metastatic carcinoid syndrome.

(217–A)   **(S&F, pp. 1839–1840)**

Treatment of metastatic carcinoid with octreotide provides relief from flushing, diarrhea, and carcinoid crisis and may result in regression of metastatic tumor. Successful octreotide therapy invariably reduces urinary 5-hydroxyindoleacetic acid levels, although usually not to normal. Serum serotonin levels may also be decreased. The effect on diarrhea is mixed. Although relief from diarrhea may occur, octreotide therapy often causes steatorrhea, which may sometimes worsen diarrheal symptoms. Octreotide markedly reduces gallbladder contractions and therefore can lead to rapid development of cholelithiasis. Unfortunately, patients with metastatic carcinoid who are being treated with octreotide often develop a tolerance to the drug, with a gradual re-emergence of symptoms despite increasing doses. The median duration of symptomatic control with octreotide is 12 months, and use of the drug should therefore be delayed until the symptoms are moderate to severe.

(218–1-D, 2-F, 3-E, 4-B, 5-A, 6-C) (S&F, pp. 1929–1930)

The sensitivity and specificity are attributes of the test itself and are the absolute percentage of cases that are true-positive or true-negative, respectively. The positive and negative predictive values take into account the false-positive and false-negative results and therefore are affected by the prevalence of the disease in the given population. For example, if prevalence of a disease in a population is low, false-positive tests will make up a greater percentage of the positive test results than when the prevalence is high.

(219–C) **(S&F, pp. 1550–1551)**
Postoperative adaptation is more prominent in the ileum than in the jejunum. Digested food, bile, and pancreatic secretions are believed to be trophic for crypt cells.

(220–D) **Small bowel obstruction (S&F, p. 1800)**
Ileus (S&F, p. 1808)
High-pitched bowel tones with gurgles and rushes distinguish the obstructed bowel from the quiet, aperistaltic bowel of adynamic paralytic ileus. Abdominal distention and vomiting are commonly present in both conditions. Fever and poor skin turgor are the result of infection and intravascular volume depletion, respectively, and can be present under both circumstances.

(221–D) **(S&F, pp. 1634–1635)**
The histologic findings of pseudomembranous colitis comprise a spectrum from focal necrosis with polymorphonuclear infiltrates to the "classic" volcanic eruption where pseudomembranes (composed of fibrin and inflammatory cells) appear to "erupt" from a necrotic focus.

(222–A, C) **(S&F, pp. 1599–1600)**
Antibiotics that are effective in treating *Aeromonas* infection include trimethoprim-sulfamethoxazole, tetracycline, and chloramphenicol, but not the beta-lactams. Diarrhea caused by this organism may be chronic, with an average duration of illness of 42 days in one study. In another study, one third of patients required hospitalization.

(223–D) **(S&F, p. 1818)**
The initial management of acute megacolon includes stopping oral feedings, parenteral hydration, and decompression using a nasogastric tube. A Hypaque (water-soluble contrast) enema is administered to rule out mechanical obstruction as well as to help evacuate the colon. Barium contrast should be avoided until colonic obstruction has been excluded. Once confirmed, acute colonic pseudo-obstruction is treated aggressively with rectal tube decompression and enemas. Any associated metabolic abnormalities or electrolyte disorders should be corrected. If the patient does not respond, and the cecum measures 11 cm or more, the next step is colonoscopic decompression. Narcotic analgesics may contribute to the development of acute colonic pseudo-obstruction in the postsurgical patient and should be discontinued if the syndrome develops.

(224–D) **(S&F, p. 1625)**
Bacillus cereus is an aerobic gram-positive rod that causes "food poisoning" syndromes, either by means of preformed toxin or by production of toxin after colonization. It is not invasive and causes acute self-limited disease characterized by prominent emetic or diarrheal components but not fever.

(225–C) **(S&F, p. 1419)**
The first inch of the duodenum is retroperitoneal and, hence, immobile. This is in contrast to the jejunum and ileum, which are suspended by an extensive mesentery and have considerable mobility within the abdominal cavity. The descending aorta is posterior to the fourth portion of the duodenum, and prosthetic grafts of this vessel may erode through the wall, causing catastrophic gastrointestinal hemorrhage.

(226–C) **(S&F, pp. 1776–1777)**
Nongranulomatous ulcerative jejunoileitis is an unusual condition characterized by unrelenting malabsorption and a rapidly fatal course. It may also be termed *unclassified sprue* but is distinct from the diffuse ulceration that complicates long-standing celiac disease.

(227–A) **(S&F, pp. 1518–1519)**
Motility disorders caused by diabetes mellitus and progressive systemic sclerosis may lead to bacterial overgrowth when normal nocturnal mechanisms for clearing of organisms from the upper tract are impaired. Surgery for peptic disease may lead to overgrowth when the normal killing action of gastric acid is reduced by vagotomy, antrectomy, and the more rapid passage of food into the duodenum. Vitamin B_{12} deficiency is common in patients with overgrowth because the bacteria take up the vitamin before it can be absorbed. However, most patients become symptomatic from other aspects of bacterial overgrowth long before vitamin B_{12} deficiency sets in. Addison's disease is not associated with bacterial overgrowth.

(228–A, D) **(S&F, pp. 1557–1559)**
The total thickness of the mucosa is usually normal because hyperplasia of the crypts compensates for the shortening of the villi. Degenerative changes, including cytoplasmic vacuolization, are usually obvious.

(229–E) **(S&F, pp. 1970–1971)**
Pruritus ani is itching of the perianal skin and is caused by many disease processes. Leakage of stool onto the perianal skin seems to be the common denominator. Careful attention should be given to rule out dermatologic diseases, contact dermatitis, pinworms, or anorectal diseases such as fistulas or fissures. Hemorrhoids do not usually produce pruritus unless they interfere with hygiene.

(230–C) *(S&F, p. 1836)*

The precise physiology of the carcinoid syndrome remains obscure. It is thought that a synergistic interaction between serotonin and bradykinin may underlie most of its features. Flushing and diarrhea are the two most common clinical manifestations. In one series, asthma was present in 8% of patients. Pellagra (diarrhea, dermatitis, and dementia) may occur in the cachectic, terminal stages of the syndrome. Valvular heart disease is a late manifestation and typically involves the right side of the heart, with tricuspid regurgitation and pulmonary stenosis most common. The aortic valve is typically not involved.

(231–D) *(S&F, pp. 1564–1567)*

Endoscopic biopsy is clearly the most valuable diagnostic test in establishing the diagnosis of celiac sprue. It may be normal or may reveal scalloping or attenuation of duodenal folds. Biopsy should be performed in the distal duodenum to avoid distortion produced by Brunner's glands, which can confuse interpretation of the mucosal architecture.

(232–C) *(S&F, pp. 1708–1709)*

Crohn's disease is a chronic transmural inflammatory process that results in disruption of crypt architecture. Although granulomas may occasionally be seen on mucosal endoscopic biopsy, they are found only approximately 50% of the time in resected specimens. Careful review of serial sections can increase the identification of granulomas.

(233–C) *(S&F, pp. 1457–1458)*

Most chloride absorption occurs by simple diffusion, reflecting the electrical potential difference across the epithelium. Cellular transport of chloride is generally linked to sodium, mostly through a dual antiport system on the apical membrane that exchanges sodium for hydrogen and chloride for bicarbonate. Whereas sodium flux provides the principal driving force for absorption of fluids, chloride provides the principal driving force for fluid secretion. Increased intestinal chloride secretion is the fundamental cause of secretory diarrheas. In the colon, short-chain fatty acids and chloride are the principal luminal anions. Short-chain fatty acids originate from bacterial metabolism of carbohydrate passing through the ileocecal valve.

(234–C) *(S&F, pp. 1894–1897)*

Turcot's syndrome is adenomatous polyposis with gliomas.

(235–A) *(S&F, pp. 1613–1617)*

Viral agents including rotavirus and Norwalk virus are the most common causes of infectious diarrhea worldwide. Whereas rotavirus is a common cause of diarrhea in children, it rarely causes diarrhea in adults.

(236–D) *(S&F, pp. 1811–1812)*

In Hirschsprung's disease (aganglionosis), the aganglionic segment always extends from the internal anal sphincter for a variable distance proximally. The most characteristic functional abnormality is failure of the internal anal sphincter to relax after rectal distention. The resting pressure in the sphincter is normal or slightly elevated. The contracted segment often fails to relax after administration of parasympathomimetic agents.

(237–1-B, 2-A, 3-B, 4-B) *(S&F, p. 1964)*

Total colonoscopy is usually indicated whenever a process is suspected that involves the entire colon. These include surveillance for neoplasms in previously detected colonic polyposis, inflammatory bowel disease, and the familial colon cancer syndromes, including Lynch syndrome. Indications for flexible sigmoidoscopy include screening for neoplasms in patients without other risk factors, complicated sigmoid diverticular disease, rectal bleeding, or suspected colitis.

(238–E) *(S&F, p. 1548)*

Congenital anomalies account for 60% of all of short bowel syndrome in children. Necrotizing enterocolitis is the most common acquired cause. The other choices are not common causes in childhood.

(239–C) *(S&F, p. 1613)*

Yersinia enterocolitica is actually much more common in Canada and Scandinavia and Europe than in the United States, perhaps owing to tolerance of the organism for cold. Indeed, several outbreaks have been due to ingestion of contaminated ice cream. Children younger than 5 years of age usually present with an acute diarrheal illness with fever and cramps. Children older than 5 may present with an acute mesenteric adenitis that mimics acute appendicitis. Infected adults may show extraintestinal manifestations similar to Reiter's syndrome with arthralgias and erythema nodosum. Culture requires special laboratory techniques.

(240–E) *(S&F, pp. 1897–1898)*

Sporadic colorectal cancer and sporadic adenomas have both been shown to have a genetic component consistent with dominant inheritance with incomplete penetrance. Lynch I, Lynch II, and Cowden's diseases all have an autosomal dominant inheritance. There is no known heritable predisposition to Cronkhite-Canada syndrome.

(241–1-A, 2-C, 3-B) *(S&F, pp. 1443, 575–577)*

During phase III of the migrating motor complex (MMC), the frequency of intestinal contractions approaches a maximum. For the antrum this is approximately 3 contractions per minute; for the duodenum, approximately 11 per minute; and for the ileum, approximately 8 per minute.

(242–D)   *(S&F, pp. 1699, 1701–1702)*

All are manifestations of acute injury except stricture formation, which is a late complication due to ischemia and progressive fibrosis.

(243–C)   *(S&F, pp. 1667–1668)*

Hookworm lacerates the bowel mucosa, causing significant bleeding. The blood loss feeds the hookworm but eventually leads to iron deficiency. Folate deficiency may also be present but is usually masked by the even more severe iron deficiency. The treatment of choice is mebendazole. Because the route of infection is penetration of the larvae through unprotected skin, use of shoes helps to prevent reinfection in endemic areas. Hookworm typically causes an eosinophilia of 7% to 15% and up to 50% in severe cases. Although with light infestations, the physical examination may be normal, heavier parasite loads characteristically cause decreased perspiration and a yellow pallor to the skin that is striking in light-skinned subjects.

(244–A)   *(S&F, pp. 1537–1539)*

Abdominal pain is an important diagnostic feature of irritable bowel syndrome (IBS). Painless diarrhea is believed to be a separate entity rather than a variant of IBS. It is a symptom that has been experienced more or less universally by a healthy population at one time or another under stressful situations and is more likely than the painful form to disappear after the stress is removed. Constipation, which at first is episodic, often becomes continuous and increasingly intractable to laxatives. Patients with all forms of IBS commonly complain of abdominal distention and increased belching or flatulence. There is mucus in the stool of most IBS patients, with the amount variable and the pathogenesis obscure.

(245–C)   *(S&F, pp. 1527–1529)*

A major function of gastric acid is to kill ingested microorganisms. Sustained hypochlorhydria (as is seen during treatment with omeprazole) may result in bacterial overgrowth. However, hyperchlorhydria is not a risk factor. Scleroderma and dysmotility predispose to bacterial overgrowth by preventing the normal cleansing of the bowel during fasting, while resection of the ileocecal valve permits reflux of cecal bacteria into the jejunum.

(246–E)   *(S&F, pp. 1979–1980)*

Pneumatosis cystoides intestinalis is an uncommon disorder characterized by multiple gas-filled cysts in the wall of the large or small intestine. Although the condition is associated with a variety of gastrointestinal diseases, the exact cause remains unknown. The mechanical theory suggests that luminal gas under pressure penetrates mucosal defects and dissects between tissue layers leading to gas-filled cysts. It has not been associated with endometriosis.

(247–C)   *(S&F, p. 1420)*

The anatomic anal canal extends from the anal verge to 2.5 to 3 cm. The surgical anal canal extends to 4 to 5 cm from the anal verge. The internal and external hemorrhoidal plexi are found in the submucosal space of the anus at the level of the columns of Morgagni and occur within 3 cm of the anal verge. On examining the rectum, it is important to palpate the ischiorectal space, because this is an area where abscess formation is prominent.

(248–A)   *(S&F, pp. 1509–1511)*

The glucose breath hydrogen test is the most reliable and simple test for bacterial overgrowth. Glucose is normally absorbed before it reaches gut bacteria. In the glucose breath test, bacterial metabolism releases hydrogen, which can be measured in expired air. Quantitative aerobic and anaerobic culture of the intestinal aspirate remains the gold standard. However, it is very difficult to perform properly and requires use of bacteriologic methods that are not readily available to the endoscopist.

(249–E)   *(S&F, pp. 1682–1683)*

The radiographic picture of eosinophilic gastroenteritis includes findings compatible with other infiltrative mucosal and muscle layer diseases. Muscle layer involvement of the lower esophageal sphincter or pyloric channel may produce findings suggestive of achalasia or pyloric stenosis. Mucosal or muscle layer involvement may produce large gastric folds and findings consistent with small bowel obstruction.

(250–C)   *(S&F, pp. 1793–1797)*

Inflammatory diarrhea is an uncommon and generally unimportant complication in diverticulitis. In contrast, all the other findings listed are routinely seen. Abscesses anywhere in the abdomen may occur, including the subphrenic location. Colovesical fistulas are a major complication and are more common in men than women. Obstruction can occur due to contraction, inflammation, and thickening of the bowel wall. Generalized peritonitis may occur as a result of a macroperforation.

(251–C)   *(S&F, pp. 1690–1691)*

Food-induced colitis is not mediated by IgE, which sets it apart from most other food allergies. Oral allergy syndrome involves swelling around the mouth, often with angioedema and pruritus. It is IgE mediated, as is gastrointestinal anaphylaxis. Eosinophilic gastroenteritis may or may not occur in the setting of other atopic illness. When it is related to food (up to half of the cases), the mechanism involves IgE. Double-blind crossover trials have shown that about 15% of infantile colic is due to food allergy.

(252–A, B, D)   *(S&F, pp. 1616–1618)*

Traveler's diarrhea is almost always caused by ingestion of bacterially contaminated food or drink. Antimotility drugs are effective for symptomatic relief, and approximately 80% of cases can be prevented by prophylactic use of either trimethoprim-sulfamethoxazole or ciprofloxacin, although prophylactic use should be discouraged unless the risk and consequences of infection are high. Approximately 90% of identifiable causes of traveler's diarrhea are due to bacterial pathogens, most notably enterotoxigenic *Escherichia coli*; *Entamoeba histolytica* is present in less than 5%, and thus empirical treatment with metronidazole is not warranted. Students and itinerant tourists have the highest risk, and persons visiting relatives have the lowest risk.

(253–C)   **(S&F, p. 1637)**

The presence of a debilitating condition or immunosuppression is not necessary for the clinical manifestation of *Clostridium difficile* colitis. Healthy children and adults are also at risk.

(254–A, C)   **(S&F, pp. 1655–1657)**

The diagnosis of amebic abscess can usually be established on the basis of a characteristic sonographic appearance in the setting of a positive serologic test, and aspiration is not required. Three negative stool examinations rule out colonic disease but are negative in half of the patients with amebic abscess. Amebic liver abscess is much more common in men than in women despite equal rates of colonic disease. Although amebic liver abscess is readily curable, it is life-threatening without prompt treatment. Patients generally have leukocytosis, but eosinophilia is quite uncommon.

(255–A, B)   **(S&F, pp. 1990–1992)**

Fecal impaction is usually seen in chronically debilitated or institutionalized individuals. The primary defect is impaired sensation of (or apathy to) rectal distention. Although incontinence of stool often accompanies an impaction, anal sphincter squeeze pressures are actually normal. Medications that predispose to impaction include those that inhibit normal colonic motility or bind to bile acids. Upper gastrointestinal barium studies should be avoided in patients with colonic obstruction and may actually precipitate fecal impaction in patients with chronic constipation. Likewise, soapsuds, hydrogen peroxide, or warm oil enemas should be avoided, as should lactulose or other fermentable laxatives. Hypaque, Phospho-Soda, and mineral oil enemas may be helpful and safe, and magnesium citrate or polyethylene glycol colon lavage solutions can be given by mouth to cleanse the rectosigmoid after disimpaction.

(256–D)   **(S&F, p. 1618)**

Although *Giardia lamblia* is commonly acquired by drinking contaminated mountain stream water, giardiasis is rarely associated with bloody diarrhea. The other agents listed frequently cause bloody diarrhea.

(257–A)   **(S&F, pp. 1749–1751)**

Ankylosing spondylitis affects 1% to 2% of patients with ulcerative colitis, and 80% of these have the HLA-B27 phenotype. The natural history of the spondylitis is completely independent of the colitis and may present years before or long after the onset of the colitis.

(258–D)   **(S&F, p. 1831)**

Gastrointestinal carcinoids have been found in most areas of the gastrointestinal tract, including esophagus, bile duct, ampulla of Vater, and Meckel's diverticulum. However, over 95% of all gastrointestinal carcinoids originate from three sites: small bowel, appendix, and rectum.

(259–B)   **(S&F, pp. 1914–1916)**

Although the term *nonpolyposis* is used in the name for hereditary nonpolyposis colorectal cancer (HNPCC), this refers to the absence of hundreds to thousands of polyps, which are commonly seen in other polyposis syndromes, such as familial adenomatous polyposis. Despite the name, the colon cancers in HNPCC are believed to arise from adenomas. The disorder reflects failure of DNA to replicate accurately during cell division.

▬▬ Reference

Lynch, H. T., Smyrk, T. C., Watson, P., et al. Genetics, natural history, tumor spectrum, and pathology of hereditary nonpolyposis colorectal cancer: An updated review. Gastroenterology *104*:1535, 1993.

(260–E)   **(S&F, p. 1849)**

Many staging systems have been used to determine the prognosis of gastrointestinal lymphoma. None is completely satisfactory. The most important prognostic factor is the stage of the disease at the time of diagnosis. Others include cell type, size of the tumor, constitutional symptoms, level of lymph node involvement, number of anatomic sites involved, patient age, and various histochemical cell markers. The peripheral white blood cell count appears unrelated to the overall prognosis.

(261–C)   **(S&F, p. 1799)**

Abdominal adhesions are the most common cause of small bowel obstruction, accounting for 50% to 70% of all cases. Other common causes of small bowel obstruction are hernias and neoplasms. Intussusception and volvulus are less common causes.

(262–C)   **(S&F, pp. 1779–1780)**

Fecaliths or viscid fecal masses are found obstructing the appendiceal lumen in only approximately 35% of cases of acute appendicitis. Viruses, bacteria, or parasites have been implicated in some of the remaining cases.

(263–1-A, 2-D, 3-B, 4-C)   **(S&F, pp. 1973–1974)**

Anal or perianal pain usually has an obvious cause such as abscess or fissure. Four different perianal pain syndromes have been described in which visible disease is absent. Proctalgia fugax is episodic rectal pain of varying severity. It has been associated with spasm of the levator muscles as well as myopathy of the internal anal sphincter. Coccygodynia is a throbbing or aching pain in the coccygeal region. Organic causes include fracture of the coccyx and arthritis of the sacrococcygeal joint. The descending perineum syndrome is often associated with straining at stool. Chronic idiopathic anal pain is a syndrome that has features overlapping the others. It is associated with pelvic or spinal surgery, sitting, and perineal descent.

(264–1-B, 2-B, 3-A, 4-A)   **(S&F, pp. 929, 1443)**

During phase II of the migrating myoelectric complex (MMC), the sphincter exhibits decreased phasic wave activity and baseline pressures, allowing bile to flow into the duodenum. During phase III of the MMC, the sphincter of Oddi exhibits the highest frequency of phasic wave activity and maximum resistance to bile flow, causing the gallbladder to fill with bile.

(265–B)   **(S&F, pp. 1553–1554)**

Proctocolectomy with extensive ileal resection usually produces fat malabsorption due to the bile salt malabsorption with its associated reduction in the bile salt pool. Bile salt deficiency increases the likelihood of cholesterol gallstone formation. Fat malabsorption is also associated with malabsorption of fat-soluble vitamins and calcium. In normal individuals, fat malabsorption leads to formation of calcium–fatty acids soaps in the colon. The lower level of free calcium allows more absorption of oxalate from the colon, leading to renal stones. Because the colon is absent in this case, this is not a problem.

(266–B)   **(S&F, pp. 1908–1911)**

Although some epidemiologic evidence suggested that antioxidants may have some protective effect in colorectal cancer, a recent trial found no effect on adenomatous polyp formation, suggesting that the protective effects, if any, are very small. All of the other measures are being investigated as dietary or chemopreventive measures, and their efficacy is not yet known.

■■■■ **References**

Giovannucci, E., Rimm, E. B., Stampfer, M. J., et al. A prospective study of cigarette smoking and risk of colorectal adenoma and colorectal cancer in United States men. J. Natl. Cancer Inst. *86*:183, 1994.
Greenberg, E. R., Baron, J. A., Tosteson, T. D., et al. A clinical trial of antioxidant vitamins to prevent colorectal adenoma: Polyp Prevention Study Group. N. Engl. J. Med. *331*:141, 1994.

(267–D)   **(S&F, pp. 1977–1979)**

Endometriosis affects 15% of menstruating women and up to 30% of infertile women. The endometrial implants most often involve the rectosigmoid colon, but endometriosis may also involve the terminal ileum, appendix, and cecum. Involvement can be detected by all of the mentioned test modalities with the exception of esophagogastroduodenoscopy.

(268–C)   **(S&F, pp. 1501–1502)**

All four of the options listed may cause detectable steatorrhea. However, severe malabsorption of fat virtually always indicates exocrine pancreatic disease with secretion of inadequate amounts of pancreatic lipase.

(269–A, B, C, D, E)   **(S&F, p. 1587)**

Whipple's disease is a systemic disease that involves essentially all organs, as is reflected by involvement of all of the listed organs with periodic acid–Schiff (PAS)-positive macrophages.

(270–1-E, 2-C, 3-B, 4-D, 5-A)   **(S&F, p. 1974)**

Epidermoid carcinomas constitute about 2% of cancers of the large bowel. Management depends on the location of the tumor, depth of invasion, and the presence of metastasis. These tumors spread into the sphincters as well as hematogenously. There is a strong association with human papillomavirus infection. Bowen's disease is an intraepithelial squamous cell carcinoma associated with pruritus ani. Conservative fixation of the grossly affected areas is as effective as wide excision. Paget's disease can involve the apocrine glands and involve the epidermis secondarily. Wide excision is the usual treatment. Malignant melanoma is a rare pigmented lesion that may resemble a thrombosed hemorrhoid or polyp. Although causing trivial symptoms, melanomas metastasize early and are highly lethal. About 10% of anorectal carcinoid tumors are malignant. For this reason, local excision is recommended regardless of size. Malignant lesions are uniformly fatal no matter what is done.

(271–B)   **(S&F, pp. 1746–1749)**

This patient's living conditions put him at risk for contracting amebiasis, and his worsening clinical condition could be due to corticosteroid therapy. A single stool sample is not sufficient to exclude amebiasis. Three samples and a serum amebic titer should have been obtained before beginning prednisone. A high titer always indicates active disease. Further corticosteroid therapy should be withheld until amebiasis has been definitively excluded. An abdominal film should be performed to assess the degree of colonic dilation whereas a colonoscopy is contraindicated because it may precipitate a toxic megacolon in patients with severe colitis.

(272–A)   **(S&F, p. 1777)**

Multiple diaphragmatic strictures in an adult are almost pathognomonic of NSAID damage. Congenital stenosis may also be diaphragm-like but rarely presents in adults.

(273–B)   *(S&F, p. 2002)*

Lipomas are benign small intestinal and colonic tumors. They usually occur in the colon or distal ileum, often near the ileocecal valve. Most are discovered incidentally at colonoscopy. They may cause intussusception or obstruction when large but are usually asymptomatic. They can usually be identified by colonoscopic appearance with their characteristic yellow tinge and soft, indentable texture yielding the typical "cushion" sign. They have no malignant potential and should not be removed unless they are causing symptoms. Because they conduct electricity poorly, snare cautery should be avoided.

(274–E)   *(S&F, p. 1525)*

Intestinal bacteria are capable of each of the listed metabolic conversions.

(275–C)   *(S&F, pp. 1728–1729)*

Adenocarcinoma of the small intestine usually occurs in a grossly involved segment. Although there is a high relative risk, the absolute risk is quite small and would not justify a surveillance program. When they occur, small bowel cancers are usually advanced at the time of diagnosis.

(276–D)   *(S&F, p. 1969)*

Anorectal fistulas are hollow fibrous tracts lined with granulation tissue. Their pathogenesis is believed to involve infection of a crypt with subsequent preservation of a tract as the abscess cavity heals. They arise in association with all the entities listed except external hemorrhoids. Few fistulas heal spontaneously, and surgical treatment is usually indicated. Recurrent fistula after surgery should prompt the physician to look for inflammatory bowel disease, particularly Crohn's disease.

(277–D)   *(S&F, p. 1758)*

Sulfasalazine may decrease sperm count in men with ulcerative colitis, but ovulation in females is not affected. Sulfasalazine is not teratogenic, nor for that matter is there any evidence that corticosteroids or azathioprine have an adverse effect on fetal health. Women with ulcerative colitis have no difficulty conceiving or bearing a child and, for women in remission, pregnancy is not a risk factor for relapse.

(278–C)   *(S&F, pp. 1967–1968)*

An anal fissure is a defect in the anoderm extending from the anal verge to the pectinate line. It usually occurs in the posterior midline and is very painful. Chronic fissures are usually accompanied by a "sentinel" pile or tag at the anal verge. Treatment consists of decreasing straining and easing passage of stool. Surgical therapies are aimed at improving anal stretching during defecation, not retarding it.

(279–C)   *(S&F, pp. 1801–1802)*

High-pitched bowel tones with gurgles and rushes distinguish the obstructed bowel from the quiet, aperistaltic bowel of adynamic paralytic ileus. The presentation and findings in this patient suggest bowel obstruction, of which internal hernias, adhesion from prior surgery, tumors, and volvulus are common causes.

(280–D)   *(S&F, pp. 1801–1802)*

Laboratory evaluation is useful in determining the severity of physiologic derangement in bowel obstruction. Because of the potential for rapid change, serum electrolytes, acid-base status, and the hemogram must be continuously monitored. Metabolic acidosis with leukocytosis suggests a strangulated obstruction. Upright abdominal films identify air-fluid levels confirming the obstruction and may provide clues to the site of obstruction, whereas an upright chest film may detect free air under the diaphragm resulting from perforation. Peritoneal lavage is of greatest value in cases of blunt trauma to the abdomen when damage to intra-abdominal organs is suspected.

(281–C)   *(S&F, p. 1803)*

The radiographic findings of dilated small bowel with a paucity of colon gas suggest a small bowel obstruction. The initial management of intestinal obstruction is to correct fluid, hematocrit, and electrolyte deficits; optimize cardiopulmonary and renal functions; and assess nutritional status. Many patients with small bowel obstruction can be successfully treated without surgery, but this patient has warning signs of a strangulated small bowel. Although the diagnosis of strangulation is problematic even with the most experienced physicians (accuracy of 70% at best), the findings of leukocytosis, acidosis, fever, tachycardia, and localized tenderness all point to strangulation.

(282–1-B, 2-D, 3-A, 4-E, 5-C)   *Adenoma (S&F, p. 1866)*
              Non-neoplastic polyps (S&F, pp. 1881–1883)

Adenomas are benign neoplastic epithelium that displays abnormal glandular architecture, often including long, branching glands and basophilic crypts. The crypts are dysplastic, often with hypercellularity and hyperchromatic, elongated nuclei arranged in a "picket fence" pattern. Hyperplastic polyps are the most common non-neoplastic polyp in the colon. They are commonly less than 5 mm and are grossly indistinguishable from small adenoma. Microscopically, the colonic crypts are elongated and the epithelial cells assume a characteristic papillary configuration. Juvenile polyps are hamartomas, which are benign mucosal tumors that consist primarily of an excess of lamina propria and dilated cystic glands. They are more common in children and often regress spontaneously. Peutz-Jeghers polyps are a form of hamartomas characterized by prominent branching bands of smooth muscle within the lamina propria. Pneumatosis cystoides intestinalis is characterized by gas in the intestinal wall with otherwise normal mucosa.

(283–A, B, C)   **(S&F, pp. 1622–1624)**

Gastrointestinal involvement is most commonly due to *Mycobacterium tuberculosis,* although *Mycobacterium bovis* is more common in areas where milk is not pasteurized. It often involves the ileocecal region and may be clinically indistinguishable from Crohn's disease. Histologic examination, usually with special stains, is almost always required to make the diagnosis of tuberculosis. Stool examination has little or no value. With currently available antibiotics, surgical intervention is almost never required.

(284–D)   **(S&F, pp. 1715–1716)**

Extraintestinal manifestations related to Crohn's colitis include all except clubbing. Clubbing, when present, is most often associated with extensive small bowel disease.

(285–C)   **(S&F, pp. 1663–1669)**

Strongyloides does not lay large number of eggs in the stool; therefore, negative stool examinations do not exclude *Strongyloides* infection. Definitive diagnosis requires examination of duodenal secretions. One examination of duodenal contents is equal in usefulness to ten concentrated stool specimens in diagnosing this difficult disease.

(286–B)   **(S&F, pp. 1639–1641)**

Although pseudomembranes are common, *Clostridium difficile* colitis may also present with erythema, edema, friable mucosa, ulceration, or hemorrhage. The most widely available diagnostic test detects stool toxin by its damaging effects on cells in tissue culture. No correlation is seen between toxin titers and the severity of clinical disease. Because *C. difficile* may be found in the stool of normal persons, the gold standard is the cytotoxicity assay.

(287–A, B, C)   **(S&F, pp. 1858–1863)**

The three most common primary benign tumors of the small intestine are adenomas, leiomyomas, and lipomas. Hematomas, fibromas, angiomas, and neurogenic tumors are much less common, accounting for less than 15% of these tumors. Benign tumors often remain asymptomatic and are often found only incidentally. When they do become symptomatic, the clinical picture is usually determined by the structures affected. Tumors arising in the duodenum may produce nausea and vomiting. Distal tumors are much more likely to produce intussusception or intermittent intestinal obstruction. Because their symptoms are often nonspecific, diagnosis is often delayed. Benign small intestinal tumors are seen in all age groups, but the peak incidence is in the seventh decade.

(288–D)   **(S&F, pp. 1833–1835)**

The small intestine is the most common location of gastrointestinal carcinoids. Almost 40% are located within 2 feet of the ileocecal valve. Small bowel carcinoids are frequently multicentric, sometimes presenting with as many as 100 or more lesions. The likelihood of metastases is proportional to the size of the tumor, with almost all lesions over 2 cm in diameter causing metastatic disease. Hepatic metastases are relatively benign. Their rate of growth is very slow, and the patient may have no symptoms even when the liver is grossly enlarged and nodular. The median survival of patients with liver metastases is three years, and 30% are alive five years or more.

(289–C)   **(S&F, p. 1591)**

Tropical sprue is not associated with periodic acid–Schiff (PAS)-positive macrophages. The other diseases may all have PAS-positive macrophages, generally in the lamina propria. The most common disorders associated with PAS-positive macrophages are Whipple's disease and *Mycobacterium avium-intracellulare* infection.

(290–C)   **(S&F, pp. 1744–1746)**

Patients with ileal involvement by Crohn's disease often have proctitis and may present with symptoms of this disorder. Thus, it is advisable to obtain radiologic assessment of the small intestine in all patients with colonic disease because ileal involvement would argue against topical therapy alone for the proctitis. The other tests are not indicated.

(291–A)   **(S&F, pp. 1914–1916)**

Because the genetic defect in hereditary nonpolyposis colorectal cancer (HNPCC) involves a germline mutation in DNA proofreading genes, it is thought that these cancers require less time to accumulate the genetic abnormalities necessary to develop colorectal cancer. The mechanisms by which the genetic abnormalities occur differ in that the majority of sporadic colorectal cancers seem to occur by means of loss of pieces of DNA rather than by point mutations as in HNPCC. Nevertheless, both mechanisms play an important role in sporadic colon cancer. Accumulating point mutations appears to preserve the content of DNA, thus making replication error–positive colorectal cancers mainly diploid. This may account for the better prognosis in the colorectal cancers of HNPCC. The frequency of metachronous malignancies is five- to six-fold greater in HNPCC. Both arise in adenomas.

References

Bronner, C. E., Baker, S. M., Morrison, P. T., et al. Mutation in the DNA mismatch repair gene homologue hMLH1 is associated with hereditary nonpolyposis colon cancer. Nature *368*:258, 1994.

Leach, F. S., Nicolaides, N. C., Papadopoulos, N., et al. Mutations of a mutS homolog in hereditary nonpolyposis colorectal cancer. Cell *75*:1215, 1993.

Lynch, H. T., Smyrk, T. C., Watson, P., et al. Genetics, natural history, tumor spectrum, and pathology of hereditary nonpolyposis colorectal cancer: An updated review, Gastroenterology *104*:1535, 1993.

Nicolaides, N. C., Papadopoulos, N., Liu, B., et al. Mutations of two PMS homologues in hereditary nonpolyposis colon cancer. Nature *371*:75, 1994.

(292–E)   **(S&F, pp. 1871–1874)**

Ureterosigmoidoscopy is strongly associated with development of neoplasms at the implantation site, with a mean delay of 20 and 26 years for adenoma and carcinoma formation, respectively. High levels of growth hormone are a direct risk factor, whereas the presence of *Streptococcus bovis* bacteremia points to the presence of a colonic lesion. The risk of adenomas is strongly associated with age. More than half of patients older than 65 years of age may harbor adenomas.

(293–1-B, 2-E, 3-A, 4-F)   ***Gonorrhea***
(S&F, pp. 1950–1951)
Syphilis (S&F, p. 1950)
Chlamydia (S&F, p. 1955)

The recommended treatment for rectal gonorrhea is ceftriaxone, 250 mg intramuscularly, and doxycycline, 100 mg b.i.d. for 7 days. If the patient is allergic to tetracycline, erythromycin stearate, 500 mg q.i.d. for 7 days, is an alternative. Syphilitic hepatitis occurs in secondary syphilis, and the recommended treatment is benzathine penicillin G, 2.4 million units intramuscularly once a week for three weeks. If the patient is allergic to penicillin, tetracycline or erythromycin can be given orally for 30 days. In acute infection with *Chlamydia trachomatis,* azithromycin is the drug of choice because treatment can be accomplished with a single dose. Doxycycline may be also be given. Only supportive treatment is recommended in acute hepatitis B infection. Interferon alfa may be used to treat patients with chronic hepatitis B. It can eliminate HBeAg in approximately 33% of patients with chronic hepatitis. Eventual clearance of HBsAg occurs in most responders.

(294–D)   **(S&F, p. 1548)**

Crohn's disease accounts for 60% to 75% of the cases of short bowel syndrome found in adults. Other causes in adults include mesenteric infarction, radiation enteritis, and volvulus. In children, congenital abnormalities account for two thirds and the remainder are caused by necrotizing enteric infection.

(295–D)   **(S&F, pp. 1681–1685)**

The diagnosis of eosinophilic gastroenteritis rests on demonstration of tissue eosinophilia in the gastrointestinal tract. Peripheral blood eosinophilia is absent in at least 20% of cases. Peripheral blood eosinophilia is not required for diagnosis.

(296–D)   **(S&F, pp. 1844–1845)**

The association between celiac sprue and gastrointestinal lymphoma has been known for many years. Usually, lymphoma is seen as a complication of celiac sprue. However, there are multiple case reports of patients with gastrointestinal lymphomas who were found to have asymptomatic celiac sprue at the time of staging laparotomy. The association between the Epstein-Barr virus and the human immu-nodeficiency virus and certain types of lymphoma is also well described. In general, patients with congenital or acquired immunodeficiency states seem to be at increased risk of developing lymphomas at all sites, especially the gastrointestinal tract. Nodular lymphoid hyperplasia may be seen with primary immunoglobulin deficiency and also predisposes to lymphoma.

(297–D)   **(S&F, p. 1550)**

Assuming that infectious causes have been excluded, the fecal fat test would be most useful. If fecal fat is in the normal range, it is likely that the patient has a bile salt diarrhea that would respond to bile acid binders. An elevated fecal fat value would suggest fat malabsorption that may best respond to a low-fat diet supplemented with medium-chain triglycerides.

(298–B)   **(S&F, p. 1695)**

Virtually all therapeutic approaches to food allergies have failed, with the exception of eliminating the offending allergen from the diet. Although dapsone is frequently effective in treating dermatitis herpetiformis, it is not usually helpful for food allergies. Desensitization also has not been effective, although food allergies tend to decrease with age.

(299–B)   **(S&F, pp. 1603–1606)**

The major site of attack of *Shigella dysenteriae* is the colon, although ulcerations in the terminal ileum may also be seen. Humans are the only known host for this organism, which produces an acute dysentery characterized by multiple small, bloody stools. Mild cases that are already resolving need not be treated with antibiotics; in more serious cases in which antibiotics are indicated, it is useful to know beforehand what the drug resistance patterns are in the community. Ampicillin is the drug of choice for susceptible strains, and trimethoprim-sulfamethoxazole is useful in cases of ampicillin resistance. Ciprofloxacin is also extremely effective.

(300–B, C, D)   **(S&F, pp. 1638–1639)**

Although *Clostridium difficile* can be cultured from the stools of normal persons, the recovery rate for healthy adults is only 2% to 3%. In contrast, carriage rates in infants range from 5% to 70%. For reasons that are not clear, infants appear to be protected from *C. difficile* and its toxin. Colitis is caused by bacterial production of a toxin. The bacterium or its spores can be transferred from one hospitalized patient to another via hospital personnel, toilets, bedpans, and so forth, and may be epidemic or endemic in hospitals. Although different strains exist, all strains are equally capable of causing severe disease.

(301–D)   **(S&F, p. 1536)**

The irritable bowel syndrome (IBS) is a motor disorder defined clinically as altered bowel habits and abdominal pain in the absence of detectable organic pathology. With new scientific advances, disorders formerly included in this syndrome, such as lactose intolerance, have been clearly distinguished from IBS.

(302–B)   **(S&F, p. 1755)**

Cyclosporine has been used to treat severe, refractory ulcerative colitis in clinical trials and does not increase the risk of toxic megacolon. Each of the other options increases the risk of toxic megacolon in patients with severe ulcerative colitis.

(303–B)   **(S&F, pp. 1793–1794)**

The size of the diverticula has not been shown to clearly correlate with the risk of developing diverticulitis. In contrast, large numbers, wide distribution, and long duration of diverticulosis have all been shown to correlate with increased risk of diverticulitis.

(304–A, B, C, D)   **(S&F, pp. 1571–1572)**

All of the problems listed are important complications of celiac sprue.

(305–D)   **(S&F, pp. 1570–1571)**

When a patient with celiac sprue who has been doing well suddenly worsens (while complying with his or her diet), three major complications must be considered: lymphomatous transformation, ulcerative "jejunoileitis," or "refractory sprue." The best initial test in this setting is small bowel examination with biopsy, which can help confirm or exclude all three diagnoses. If endoscopy with biopsy is negative, computed tomography may be helpful to assess the possibility of lymphoma. Endoscopic retrograde cholangiopancreatography would help exclude superimposed pancreatic disease but would not be the first examination considered.

(306–C)   **(S&F, pp. 1567–1568)**

Foods containing wheat, rye, and barley should be removed from the diet of patients with celiac sprue. Rice, corn, and soy contain no gliadin and are not toxic to patients with celiac sprue.

(307–A, B, C, D, E)   **(S&F, pp. 1751–1752)**

Sulfapyridine is rapidly absorbed from the gastrointestinal tract after cleavage from sulfasalazine and is responsible for most of the side effects of sulfasalazine. Idiosyncratic effects include male infertility, hypersensitivity rashes, and hemolytic anemia, as well as occasional dose-dependent headache, nausea, and vomiting. The dose-dependent side effects can sometimes be overcome by starting at a low dose of 500 mg/day and slowly increasing to the full dose of 3 g/day over a period of one week.

(308–C)   **(S&F, p. 1536)**

Female patients with clinically diagnosed irritable bowel syndrome (IBS) outnumber males 2:1, but the prevalence of symptoms is similar in each sex. The incidence is higher in whites than in nonwhites. IBS is the most common cause for referral to gastroenterologists, constituting 20% to 50% of referred patients. Between 32% and 44% of IBS patients report sexual abuse as children. Symptoms begin before age 35 in 50% of the patients, whereas 40% of patients are 35 to 50 years of age.

(309–A)   **(S&F, p. 1894)**

Peutz-Jeghers syndrome is associated with distinctive ovarian sex cord tumors in 5% to 12% of the affected females with a median age at diagnosis of 50. Approximately half of these patients will develop a malignancy of some type during their lifetime.

(310–B, C, D)   **(S&F, p. 1979)**

Medical treatment of endometriosis is based on the well-founded premise that growth and regression of the ectopic endometrium are governed by the ovarian hormones. Low-dose estrogen-progestin compounds, danazol, gonadotropin-releasing hormone (GnRH) agonists, and progesterone are all useful in treating endometriosis. Most effective are danazol and GnRH. However, both are associated with moderate androgenic and anabolic properties as well as bone loss. Surgery should be strongly considered for patients whose symptoms do not promptly improve on medical treatment.

(311–A)   **(S&F, p. 1946)**

In a prospective study, 20% of 89 homosexual men carried *Entamoeba histolytica.* The gastrointestinal symptoms in this setting are relatively nonspecific and include diarrhea, cramping, and flatulence. The relatively mild clinical presentation of venereally transmitted amebic infection appears to reflect the noninvasive zymodemes of *E. histolytica* strains carried by homosexual men. Systemic complications of sexually transmitted amebiasis are uncommon, although liver abscesses have been reported. The mechanism of transmission in sexually acquired amebiasis is ingestion of amebic cysts during oral-anal contact. Both cysts and trophozoites are found within the rectal ampulla and may be carried directly from one anus to the next. *E. histolytica* has caused few problems in homosexual acquired immunodeficiency syndrome (AIDS) patients, possibly because the isolates found in this group are usually commensal noninvasive strains.

(312–B)   **(S&F, p. 1774)**

Lymphoma should be high on the differential list in patients with extensive small bowel ulceration. These lymphomas are most often T-cell lymphomas. The other choices are possible but unusual. *Yersinia* typically affects the terminal ileum.

(313–A, C, E)   *(S&F, pp. 1641–1643)*

Although the greater clinical experience exists with oral vancomycin, comparative clinical trials indicate that metronidazole, which is much less expensive, is therapeutically equivalent. Both antibiotics have similar relapse frequencies. Antibiotic treatment is not recommended for patients who are spontaneously improving, because there is little benefit and the risk of relapse may be increased. Relapses can be managed in many ways, including careful observation without specific treatment, a repeat course of antibiotics using either the same or a different drug, treatment with resins that bind bacterial toxins, or by a combination of these. Cholestyramine has been used in the treatment of relapse alone or in combination with vancomycin. It appears to bind toxins A, B, and C. One potential disadvantage of combination therapy is the fact that cholestyramine can also bind vancomycin, reducing the levels of this antibiotic in the colonic lumen.

(314–D)   *(S&F, pp. 1933–1935)*

Sphincter-saving operations can be performed with as little as 2 cm of tumor-free margin.

(315–C)   *(S&F, pp. 1423–1430)*

Meckel's diverticulum is the most frequent congenital anomaly of the intestinal tract, having an incidence of 0.3% to 3.0%. It most commonly remains asymptomatic through life; however, complications include ulceration, hemorrhage, intestinal obstruction, diverticulitis, intussusception, perforation, and peritonitis. The most common complication is painless bleeding from ulceration of the ileal mucosa adjacent to the ectopic gastric mucosa. Meckel's diverticulum is the most common diagnosis in children younger than age 2 who present with either tarry stools or "currant jelly" hemorrhage.

(316–A)   *(S&F, p. 1698)*

Chronic radiation injury to the bowel is rare with total doses lower than 4000 rads. The risk of chronic injury is dependent on the total dose and the site irradiated.

(317–C)   *(S&F, pp. 1472–1473)*

Several factors can delay gastric emptying. Duodenal mucosal receptors for pH and osmolality trigger a delay in gastric emptying when gastric effluent is acidic, hypertonic, or hypotonic. Gastric emptying is also controlled by a mechanism involving the ileum. If fat escapes digestion and absorption in the jejunum, its presence in the ileum delays gastric emptying and gastrointestinal transit. This "ileal brake" is probably mediated by a neural-hormonal mechanism. Adequate lipid digestion is critically dependent on the presence of bile salts, but they do not otherwise affect gastric emptying.

(318–A)   *(S&F, p. 1816)*

The differentiation of congenital from acquired megacolon is difficult, and the history and physical examination may be inadequate to distinguish between them. When the aganglionic segment is short, the narrowed segment characteristic of Hirschsprung's disease may not be evident on barium enema. In these cases, the diagnosis is also likely to be missed by superficial rectal biopsy. Moreover, transit studies may show no difference between the two forms. Anorectal manometry, which shows an intact rectoanal response only in acquired megacolon, is the most useful method available to distinguish acquired from congenital megacolon.

(319–C)   *(S&F, p. 1423)*

Cell renewal in the small intestine is a dynamic process involving rapid maturation of crypt cells as they progress toward the villous tip. The entire process takes from four to six days. As cells advance toward the villous tip, they differentiate into absorptive cells, gaining the necessary enzymes and transport proteins. After reaching the extreme villous tip, they degenerate, lose their absorptive capacity, and are sloughed into the lumen of the intestine. Because of this rapid proliferation, intestinal cells are particularly susceptible to abdominal radiation or cancer chemotherapeutic agents.

(320–B)   *(S&F, pp. 1964–1967)*

Treatment of first-degree hemorrhoids is aimed at reducing the downward pressure. This is most easily accomplished by adding bulk agents to the diet and avoiding prolonged sitting at the stool. Injection of sclerosants, rubber band ligation, and photocoagulation are all accepted methods for the treatment of first- and second-degree hemorrhoids. Fourth-degree prolapsed hemorrhoids are not suitable for rubber band ligation. Reports of fatal sepsis after rubber band ligation caused many surgeons to abandon this technique in the 1980s, although more recent reports have demonstrated few serious side effects.

(321–B)   *(S&F, pp. 1995–1996)*

Nonspecific ulcerative proctitis is a variant of diffuse ulcerative colitis characterized by a more favorable clinical course and a relatively benign prognosis. Approximately one third of patients with ulcerative colitis will have disease limited to their rectum. Other causes of ulcerative proctitis that need to be excluded include infection with *Clostridium difficile,* Crohn's disease, infection with bacteria such as *Shigella* and *Salmonella,* viral infections with herpes simplex or cytomegalovirus, and traumatic proctitis. Histologic examination of the rectal mucosa may help distinguish nonspecific ulcerative proctitis from proctitis due to specific infectious agents but not from ulcerative colitis, which has similar findings of distorted crypt architecture, lamina propria inflammation, and goblet cell depletion. The proctitis usually follows a benign course, and up to 75% of patients experience no further relapses. Treatment is aimed at mitigating symptoms using topical therapy with corticosteroids or mesalamine enemas.

(322–C)   **(S&F, pp. 1877–1878)**

The primary difference between carcinoma in situ and a malignant polyp is that the carcinomatous focus in the latter extends beyond the muscularis mucosa. There are no lymphatics in the mucosa, and therefore a carcinomatous focus confined to the mucosa has no metastatic potential.

(323–D)   **(S&F, pp. 1693–1695)**

Prick skin test and food elimination diets can be very useful in diagnosing food allergies. The double-blind placebo-controlled oral food challenge is the gold standard for most food allergy diagnoses. Medical history is useful about half of the time but is frequently misleading. Food-specific IgG has no diagnostic value.

(324–C)   **(S&F, p. 1958)**

Cytomegalovirus (CMV) is transmitted during sexual contact by ingestion of virus particles that are found in urine, semen, or cervical secretions. Ingestion of semen during sexual contact carries the highest risk. Asymptomatic infections are more common than symptomatic infections. Symptomatic infections can produce a syndrome resembling infectious mononucleosis, with liver function test abnormalities and hepatosplenomegaly. Acute CMV infections do not commonly produce gastrointestinal symptoms, but acute ulcerative proctocolitis has been reported. Latent infections reactivated by immunosuppression tend to cause more severe and diverse symptoms. After acute infection, the virus may be shed into urine and semen for several years.

(325–B)   **(S&F, p. 1954)**

Many infectious diseases can mimic inflammatory bowel disease, including tuberculosis, lymphogranuloma venereum (LGV), and *Entamoeba histolytica*. Infectious causes must be excluded before the diagnosis of inflammatory bowel disease is made and treatment initiated. Thus, starting this patient on prednisone or sulfasalazine is premature and may be harmful if infection is present. The patient's human immunodeficiency virus status and LGV titers should be determined. At present, the best methods for diagnosing chlamydial infections are isolation of the organism and serologic examination. A complement fixation titer of more than 1:16 is generally accepted as evidence of LGV infection. LGV proctocolitis often presents as symptoms similar to those in this case. Biopsy specimens can show diffuse inflammation with crypt abscesses, granulomas, and giant cells consistent with the appearance of Crohn's disease. Radiographically, LGV can resemble ulcerative colitis with a similar mucosal pattern, poor distensibility, and loss of haustration. Multiple strictures with normal intervening portions similar to skip lesions have also been described.

(326–1-D, 2-E, 3-A, 4-C, 5-B)   **(S&F, p. 1866)**

Patients with Peutz-Jeghers syndrome display characteristic mucocutaneous pigmentation due to melanin deposits around the mouth, nose, lips, buccal mucosa, hands, and feet. Patients with Muir-Torre syndrome have multiple skin lesions, including sebaceous adenomas and carcinomas, basal cell and squamous carcinomas, and keratoacanthomas in conjunction with adenomas and adenocarcinomas of the colon. Gardner's syndrome consists of familial polyposis and osteomas of the mandible, skull, and long bones associated with a variety of benign soft tissue neoplasms, including desmoid tumors. Cowden's syndrome consists of multiple orocutaneous hamartomas with fibrocystic disease of the breast, nontoxic goiter, thyroid and breast cancer, and hamartomatous polyps of the stomach, small intestine, and colon. The hallmark is the presence of multiple facial trichilemmomas, which arise from follicular epithelium and typically occur around the eyes, nose, and mouth. Patients with neurofibromatosis (von Recklinghausen's disease) can develop multiple submucosal neurofibromas of the upper digestive tract that may cause dyspepsia, abdominal pain, or hemorrhage.

(327–E)   **(S&F, p. 1536)**

Available data suggest that 50% of women with functional gastrointestinal disorders are victims of sexual abuse. Most of the time the gastroenterologist is not aware of this history. Irritable bowel syndrome is the most frequent diagnosis among these patients, but constipation is also a common feature. Somatic reactions to sexual abuse include abdominal pain, constipation, and appetite disturbance. Twenty percent of children who have been sexually abused present to the emergency department for abdominal pain or constipation. Female victims of full coitus during childhood or adolescence frequently see gastroenterologists or surgeons for consultation later in life and often undergo unnecessary surgery in search of an organic diagnosis.

(328–D)   **(S&F, pp. 1845–1846)**

Mucosa-associated lymphoid tissue (MALT) lymphomas are tumors of B-cell lineage. They arise in the gut as well as in the lungs, thyroid, and salivary glands. Histologically, they are characterized by the lymphoepithelial lesion formed by centrocyte-like cells. Plasma cell infiltrates usually lie deep in the epithelium. Within the gastrointestinal tract, the stomach is the most common site of involvement. Treatment of gastric *Helicobacter pylori* infection has been associated with regression of the lesion. Pseudolymphoma has been considered a benign condition until recently. Many of these lesions appear malignant on the basis of their clinical behavior and behave like some cases of MALT lymphoma. Most pathologists now consider the pseudolymphoma as a slowly progressive variant of MALT lymphoma.

(329–1-C, 2-A, 3-B)   **(S&F, pp. 1488–1489)**

Vitamin E comprises a group of eight tocopherols, the most potent of which is alpha-tocopherol. Although various diseases can result from deficiency in animals, it has proved difficult to ascribe a human disease to vitamin E deficiency. Beta-carotene is a precursor of vitamin A that consists of two conjoined molecules of retinal. Beta-carotene is split by an oxygenase in the brush border yielding two molecules of retinal. Vitamin D_2 and vitamin D_3 are produced by ultraviolet irradiation of their precursor sterols ergosterol and 7-dehydrocholesterol *in vivo*. Adults with normal exposure to sunlight do not require any intake of vitamin D.

(330–D)   **(S&F, pp. 1781–1782)**

The history is not suggestive of a typical presentation of simple appendicitis but may be consistent with a perforated appendiceal abscess. The antecedent history of diarrhea and weight loss may suggest Crohn's disease, now possibly complicated by an abscess. Abdominal computed tomography would be most useful to evaluate for the presence of an intra-abdominal abscess.

(331–B, C)   **(S&F, pp. 1538–1540)**

The reduced motor activity of the colon during sleep may result from a reduction of psychologic and physiologic stimuli. This may account for the infrequency with which patients with irritable bowel syndrome (IBS) are awakened from sleep by their symptoms. In patients with IBS, food induces colonic hypermotility. This response is blunted compared with that in normal subjects but continues postprandially for a longer time and gradually gets stronger. Balloon distention of the rectosigmoid and rectum induces spastic contractions that are significantly greater in patients with IBS than in normal subjects. Cholinergic agents produce colonic hyperactivity in both normal individuals and in patients with IBS, but the response is more pronounced in the latter.

(332–C)   **(S&F, pp. 1669–1672)**

The first three statements are true. Although cysticercosis may be acquired though the ingestion of inadequately cooked pork by the mechanism of hyperinfection, it is usually acquired by the inadvertent ingestion of eggs shed in the feces by human or porcine carriers of adult worms.

(333–A)   **(S&F, pp. 1482–1483)**

Each of the pancreatic proteases is secreted as a proenzyme and must be activated in the lumen. Enterokinase plays a critical role in activation of proteases because it converts trypsinogen to trypsin. Trypsin, in turn, activates other proteases and can also convert trypsinogen to trypsin. Trypsin, chymotrypsin, and elastase are all endopeptidases and have a specificity for peptide bonds adjacent to certain specific amino acids. Exopeptidases (e.g., carboxypeptidase A and B) remove a single amino acid from the carboxyl terminal end. In contrast to carbohydrate absorption, amino acids can be absorbed as monomers, dipeptides, or tripeptides. This explains why patients with cystinuria or Hartnup's disease, who have specific defects in absorption of basic and neutral amino acids, respectively, do not develop essential amino acid deficiency states.

(334–C)   **(S&F, pp. 1996–1997)**

Escherichia coli serotype 0157:H7 may cause acute hemorrhagic colitis. Patients typically have watery diarrhea

followed by several days of bloody diarrhea. The disease usually runs a self-limited five- to seven-day course. Complications typically arise from dehydration. The bacteria bind to epithelial cells and produce two distinct toxins similar to those produced by *Shigella*. Mucosal disease is usually right-sided. Other causes of bloody diarrhea need to be ruled out. Confirmation of 0157:H7 is not possible on a routine microscopic examination of stool, though erythrocytes and some leukocytes may be seen. Because virtually all stool contains *E. coli*, and most strains of *E. coli* except for 0157:H7 ferment sorbitol, the absence of this reaction in stool cultures grown in sorbitol-containing MacConkey medium provides a presumptive diagnosis. Subsequent confirmation is performed serologically. Treatment is supportive, because antibiotics neither shorten nor attenuate the illness.

(335–D, E, A, C, B)   **(S&F, pp. 1877–1878)**

Hyperplastic polyps are believed to have no malignant potential. Similarly, hamartomas are thought to have no malignant potential. Although certain hamartomatous conditions such as Peutz-Jeghers syndrome are associated with an increased risk of developing colorectal cancer, this risk is due to adenomatous tissue that is occasionally found in the hamartomas rather than to the hamartomas themselves. Adenomas discovered in the setting of familial adenomatous polyposis are believed to be at only slightly greater risk of developing malignancy than are sporadic adenomas. The near 100% risk of developing colon cancer in these patients is due more to the large number of adenomas present than to an increased risk in a given polyp. In contrast, adenomas seen in patients with hereditary nonpolyposis colorectal cancer are much more likely to degenerate into malignancy because they lack DNA proofreading functions. As a result, they accumulate genetic abnormalities much more rapidly.

■■■**Reference**

Bronner, C. E., Baker, S. M., Morrison, P. T., et al. Mutation in the DNA mismatch repair gene homologue hMLH1 is associated with hereditary nonpolyposis colon cancer. Nature *368*:258, 1994.

(336–C)   **(S&F, p. 1784)**

Children with cystic fibrosis can have chronic appendicitis due to mucus engorgement of the lumen. Otherwise, it is a rare entity and an unlikely cause of symptoms in otherwise healthy individuals.

(337–B)   **(S&F, pp. 1663–1664)**

In general, the physical examination is completely normal in patients with *Ascaris* infection. Pyrantel pamoate is the best drug for treating *Ascaris*, but mebendazole is often used because patients who have *Ascaris* are at risk for other intestinal parasites for which pyrantel pamoate is not as effective. *Ascaris* is not limited to the lumen of the intestine. Larval forms penetrate the wall of the duodenum and pass through the liver and into the lungs where they eventually cause cough, sputum production, and pulmonary infiltrates before their migration into the pharynx. Abdominal discomfort and malnutrition are major symptoms, but patients may have many other problems, including allergic reactions, cough, and pneumonitis. A large organism burden may cause diarrhea in children but generally does not cause symptoms in adults.

(338–A) **(S&F, p. 1643)**

No evidence exists that treatment of asymptomatic carriers results in eradication of the carrier state. Theoretically, treatment with antibiotics may result even in the clinical expression of disease in these individuals.

(339–D) **(S&F, p. 1507)**

Vitamin B_{12} is normally bound to R proteins that must be degraded by pancreatic enzymes before the vitamin can bind to intrinsic factor produced by the stomach. The B_{12} intrinsic factor complexes are absorbed by the ileum. Thus, disease of the exocrine pancreas or disease processes involving gastric or ileal mucosa may produce an abnormal Schilling test. Bacterial overgrowth may also produce an abnormal test because bacterial uptake of vitamin B_{12} prevents its absorption in the ileum.

(340–A) **(S&F, pp. 1793–1795)**

Acute suppuration in the lumen is the hallmark first event in appendicitis but not in diverticulitis. More commonly, microperforation (rather than luminal disease) occurs early in diverticulitis, producing the inflammatory response. Both syndromes may present with lower abdominal pain, although appendicitis usually causes pain on the right and diverticulitis on the left. Both microperforation and peritonitis may complicate either diverticulitis or appendicitis. However, microperforation is more common in diverticulitis, whereas peritonitis is more common in appendicitis.

(341–D) **(S&F, pp. 1950–1951)**

The most likely scenario is that this patient is an asymptomatic rectal carrier of gonorrhea who has developed endocarditis. Rectal carriers serve as a reservoir for perpetuation and spread of gonorrheal urethritis. These carriers are not only a risk to others, but they are also at risk of developing gonococcal sepsis, endocarditis, meningitis, and arthritis. Given this patient's history, symptoms, and signs, one must be very suspicious of gonococcal endocarditis.

(342–D) **(S&F, p. 1697)**

Adequate rest between doses of radiation is required to allow recruitment of noncycling stem cells into actively proliferating stem cells needed for regrowth of the normal epithelium.

(343–B) **(S&F, pp. 1536–1538)**

Irritable bowel syndrome (IBS) is one of the most commonly encountered gastrointestinal disorders. It is a motor disorder manifesting irritability that involves many areas of the gut other than the colon. The terms *nervous colitis* and *spastic colitis* are physiologically incorrect because inflammation is not present. Although it may be associated with severe pain and discomfort, IBS does not predispose to other chronic or life-threatening conditions such as inflammatory bowel disease or cancer. Four symptoms that help distinguish IBS from organic disease are visible distention, relief of pain with bowel movements, more frequent bowel movements with the onset of pain, and looser stools with the onset of pain. More than 90% of IBS patients have two or more of these symptoms.

(344–C) **(S&F, pp. 1445–1446)**

Multiple small molecules serve as neurotransmitters in the enteric nervous system. They come from a wide variety of categories, including catecholamines, amino acids, purines, and peptides. Many are also found in the central nervous system. The importance of many of these is not clearly defined. Although gastrin plays an important role in regulating acid secretion by parietal cells, this hormone plays no known role in the enteric nervous system.

(345–C) **(S&F, pp. 1672–1674)**

Long-term *Schistosoma* infection can produce dysfunction of many organ systems. Chronic inflammation of the colon wall predisposes chronically infected patients to colon cancer. Similarly, inflammation in the small intestine can produce chronic protein-losing enteropathy. When fluke burdens are heavy, *Schistosoma japonicum* may cause intestinal obstruction. There may be extensive portal fibrosis leading to portal hypertension and bleeding esophageal varices, but the parenchymal cells are spared. Thus, hepatic synthetic and detoxification functions remain intact and encephalopathy does not occur.

(346–B) **(S&F, pp. 1765–1766)**

Patients with inflammatory bowel disease are significantly more likely to have pouchitis than are patients with familial polyposis. Extraintestinal manifestation including arthritis can be seen with pouchitis.

(347–B) **(S&F, p. 1783)**

Appendiceal perforation is common in all children: 90% in children younger than age 2, 55% to 70% in children younger than 6, and 35% overall.

(348–A) **(S&F, pp. 1503–1504)**

Carbohydrate malabsorption is virtually always associated with diminution in the brush border enzymes responsible for digesting oligosaccharides into simple sugars. Enzyme deficiency may reflect generalized mucosal diseases such as celiac sprue or specific defects such as lactase deficiency. Although pancreatitis commonly reduces amylase output, amylase levels rarely fall low enough to cause carbohydrate malabsorption. Excess acidity may inactivate pancreatic enzymes and precipitate bile acids, but this commonly causes malabsorption of fat rather than carbohydrates.

(349–C) *(S&F, pp. 1811–1814)*

Hirschsprung's disease has been diagnosed as late as age 69, despite the fact that it is a congenital disease. Spontaneous remissions can occur. Clinical features may overlap with those of idiopathic constipation. In 10% of the cases, distal narrowing is absent on barium enema, rendering diagnosis difficult.

(350–A, C) *(S&F, p. 1737)*

The incidence of ulcerative colitis is clearly higher in nonsmokers, whereas the opposite is true with respect to Crohn's disease. Heavy smokers who quit are at a particularly high risk of developing ulcerative colitis for two years after smoking cessation. The active principal agent in cigarette smoke is unknown but does not appear to be nicotine.

(351–A) *(S&F, pp. 1478–1482)*

Fifty percent of digestible carbohydrates in an average western diet is in the form of starch derived from cereals and plants. Starch is composed of long chains of glucose molecules as either amylose or amylopectin. Glucose, galactose, and fructose are the three major dietary-derived monosaccharides. Lactose is a disaccharide that must be hydrolyzed to glucose and galactose before absorption can occur. Glucose and galactose are actively absorbed by sodium-coupled cotransport across the brush border membrane. Energy for this process is derived from the sodium gradient across the apical cell membrane. Fructose absorption occurs by passive diffusion through a membrane carrier protein.

(352–A) *(S&F, p. 1784)*

After medical treatment of appendiceal abscess, recurrent appendicitis occurs in about 20% of patients. When the appendix is not removed during the initial presentation, it is most reasonable to perform an elective appendectomy in six weeks to three months.

(353–B) *(S&F, p. 1464)*

Vasoactive intestinal peptide increases intracellular cyclic adenosine monophosphate, which inhibits electroneutral sodium chloride absorption and stimulates chloride secretion. Serotonin (produced by carcinoid tumors) increases intracellular calcium in enterocytes, which also inhibits electroneutral sodium chloride absorption and stimulates chloride secretion.

(354–B) *(S&F, pp. 1664–1666)*

Ascaris infection is acquired by ingestion of eggs, whereas hookworms shed eggs into the lumen that hatch

in the soil. Filariform larvae then invade the skin. In contrast, *Strongyloides* eggs develop into noninfectious larvae while still in the host. These are then shed into the environment where they develop into free-living adults or infectious filariform larvae. Skin manifestations are a common symptom in *Strongyloides* infection and are more common than gastrointestinal symptoms. In acute infections patients may have a maculopapular rash, whereas in chronic infections they may develop cutaneus larval tracts. *Ascaris,* hookworm, and whipworm are debilitating but rarely fatal. *Strongyloides,* on the other hand, is capable of disseminating into a systemic hyperinfection that is often fatal.

(355–C) *(S&F, p. 1487)*

Foodbound cobalamin is initially released by hydrochloric acid in the stomach and preferentially bound by salivary R protein, which is later hydrolyzed by proteolytic enzymes from the pancreas. It is then bound by intrinsic factor (secreted by the parietal cell), and the intrinsic factor–cobalamin complex is bound and transported into the enterocyte by ileal receptors. On release from the enterocyte, cobalamin is bound to the plasma protein transcobalamin and transported to the liver.

(356–E) *(S&F, p. 1758)*

Women with ulcerative colitis have no difficulty in conceiving and are not at increased risk for spontaneous abortion. Moreover, there is no good evidence that pregnancy is a risk factor for relapse. Women with ulcerative colitis usually produce healthy newborns, with no adverse effect on the developing fetus. Sulfasalazine, corticosteroids, and even azathioprine appear to be safe to use in pregnancy. If the disease should relapse during pregnancy, it must be aggressively treated to establish a quick remission. The mother's health is the most important determinant of fetal health.

(357–D) *(S&F, pp. 1851–1853)*

Immunoproliferative small intestinal disease is usually found in persons from the Mediterranean basin, Iran, and South Africa. It is associated with lower social and economic status. An initial insult to the intestinal mucosa is believed to stimulate the enteric immune system, which, when chronic, leads to malignant degeneration into an immunoblastic lymphoma. In contrast to nonimmunoproliferative small intestinal disease, there is a dense compact mucosal cellular infiltrate that is diffuse, continuous, and uninterrupted along the entire length of the small intestine. This leads to marked involvement of the entire small intestine, subsequently reducing the absorptive capacity and resulting in chronic diarrhea, malabsorption, and weight loss.

(358–A) *(S&F, p. 1710)*

Approximately 50% of patients with Crohn's disease display an ileocolonic distribution. Small bowel involvement alone is seen in about a third of patients, and colonic disease alone is seen in approximately 20%.

(359–C)   **(S&F, pp. 1473–1474)**

In most developed countries, about 40% of adult energy requirements are met by lipids, the majority of which are triglycerides. The most common fatty acids in triglycerides are oleate and palmitate. In animal fat, most of the fatty acids are long-chain fatty acids (i.e., longer than 14 carbons). Polyunsaturated fatty acids such as linoleic and linolenic acids are derived from phospholipids of vegetable origin. They cannot be synthesized *de novo* and are thus essential fatty acids. Most dietary lipid is absorbed by the middle third of the jejunum. Ingested triglycerides are broken down to glycerol and fatty acids. Movement across the brush border membrane occurs by passive diffusion for the vast majority of lipids.

(360–A, B, C, D, E)   **(S&F, pp. 1608–1609)**

All of the diseases listed are predisposing factors for salmonellosis. Sickle cell disease and malaria may block reticuloendothelial clearance of the organism, whereas malignancies, corticosteroid treatment, and acquired immunodeficiency syndrome (AIDS) predispose by immunosuppression.

(361–C)   **(S&F, pp. 1774–1776)**

Diffuse ulceration complicating celiac sprue does not typically respond to gluten withdrawal. The remaining statements are true.

(362–D)   **(S&F, pp. 1681–1682)**

Eosinophilic gastroenteritis is a rare disease involving eosinophilic infiltration of different layers of the gut wall in any area of the intestinal tract. The term is a misnomer because, like Crohn's disease, eosinophilic gastroenteritis can involve any portion of the gastrointestinal tract from the esophagus to the rectum. The stomach and the small bowel are most commonly affected.

(363–A, D)   **(S&F, p. 1967)**

A thrombosed external hemorrhoid is a blood clot within a subcutaneous hemorrhoidal vein. It is most often noted by the patient as a painful lump that appears suddenly. Bleeding occurs only if the skin ulcerates. The lesion is normally external and should not be further manipulated. The pain reaches a peak in two to three days and disappears in about one week. Analgesics, sitz baths, stool softeners, and topical emollients are the treatment of choice.

(364–B, C, D)   **(S&F, p. 1881)**

Although the endoscopic appearance of hyperplastic polyps may differ from that of adenomas, the difference is not consistent enough to reliably differentiate among them. Hyperplastic polyps predominate in the rectum and sigmoid colon, whereas adenomas are usually found more proximally.

(365–C)   **(S&F, p. 1820)**

A diagnosis of chronic intestinal pseudo-obstruction requires symptoms of intestinal obstruction, the absence of any mechanical obstruction, and radiographic evidence of ineffective intestinal propulsion. Hence, all of the listed findings are consistent with chronic intestinal pseudo-obstruction except for normal results of examination.

(366–1-C, 2-B, 3-D)   **(S&F, pp. 1486–1488)**

Folic acid consists of a pterin molecule conjugated to *p*-aminobenzoic acid and glutamic acid. It is widely distributed in the diet, with spinach, liver, and peanuts being particularly rich sources. The recommended intake is doubled during pregnancy because deficiency may cause neural tube birth defects. Vitamin B_{12} is taken up in the terminal ileum and leaves the cell as free cobalamin where it immediately binds transcobalamin II in the portal blood. Thiamin is widely distributed, but the only important dietary sources are seeds of plants, including cereal germ, nuts, peas, and beans. All vitamins listed are water soluble. Vitamin C can be synthesized by most species except primates, guinea pigs, and some birds. As little as 10 mg/day will prevent scurvy, but recommended daily intake is 40 mg/day.

(367–D)   **(S&F, pp. 1781–1782)**

In clinical settings when the diagnosis is in doubt, ultrasonography is a useful aid in diagnosis. In acute appendicitis, ultrasound evaluation has an overall accuracy that exceeds 85%. It is particularly helpful in women when tubo-ovarian pathology is possible. Computed tomography is most helpful in patients suspected of appendiceal perforation.

(368–E)   **(S&F, pp. 1679–1681)**

The pathogenesis of eosinophilic gastroenteritis involves disruption of mucosal tissue integrity, antigen presentation, and mast cell degranulation. Eosinophilic infiltration of tissue follows, triggered by a type 1 hypersensitivity reaction. Histamine receptors do not play a role in type 1 hypersensitivity reactions and would not be expected to respond to therapy with H_2 receptor antagonists.

(369–D)   **(S&F, p. 1686)**

The prognosis of eosinophilic gastroenteritis is good, although fatal outcomes have rarely been reported. Prognosis is not related to the degree of peripheral eosinophilia or the tissue layer involved. The risk of malignancy is not increased in these patients. Obstruction and malnutrition are the most common complications.

(370–D)   **(S&F, pp. 1793–1794)**

Plain films are helpful in assessing the degree of ileus or obstruction and in diagnosing a free perforation but are frequently nonspecific in uncomplicated diverticulitis. Although barium contrast studies may be helpful by demonstrating the presence of diverticula and may occasionally demonstrate contrast outside the lumen of the bowel or an inflammatory narrowing with intact mucosa characteristic of diverticulitis, the risk of disrupting a localized, contained perforation and causing peritonitis argues against using this test. Endoscopic examination may be helpful in establishing the presence of diverticula and in excluding a mucosal tumor but has the same risk as a barium enema of disrupting a contained perforation. Computed tomography is more sensitive and specific than sonographic imaging in evaluating the lower abdomen and is the most reliable test currently available.

(371–D)   **(S&F, p. 1674)**

Needle biopsy of the liver can be particularly helpful in identifying eggs in patients at risk for liver involvement. Rectal biopsy has a high diagnostic yield, particularly in *Schistosoma mansoni* infections. Examination of concentrated stool specimens is quite helpful because the eggs are almost invariably present in acute disease. Reliance on serologic testing alone is hazardous because false-positive reactions may occur, owing to cross-reacting antibodies to other parasites.

(372–C)   **(S&F, pp. 1477–1478)**

Absorbed fatty acids are converted back into triglycerides in the endoplasmic reticulum of the enterocyte. These triglycerides are then packaged with cholesterol and cholesterol esters for export in the form of chylomicrons. Chylomicrons are composed of a core of triglycerides with cholesterol ester and phospholipid forming more than 80% of the surface coat. During fasting, chylomicrons are not made and very low density lipoproteins (VLDLs) become the major lipoprotein in blood. Fatty acids from dietary triglycerides go predominantly into the formation of chylomicrons, whereas those derived from phospholipids appear to be utilized in the formation of VLDLs. Thus, VLDLs and chylomicrons have very different fatty acid compositions. An essential component on the surface of chylomicrons is apo B. The absence of apo B prevents the synthesis and secretion of chylomicrons, as occurs in congenital abetalipoproteinemia.

(373–E)   **(S&F, pp. 1914–1915)**

A young age at first diagnosis of colon cancer strongly suggests an inborn error in DNA replication, resulting in more rapid accumulation of the genetic defects that combine to produce a malignant cell.

(374–A)   **(S&F, pp. 1682–1684)**

The differential diagnosis of large gastric folds includes lymphoma, carcinoma, Ménétrier's disease, granulomatous gastritis, and hypersecretory states such as Zollinger-Ellison syndrome.

(375–D)   **(S&F, pp. 1684–1685)**

The differential diagnosis of eosinophilic gastroenteritis includes parasitic infestation, drug allergy, connective tissue disease, vasculitis, and systemic mastocytosis. Also included are celiac disease, carcinoma or lymphoma, eosinophilic granulomas, hypereosinophilic syndrome, and the inflammatory bowel diseases.

(376–A, C, D)   **(S&F, pp. 1651–1655)**

Although giardiasis is frequently missed by stool examinations, three negative stool examinations for ova and parasites are generally sufficient to exclude amebic infection. Colonic disease is equally common in men and women. Amebae seem to benefit from the presence of certain bacteria in the colon, and thus the parasitic infection may respond partly to antibiotic therapy. It is important to exclude amebiasis before treating patients with corticosteroids, because life-threatening dissemination of the parasite may otherwise occur. Metronidazole has developed a fairly high failure rate, and other drugs may be required to eradicate the organism.

(377–A)   **(S&F, p. 1635)**

Sulfonamides have rarely been implicated in cases of *Clostridium difficile* colitis. One possible explanation is the low activity of sulfonamides on anaerobic gut flora. Lack of competition from other bowel flora is responsible for the emergence of vegetative forms of *C. difficile*.

(378–B)   **(S&F, pp. 1536–1539)**

The diagnosis of irritable bowel syndrome (IBS) relies on a recognition of positive clinical features as well as on the meticulous exclusion of the many other disorders that have similar manifestations. Some of the more reliable positive features are the presence of lower abdominal pain, small stools, and persistence of symptoms that are fairly constant in their pattern but variable in their severity. The intensity of symptoms is not a differentiating feature, and even extremely severe pain, constipation, or vomiting is compatible with the diagnosis. Supporting the diagnosis of IBS is a lower abdominal pain that is aggravated by meals and relieved by defecation, more frequent and looser stools with the onset of pain, and the fact that the patient is not awakened by pain. Visible abdominal distention and symptoms getting worse with periods of stress are also characteristic. Against the diagnosis of IBS are onset in old age, fever, weight loss, rectal bleeding, steatorrhea, dehydration, and new symptoms appearing after a long period of an established pattern.

(379–E)   **(S&F, pp. 1541–1543)**

Because irritable bowel syndrome (IBS) is largely a diagnosis of exclusion and the differential diagnosis is broad, certain diagnostic tests should be performed routinely. At a minimum, it is desirable to obtain a complete blood cell count (CBC) and differential, erythrocyte sedimentation rate, stool Hemoccult test, stool for ova and parasites (with specific request to search for *Giardia*), and flexible sigmoidoscopy. If these are negative, a therapeutic trial on a lactose-free diet for two weeks or a lactose tolerance test (or breath hydrogen) may be performed. In the IBS patient who also has dyspepsia (not a problem in the current patient), an upper gastrointestinal evaluation should be obtained.

(380–C) (S&F, pp. 1544–1546)

Reassurance and psychological support are key factors in dealing with anxiety and stress. In the treatment of irritable bowel syndrome (IBS), emotional catharsis often is more beneficial than physical catharsis. In the current case, there appears to be a precipitating emotional factor. The effectiveness of fiber in IBS is not well documented. Indeed, 15% to 25% of patients complain that a high-fiber diet aggravates symptoms. Oral antibiotics and colectomy have no role in the management of IBS. Antispasmodics such as dicyclomine may provide temporary relief, but the relief is neither dramatic nor permanent. They are most effective when used in anticipation of predictable pain. A trial of lactose-free diet for two weeks is recommended in all patients who complain of distention, bloating, or diarrhea. To conclusively establish the diagnosis of IBS, lactose intolerance should already have been ruled out.

(381–C) (S&F, p. 1443)

The migrating motor complex (MMC) refers to the characteristic pattern of electrical activity that migrates along the length of the gut during fasting. Each phase is first seen at proximal sites and is then observed more distally, hence the "migration" of the activity. This pattern usually occurs during fasting and is interrupted by meals. It is thought to serve a "housekeeper" function by clearing the intestinal lumen of bacteria and useless cellular debris. The neurotransmitters involved in control of the enteric nervous system are not well characterized.

(382–1-A, 2-C, 3-B, 4-D, 5-E) (S&F, pp. 1624–1627)

Bacillus cereus is often associated with uncooked rice. *Vibrio parahaemolyticus* is often associated with uncooked seafood including shellfish. *Staphylococcus aureus* food poisoning usually has a very short (one- to six-hour) incubation period. *Listeria monocytogenes* food poisoning has been associated with unpasteurized milk or cheese. *Clostridium perfringens,* the most common form of bacterial food poisoning, is usually associated with roasted, boiled, stewed, or steamed meats.

(383–A) (S&F, pp. 1935–1938)

Levamisole plus 5-fluorouracil has been shown to increase both time to tumor recurrence and the five-year survival of patients with stage C colon cancers. It is the first-line therapy in Dukes' B2 and C stage cancers. Because of the high frequency of local recurrence, treatment for rectal cancer includes adjuvant radiation. Levamisole plus 5-fluorouracil appears to be more effective than 5-fluorouracil alone for distant metastatic disease. It has not been convincingly demonstrated that portal infusion of chemotherapeutic agents as adjuvant therapy reduces liver metastasis. Only 5% to 10% of hepatic metastases are believed to be amenable to surgical resection.

■ **Reference**

Francini, G., Petrioli, R., Lorenzini, L., et al. Folinic acid and 5-fluorouracil as adjuvant chemotherapy in colon cancer. Gastroenterology *106*:899, 1994.

(384–C) (S&F, pp. 1663–1669)

Ascaris is a large roundworm that can be more than 20 cm long. Infections are frequently complicated by obstruction as listed. *Strongyloides* has been reported to cause intestinal obstruction, but this is uncommon. Hookworm generally produces none of these findings and is a more common cause of severe iron-deficiency anemia. Whipworm is much smaller than *Ascaris* and occasionally produces appendicitis but rarely causes obstructions.

(385–C) (S&F, p. 1750)

Ankylosing spondylitis, not sacroiliitis, is associated with HLA-B27. The natural history of ankylosing spondylitis is independent of the ulcerative colitis, and hence colectomy has no effect on the natural history of ankylosing spondylitis. The acute arthropathy of ulcerative colitis has an asymmetric distribution that affects larger joints, such as the knees, hips, and wrists. Symptoms of ankylosing spondylitis may precede symptoms of colitis by years.

(386–C) (S&F, pp. 1751–1753)

Corticosteroids are effective for controlling active disease but are ineffective in maintaining long-term remission. Prolonged therapy with corticosteroids also has an unacceptable side-effect profile. The others have all proven to be useful in maintaining remissions.

(387–E) (S&F, p. 1554)

Patients with ileal resection are at high risk for the development of gallstones due to depletion of the bile salt pool. An abdominal ultrasonogram is the best option to detect the presence of gallstones.

(388–B) (S&F, pp. 1662–1663)

Blastocystis hominis is not rare. It is present in up to 20% of stool specimens examined in parasitology laboratories. *B. hominis* is commonly present without producing symptoms. It is more prevalent in immunosuppressed patients but usually produces symptoms in this population. Because *B. hominis* often causes no symptoms, the question often arises as to whether it should be treated. Studies suggest that stool examinations with five or fewer organisms per high-power ($40\times$) field are usually associated with no symptoms. Stools with more than five organisms per high-power field are more likely to be associated with diarrhea and should therefore be treated. The drug of choice is metronidazole.

(389–D)   **(S&F, pp. 1704–1705)**

Although there are numerous reports of improvement with various preparations, few data demonstrate consistent improvement after treatment with the widely available agents used to treat idiopathic proctitis. Symptoms of chronic radiation proctitis rarely remit but may be reduced somewhat by medical therapy.

(390–A)   **(S&F, pp. 1887–1888, 1894)**

The Muir-Torre syndrome has been linked to chromosome 2. Colon cancers associated with this syndrome are known to have microsatellite instability, strongly suggesting that this disorder is a variant of hereditary nonpolyposis colorectal cancer. All of the other syndromes have been linked to the adenomatous polyposis coli gene.

(391–C)   **(S&F, pp. 1672–1673)**

The major *Schistosoma* species are *S. japonicum, S. haematobium,* and *S. mansoni. S. mekongi* is assuming greater importance as refugees from the Mekong river valley in Southeast Asia emigrate to the United States. In general, this disease is less severe, but these patients can present with bleeding esophageal varices even at a young age. *S. amazoni* is a fictitious species name.

(392–D)   **(S&F, pp. 1765–1769)**

Ileorectal anastomosis is preferred. Crohn's disease is a contraindication to creating an ileal pouch. An ileoanal anastomosis would be associated with an unacceptably high bowel movement frequency and incontinence. With normal rectum and ileum, an ileorectal anastomosis is usually preferred over a Brooke ileostomy.

(393–D)   **(S&F, p. 1693)**

Peripheral eosinophilia is common in eosinophilic gastroenteritis but is not always present. Intense infiltration of the gastric and small bowel mucosa with eosinophils is the hallmark of this illness. Infiltration in the distal stomach and duodenum may cause dysmotility and vomiting. In general, elimination diets will help eosinophilic gastroenteritis, but the response is often quite slow. Although most food allergies respond to elimination diets within 1 week, eosinophilic gastroenteritis may not respond for up to 12 weeks after discontinuation of the offending food. The clinical response to corticosteroid treatment is prompt, but symptoms usually relapse when the dosage of corticosteroids is tapered.

(394–C)   **(S&F, p. 1955)**

Sexual transmission of herpes simplex virus (HSV) occurs by direct skin-to-skin contact. HSV is divided into two serotypes: HSV-1, predominantly affecting the oral cavity, and HSV-2, principally affecting the anogenital area. HSV-1 is a common cause of nonbacterial acute pharyngitis, but HSV-2 can also cause acute pharyngitis and tonsillitis after oral-genital contact. Patients may present with odynophagia, dysphagia, malaise, fever, and myalgias. Physical findings include marked pharyngeal erythema and ulcers over gingiva, palate, tonsils, and posterior pharynx. Virus carried into the esophagus can produce vesicles and painful swallowing. Infection may occur even when no herpes lesion is visible on the sexual partner because of asymptomatic viral carriage in the prostate, seminal vesicles, or cervix. The other listed infections may also be isolated from the pharynx but usually produce relatively mild symptoms without esophageal involvement in immunocompetent hosts.

(395–B)   **(S&F, p. 1633)**

Staphylococcus aureus was believed to be the cause of pseudomembranous enterocolitis on the basis of Gram's stain and cultures of the stool. This idea was reinforced by the success obtained with treatment with oral vancomycin.

(396–E)   **(S&F, pp. 1919, 1926–1927)**

Colorectal cancers in the right colon are larger at the time of diagnosis and tend to bleed more, therefore causing more constitutional symptoms associated with anemia. The lumen of the distal colon is smaller than the proximal colon, thereby making it more prone to obstruction and circumferential lesions. As a result, masses in the right colon stay asymptomatic longer and are more often palpable.

(397–C)   **(S&F, pp. 1486–1488)**

Vitamin B_{12} is found almost entirely in animal sources, and strict vegetarians will have an inadequate intake. The first protein to bind vitamin B_{12} is R protein, which is secreted in saliva. At a gastric pH of less than 3, intrinsic factor has a much poorer affinity for the vitamin than for R protein. It is only in the duodenum when the R protein is hydrolyzed by pancreatic enzymes that intrinsic factor is able to bind the cobalamin. Intrinsic factor is secreted by parietal cells in humans. The intrinsic factor/vitamin B_{12} complex binds specific receptors in the terminal ileum and enters the cell by endocytosis.

(398–B)   **(S&F, pp. 1532–1533)**

The ^{14}C-xylose breath test has a sensitivity of 90%. The sensitivity of the ^{14}C-bile acid breath test is only 60% to 70%. The latter test is also unable to differentiate bacterial overgrowth from ileal injury.

(399–B)   **(S&F, pp. 1456–1457)**

Nutrient absorption is generally linked to uptake of sodium, which provides the driving force for accumulation of intracellular nutrients against a concentration gradient.

Most cells, including those in the intestinal mucosa, maintain a low intracellular sodium concentration and a negative internal electrical potential. The movement of extracellular sodium down this electrochemical gradient provides the driving force for accumulation of intracellular glucose and certain amino acids against a concentration gradient. This process does not require hydrolysis of adenosine triphosphate (ATP), except indirectly to maintain the sodium gradient. Cytoplasmic sodium is pumped back out of the cell by the sodium/potassium ATPase. Sodium channels also exist in the apical membrane that permit the entry of sodium into the cell without any cotransported molecule.

(400–C)   **(S&F, pp. 1668–1669)**

More than 2 million people in the United States (1%) harbor whipworm. Although microscopic examination of the stool may be helpful in diagnosing whipworm, the worms are 3 to 5 cm long and can often be seen by the naked eye, especially when writhing in the toilet bowl. No other worm is this size. The diagnosis is suggested by patients who report seeing appropriately sized worms in the stool or by visualizing the adult worms on proctosigmoidoscopy.

(401–C)   **(S&F, pp. 1960–1962)**

Innervation of the upper portion of the anal canal is autonomic only, and this area is relatively insensitive to pain. In contrast, the perianal skin is extremely sensitive to painful stimuli. The lining of the lower anal canal is squamous epithelium that is void of hair follicles, sweat glands, and sebaceous glands. The valves of Houston contribute little to continence. Inguinal lymphadenopathy is an important sign of inflammatory or malignant anal diseases.

(402–C)   **(S&F, pp. 1657–1661)**

Isospora is extremely difficult to diagnose on stool specimens, and small bowel biopsy showing histologic evidence of intracellular parasites is the most sensitive way of making the diagnosis. Trimethoprim-sulfamethoxazole is the drug of choice, and symptoms usually resolve in one to three days. Cryptosporidiosis is usually a self-limited illness in patients with an intact immune system. Eradication of *Cryptosporidium* in patients with the acquired immunodeficiency syndrome is not absolutely essential because the infection is usually not fatal. If treatment is otherwise indicated to reduce diarrhea, then paromomycin is a good choice.

(403–1-C, 2-A, 3-B)   ***Small bowel (S&F, p. 1800)***
Colon (S&F, p. 1805)

Proximal small bowel obstruction causes early onset of colicky pain after eating, prominent nonfeculent vomiting that relieves pain, and little or no abdominal distention. In contrast, abdominal distention and feculent vomiting are prominent findings in distal small bowel or colonic obstruction. Distention becomes more severe with more distal sites of obstruction.

(404–D)   **(S&F, p. 1765)**

The patient most likely has pouchitis. Obtaining biopsy specimens may be helpful to evaluate for the presence of Crohn's disease. Given the clinical likelihood of pouchitis, metronidazole is the most reasonable first-line drug because it often produces dramatic improvement. The other treatments should be reserved for cases refractory to metronidazole.

(405–B)   **(S&F, p. 1491)**

Meat-eating persons typically ingest 20 to 30 mg of iron per day. However, absorption and loss average only 1 mg/day. Menstruating females lose an additional 5 to 50 mg/month, which is normally replaced by more avid absorption. Because dietary intake may markedly exceed the body's need for iron, only a small proportion of ingested iron is normally absorbed. Most absorption occurs in the proximal small intestine, where the low pH favors iron solubility (ferric iron is essentially insoluble at pH >3.0). Ferrous iron is more efficiently absorbed than ferric iron, although the two forms interconvert in the intestinal fluid. At least three mechanisms of iron absorption exist. The primary route is regulated and appears to be dependent on metabolic energy. A small amount of inorganic iron passes through the intestinal mucosa by a paracellular route. Finally a separate transcellular route is stimulated by uptake of nonessential fatty acids. Heme iron is transported by a distinct receptor-mediated mechanism.

(406–D)   **(S&F, pp. 1972–1973)**

Solitary rectal ulcer syndrome is a chronic benign condition that affects mainly young adults, women more commonly than men. It is characterized by anal pain and bleeding and associated with excessive straining while defecating. Proctosigmoidoscopy discloses a shallow ulcer 6 to 10 cm above the anal verge. This condition can be difficult to treat, and traditional therapy is directed toward avoiding straining. Recent reports suggest that sucralfate retention enemas cause healing in the majority of patients.

(407–A)   **(S&F, p. 1578)**

Tropical sprue is unusual in its marked geographic restriction. Even within endemic areas (especially India, Southeast Asia, and the Caribbean) the disease is not pervasive, suggesting that the causal factor is geographically restricted. It is a disease acquired while living for prolonged periods of time in endemic areas; visitors staying briefly rarely are affected.

(408–C)   **(S&F, p. 1763)**

Because of the obligate sodium losses due to the lack of colonic reabsorption, patients with proctocolectomies often have a highly concentrated urine, owing to renal conservation of sodium and water. This is associated with a 5% incidence of urolithiasis.

(409–C)   **(S&F, pp. 1779–1780)**

A low-fiber diet has been associated with an increase in the incidence of acute appendicitis. In addition, the decreasing rate of acute appendicitis has been associated with improvements in hygiene. Although these are only associations and causality is not established, a low-fiber diet is the most likely explanation of the choices given.

(410–D)   **(S&F, pp. 1503–1504)**

Maldigestive and malabsorptive disorders can be classified by the site of the defect: as premucosal, mucosal, or postmucosal. Whipple's disease, lactase deficiency, and intestinal resection are all examples of mucosal defects. Zollinger-Ellison syndrome causes fat maldigestion by acidifying the intestinal fluid, a premucosal defect. Lymphatic obstruction with chylous ascites is considered a postmucosal defect.

(411–B)   **(S&F, p. 1602)**

Escherichia coli 0157:H7, prominent in Minnesota, has been associated with hemolytic uremic syndrome (HUS). In one series, this organism was isolated from 46% of patients presenting with HUS.

(412–B)   **(S&F, p. 1952)**

Syphilitic gastritis is a manifestation of secondary syphilis, and the gastric mucosa may be extensively involved, producing pain and vomiting, typically without nausea or anorexia. Barium studies show loss of normal mucosal pattern with retention of pliability. If untreated, the disorder may progress to constriction or pyloric obstruction. During gastroscopy, markedly friable, hemorrhagic mucosa with diffuse mucosal ulceration is noted. Spirochetes can be found in a saline preparation of a crush biopsy specimen. Serologic tests for syphilis are positive in secondary syphilis.

(413–A)   **(S&F, p. 1491)**

Iron in meat is in the form or myoglobin or hemoglobin, and both are more readily absorbed than the iron in vegetables. Nonetheless, because daily iron intake (5 to 30 mg/day) greatly exceeds requirements (1 mg/day), vegetarians rarely develop iron deficiency as a result of inadequate intake alone. The efficiency of iron absorption increases in states of iron deficiency, pregnancy, increased erythropoiesis, or hypoxia.

(414–B, D, E)   **(S&F, pp. 1606–1609)**

Nontypical *Salmonella* species are ubiquitous in nature, particularly in animal reservoirs. Commercially prepared food is implicated in as many as 40% of cases. There is no evidence that antibiotics accelerate the rate of clinical recovery. In fact, antibiotic therapy often increases the incidence and duration of intestinal carriage of these organisms. Antibiotics should be reserved for cases of severe illness. Although multiple drug resistance is emerging, the quinolones in general have high efficacy against *Salmonella* organisms.

(415–A, D)   **(S&F, pp. 1506–1507)**

D-Xylose is a simple sugar that is readily absorbed by the normal small bowel mucosa but is not subsequently metabolized. Absorption of D-xylose is strictly proportional to mucosal microvillous surface area. Thus, levels of D-xylose in blood or in a timed urine collection after a standardized dose provide a measure of small intestinal mucosal function. One of the major vagaries of this test is that incomplete urine collections may generate false-positive results. D-Xylose absorption is dramatically reduced by bacterial overgrowth because bacteria metabolize the xylose, impairing absorption and thereby elimination in the urine. One of the major weaknesses of the test is that patients with very mild or distal disease may have a normal D-xylose test. In contrast to xylose, lactose is a disaccharide that must be cleaved to glucose plus galactose before it can be absorbed.

(416–E)   **(S&F, pp. 1561–1563)**

Celiac sprue is associated with all findings listed except arthritis. When present, arthritis suggests the diagnosis of Whipple's disease.

(417–A)   **(S&F, pp. 1755–1757)**

The duration and extent of the colitis are each correlated with the risk of colon cancer in patients with ulcerative colitis, whereas disease severity is not.

(418–C)   **(S&F, p. 1717)**

Patients with active disease at the time of conception have an increased risk of spontaneous abortion and premature delivery. However, patients in remission at conception have no greater risk than control populations. The majority of patients in remission (75%) remain in remission throughout their pregnancy. Approximately two thirds of patients with active disease at conception do not achieve a remission despite medical therapy. There is no rationale to avoiding pregnancy unless the patient is on medications that are potentially toxic to the fetus.

(419–E)   **(S&F, p. 1764)**

The presence of "backwash ileitis" is not predictive of the development of prestomal ileitis. Output is increased due to mechanical obstruction with proximal bowel dilatation and resultant increased intestinal secretion. It is not clear whether prestomal ileitis has a different pathogenesis from the changes that follow simple mechanical obstruction.

(420–C)   **(S&F, p. 1482)**

Eight of the 22 amino acids found in human proteins cannot be synthesized endogenously unless the corresponding keto acids are available from exogenous sources. These eight (threonine, lysine, phenylalanine, leucine, isoleucine, valine, methionine, and tryptophan), along with histidine, which is required for growth in infants, are called essential amino acids. Because they can be synthesized *in vivo* when the keto acids are fed, it is really the keto acids that are essential. By contrast, the keto acids of the nonessential amino acids are available as derivatives of carbohydrate metabolism.

(421–D)   **(S&F, p. 1564)**

Both malabsorption of iron and malabsorption of vitamin B$_{12}$ can occur, leading to a mixed picture of microcytic and macrocytic anemia. Malabsorption of vitamin K leads to depletion of vitamin K–dependent clotting factors (II,VII, IX, X) and an elevated prothrombin time. Thrombocytopenia is not typical of celiac sprue. In the setting of severe iron-deficiency anemia, thrombocytosis may even occur.

(422–A, C, D, E)   **(S&F, pp. 1813–1814)**

The characteristic transition from narrowed distal rectal segment to a dilated proximal colon on barium enema confirms the diagnosis of Hirschsprung's disease. However, when the aganglionic segment is short, a narrowed segment may not be evident. The narrowed segment is best seen on a lateral view. In doubtful cases the diagnosis requires full-thickness rectal biopsy. The presence of a normal number of ganglion cells excludes the diagnosis. Immunohistochemical techniques can be helpful in highlighting the morphologic abnormalities, which feature an abundance of hyperplastic axons but absence of ganglion cells. The most important pathophysiologic test is the response of the anal sphincters to distention of the rectum. Patients with aganglionosis have elevated levels of acetylcholinesterase in superficial rectal biopsy specimens. When manometry and acetylcholinesterase levels are both abnormal, deep rectal biopsy is not needed to make the diagnosis.

(423–A)   **(S&F, p. 1817)**

Acute megacolon can occur in patients without obvious colonic disease or mechanical obstruction. This syndrome is a form of pseudo-obstruction localized to the colon. The characteristic time course is acute or subacute, and most cases are clearly related to an underlying primary process such as recent trauma or surgery. The typical patient is an older person who is often recovering uneventfully from orthopedic surgery. An abdominal film typically shows massive gaseous distention of the colon and rectum.

(424–B)   **(S&F, p. 1564)**

Diffuse small bowel disease often leads to folate deficiency. As a result, the mean corpuscular volume may go up, the hematocrit may go down, and the serum and red cell folate levels may fall. In general, no effect is seen on vitamin B$_{12}$ levels. In contrast, anorexia usually produces a decline in serum folate without a fall in the red blood cell folate, allowing discrimination between anorexia and diffuse small bowel disease.

(425–A)   **(S&F, p. 1953)**

Proctitis is associated in varying degrees of severity with many chlamydial serotypes. Infection with lymphogranuloma venereum types are the most severe. Primary lesions consisting of small vesicles develop one to two weeks after exposure. They grow into shallow ulcers and disappear. In the secondary stage, femoral or inguinal lymphadenopathy accompanies systemic symptoms of fever, chills, and headache. Abscesses and fistulas are frequent. Fibrotic changes may result in rectal strictures. Proctitis caused by *Neisseria gonorrhoeae*, *Treponema pallidum*, *Escherichia histolytica*, and cytomegalovirus can produce nonspecific symptoms such as burning, itching, bloody or mucoid discharge, and diarrhea but does not form abscesses or strictures.

(426–C-B-D-A)   **(S&F, p. 1780)**

Pain at some site in the abdomen followed by anorexia, nausea, or vomiting followed by pain over the appendix followed by fever is the typical sequence. Not all patients have all symptoms, but if the symptoms occur in a different order, then the diagnosis of acute appendicitis should be questioned.

(427–B, E)   **(S&F, pp. 1635–1637)**

Loose, watery stools are the most common feature of pseudomembranous colitis. Gross bleeding is rare. The onset of diarrhea is noted during the course of antibiotic treatment in two thirds of patients; the remaining third develop symptoms anywhere from one to six weeks after discontinuation of the offending drug. There is no relation between the dose of the antibiotic and the severity of the colitis. Although commonly present, stool leukocytes are neither sensitive nor specific for *Clostridium difficile* colitis. Pseudomembranous colitis can present with systemic signs of infection, including high fever, leukocytosis, hypoalbuminemia, and toxic megacolon.

(428–A)   **(S&F, pp. 1557, 1563)**

The prevalence of celiac disease varies throughout the world. It is most common in Europe and has the highest prevalence in West Ireland (1 in 300). In contrast, there are no more than 1000 cases of Whipple's disease worldwide. The absence of previous medical illness makes the diagnoses of bacterial overgrowth, pancreatic disease, or tuberculosis unlikely. Based solely on the epidemiologic setting, celiac sprue is the most likely diagnosis.

(429–1-B, 2-A, 3-C, 4-D)   **(S&F, p. 1539)**

Mucosal biopsy specimens are an important adjunct to cultures and smears of the rectal mucosa in detecting a variety of diseases. They can often detect infection with schistosomiasis when repeated stool examinations are negative. Various systemic diseases including amyloidosis, cystic fibrosis, tuberculosis, histoplasmosis, and gonorrhea can also be found in rectal biopsy specimens. Amyloid demonstrates a characteristic green birefringence when stained with Congo red and visualized using polarized light. The lack of ganglion cells in Hirschsprung's disease is usually accompanied by hypertrophied and disorganized nonmyelinated nerve fibers in the submucosa.

(430–C)   **(S&F, pp. 1441–1444)**

Intestinal motility involves both transit and mixing. The two types of fundamental wall motions are ring and sleeve contractions. Ring contractions are primarily propulsive. Sleeve contractions produce mixing of intestinal content by causing shifts of fluid between the center and the periphery. Both types of contractions often occur simultaneously, thus maximizing intraluminal mixing. Contractions occur most frequently in the proximal intestine and least frequently in the rectum.

(431–D)   **(S&F, pp. 1820–1821)**

Chronic intestinal pseudo-obstruction is caused by a number of primary or secondary smooth muscle disorders such as progressive systemic sclerosis. Disorders of the myenteric plexus such as familial visceral neuropathies and extraintestinal neurologic disorders such as Parkinson's disease or familial autonomic neuropathy can also cause the syndrome. Other secondary causes are metabolic disorders and drugs. *Helicobacter pylori* infection may cause a transient dysmotility of the upper gastrointestinal tract but does not cause the syndrome of chronic intestinal pseudo-obstruction.

(432–A)   **(S&F, pp. 1600–1602)**

Enteropathic *Escherichia coli* usually is not invasive; the disease is typically mild, and therapy is often not indicated. Most of the enteroinvasive *E. coli* have been identified as closely related biochemically and antigenically to *Shigella*. They also are invasive and make a shiga-like toxin. Enterohemorrhagic *E. coli* is associated with serotype 0157:H7. Ninety-five percent of infected persons have bloody diarrhea, and an increased incidence of hemolytic-uremic syndrome and thrombotic thrombocytopenic purpura occurs. Enterotoxigenic *E. coli* produce two toxins: one (LT) is heat labile and is similar but not identical to the cholera toxin; the other, a heat-stable toxin (ST), has no similarity to cholera toxin.

(433–D)   **(S&F, p. 1463)**

Aldosterone increases the sodium conductance of the apical membrane in the colon. Absence of mineralocorticoid activity may lead to diarrhea in Addison's disease. Glucocorticoids directly stimulate sodium and water absorption in the intestine, probably by stimulation of the sodium pump. Epinephrine stimulates electroneutral sodium chloride absorption and decreases net bicarbonate secretion. Somatostatin stimulates salt and water absorption in both the ileum and colon.

(434–E)   **(S&F, pp. 1876–1877)**

Despite the results from the National Polyp Study, there is still a surprising lack of consensus regarding postpoly-

pectomy surveillance. The one thing that is clear is that surveillance need not be performed more often than every three years. Evidence is mounting that a small single tubular adenoma does not confer an increased risk of having metachronous adenomas nor an increased risk of future colon cancer. This implies that this group may not need surveillance, although this issue certainly has not yet been resolved. Options B and C are routine screening regimens that might be followed if more intensive surveillance is deemed unnecessary.

(435–A)   **(S&F, pp. 1648–1651)**

The only important forms of *Giardia* are the encysted and trophozoite forms. They do not have to pass through other intermediate hosts, although some of them may afflict other mammals just as they do humans. The remaining answers are true.

(436–D)   **(S&F, pp. 1663–1669)**

The degree of eosinophilic response to worms is related to the degree of chronic tissue invasion. Whipworm generally invades the mucosa minimally, and thus eosinophilia is either not present or is mild. Strongyloidiasis has the greatest amount of tissue invasion and is most frequently associated with a severe (>50%) eosinophilia. *Ascaris* generally causes minimal tissue invasion, because the adult worms live entirely within the lumen of the bowel. Hookworm causes a modest but consistent breech of the mucosa and enters the circulation as filariform larvae, producing a moderate eosinophilia in most cases.

(437–E)   **(S&F, pp. 1771–1772)**

Long-term use of nonsteroidal anti-inflammatory drugs has been the most common cause of perforated small intestinal ulcers since the 1980s. Enteric-coated potassium supplements were associated with a high incidence of small bowel ulceration in the 1960s and were subsequently withdrawn from the market. Currently available slow-release potassium preparations are much less likely to cause small bowel perforation. The other choices are not associated with an increased incidence of small bowel ulceration.

(438–E)   **(S&F, pp. 1740–1741)**

Although all the listed features are common findings in ulcerative colitis, they may also be seen in other forms of colitis, including dysentery, Crohn's disease, and pseudomembranous colitis. Distorted crypt architecture, crypt atrophy, and a chronic inflammatory infiltrate all suggest chronicity and can help to make the diagnosis of idiopathic ulcerative colitis with an 80% probability.

(439–A)   **(S&F, pp. 1906–1908)**

The change in the colorectal cancer rate in populations that have migrated to areas with a different colorectal cancer risk is the strongest evidence for an environmental contribution. The great increase in colon cancer among

Japanese immigrants to the United States is perhaps the best documented example of this phenomenon.

(440–A)   **(S&F, pp. 1991, 1965)**

Stercoraceous perforation is a rare lethal consequence of prolonged storage of hard feces. Only 50% of patients with anterior mucosal prolapse have a history of constipation or straining. Although some studies have established a link between cancer of the large intestine and constipation, the risk is small and likely reflects uncontrolled variables such as obesity or dietary fiber. Hemorrhoids are not caused by constipation. In a prospective case-control study, diarrhea but not constipation was found to be a risk factor for developing hemorrhoids.

(441–D)   **(S&F, pp. 1681–1683)**

Eosinophilic gastroenteritis with serosal involvement typically presents as eosinophilic ascites. In contrast, mucosal layer involvement typically presents as colicky abdominal pain, weight loss, and diarrhea. Mucosal layer disease can also present as protein-losing enteropathy and malabsorption. Muscle layer involvement usually presents as crampy abdominal pain and intestinal obstruction. Nausea and vomiting are nonspecific symptoms.

(442–E)   **(S&F, pp. 1722–1725)**

This patient requires the institution of a medication that permits tapering of the prednisone so that the potentially devastating effects of long-term high-dose corticosteroids may be avoided. 6-Mercaptopurine is the drug of choice in this circumstance. Total parenteral nutrition may allow reduction of corticosteroids, but it is associated with a high complication rate and would have an unfavorable effect on the quality of life. Methotrexate is experimental and metronidazole has fairly limited efficacy in small bowel disease.

(443–A, B)   **(S&F, pp. 1812–1814)**

Hirschsprung's disease usually becomes apparent shortly after birth when the infant passes little meconium and the abdomen is distended. In about 20% of patients, diarrhea persists due to pseudomembranous enterocolitis, which develops as a complication of the obstruction. Later in life, the presentation is often less dramatic and may not mimic acute intestinal obstruction as in infants. The overall incidence among siblings of index cases is 3.6% (5% for brothers and 1% for sisters), but the risk is 10% for long segment disease irrespective of gender. Although most children have major difficulties before the second month of life, short segment aganglionosis is less severe and may not cause symptoms until later in life.

(444–D)   **(S&F, pp. 1788–1790, 1791–1792)**

Diverticula do indeed protrude through the bowel wall, but they protrude between the taenia coli, presumably because the bowel wall is weaker where the longitudinal muscle layer is less developed. They are most commonly found in the sigmoid colon, although right-sided diverticula are more likely to cause massive bleeding. Myochosis is a phenomenon characterized by excessive deposition of contracted elastin in the colon wall that tends to narrow the lumen and promote division of the colon into discontinuous chambers during contractions. The process predisposes to diverticula.

(445–D)   **(S&F, pp. 1618–1619)**

Campylobacter jejuni, like *Shigella*, involves the colon, is invasive, and may be associated with hemorrhage and/or fecal leukocytes. The other diseases listed involve only the small intestine (enterotoxigenic *Escherichia coli* is a small bowel pathogen unlike enteroinvasive or enterohemorrhagic *E. coli*), are not invasive, and are rarely associated with blood or leukocytes in the stool.

(446–D)   **(S&F, p. 1802)**

Obstruction disables digestive function by reversing the normal net positive balance of absorption. Decreased absorption and massive increases in mucosal secretion distend the bowel. The fluid deficit due to vomiting and poor oral intake combines with that due to intestinal distention and wall edema to produce hypovolemia that may produce shock if not corrected. Moreover, bacterial overgrowth proximal to the obstruction in the setting of distention results in translocation of bacteria into mesenteric lymph and ultimately the blood stream, with resulting septic shock.

(447–D)   **(S&F, pp. 1991–1992)**

Treatment of fecal impaction should be limited to digital disimpaction if possible. This may require topical anesthesia as well as lubrication of the distal rectum. Once the large mass of feces has been softened and partially removed, water or saline enemas may be given. To prevent further impaction, oral doses of a variety of preparations may be given, including citrate of magnesium, Phospho-Soda, or colonoscopy preparations such as electrolyte-polyethylene glycol solution.

(448–B)   **(S&F, p. 1526)**

Vitamin B_{12} malabsorption is one of the most common nutritional abnormalities in patients with bacterial overgrowth. Intestinal bacteria take up vitamin B_{12} and vitamin B_{12}–intrinsic factor complexes, thereby reducing intestinal uptake of the ingested vitamin. Although enteric microorganisms also synthesize vitamin B_{12}, the vitamin is unavailable to the host. In contrast, folic acid produced by intestinal bacteria is subsequently released into the lumen and absorbed by the host.

(449–D)   **(S&F, pp. 1772–1773)**

Histologically, there is evidence of chronic inflammation with an occasional prominent eosinophilic infiltrate. Granulomas generally do not occur. When they are present, a prominent granulomatous component would suggest Crohn's disease as the underlying cause.

(450–B)   **(S&F, p. 1698)**

With current dose and technique for common tumors, the overall risk of chronic radiation bowel injury is 2.5% to 25%. Rectal exposure to 55 Gy is associated with a 5%

or less risk of chronic injury at five years. This risk increases to as much as 50% with exposures of 80 Gy.

(451–C)   **(S&F, pp. 1757–1758)**

The life expectancy for patients with ulcerative colitis differs little from persons without ulcerative colitis. Patients deserve strong support from their physicians when dealing with arbitrary and uninformed decisions such as the case presented here.

452. A 43-year-old man complains of long-standing pyrosis. At endoscopy, he is noted to have Barrett's esophagus involving the distal 10 cm of the esophagus. Biopsy specimens are taken at 2-cm intervals in all quadrants and reveal mild to intermediate dysplasia with inflammation. The MOST appropriate treatment would be:
A. Treatment with H_2 blockers and repeat endoscopic biopsy in one year
B. Treatment with a proton pump inhibitor and repeat endoscopic biopsy at three months
C. Esophagectomy
D. Photodynamic therapy

453. A 45-year-old woman undergoes an upper gastrointestinal series for evaluation of dyspepsia. The examination reveals a smooth, extramural mass in the distal esophagus. At endoscopy, normal overlying mucosa is found covering an 18-mm lesion. The MOST likely histopathology is:
A. Lipoma
B. Leiomyoma
C. Squamous cell papilloma
D. Inflammatory fibroid polyp

454. Which of the following statements regarding Barrett's esophagus are TRUE?
I. Intensive medical treatment does not reverse Barrett's metaplasia.
II. Males and females are affected in equal proportions.
III. With Barrett's esophagus, the relative risk of adenocarcinoma is increased 30-fold to 40-fold.
IV. Columnar lined esophagus less than 3 cm ("short segment" Barrett's) poses little risk of developing adenocarcinoma.

A. I and III
B. II and IV
C. I, II, and III
D. All of the above

455. A 36-year-old woman with acquired immunodeficiency syndrome (AIDS) complains of persistent, severe odynophagia despite a ten-day course of oral antifungal therapy. The MOST appropriate diagnostic test would be:
A. Barium swallow
B. Computed tomography of the chest
C. Endoscopy with brushings and biopsies
D. Cytomegalovirus titers

456. Each of the following statements regarding the upper esophageal sphincter (UES) is true EXCEPT:
A. Pressures within the UES are greater in the anterior-posterior axis.
B. Inspiration decreases UES pressure.
C. Acid and slow distention of the upper esophagus increase UES pressure.
D. Upward and forward movement of the larynx is the primary mechanism for opening the relaxed UES.

457. Factors that alter peristaltic waves observed in the esophageal body during manometry include which of the following?
I. Size and temperature of swallowed bolus
II. Interval between swallows
III. Position of the patient
IV. Use of sedation

A. I and III
B. II and IV
C. I, II, and III
D. All of the above

458. Which one of the following is the LEAST common complication of esophagitis?
A. Stricture formation
B. Barrett's epithelium
C. Hemorrhage
D. Perforation

459. For the treatment of esophageal varices that have bled, both sclerotherapy (EST) and variceal ligation (EVL) have been used successfully. Which of the following complications is seen more frequently with EVL than EST?
A. Esophageal strictures
B. Bleeding from treatment-induced ulcers
C. Esophageal tears from overtube trapping of mucosa
D. Pulmonary infection
E. Bacterial peritonitis

460. Each of the following statements regarding esophageal anatomy is true EXCEPT:
A. The esophagus passes through a horizontally oriented diaphragmatic hiatus 1 to 2 cm in vertical height.
B. The venous drainage includes the superior vena cava, azygous system, and the portal vein.
C. Innervation derives from both the sympathetic and parasympathetic systems.
D. The esophagus is lined by stratified squamous epithelium.

461. Which of the following statements about patients with disorders of the oropharyngeal phase of swallowing are TRUE?
I. They respond affirmatively when asked, "Do you have difficulty swallowing?"
II. They have tracheobronchial aspiration and nasopharyngeal regurgitation.
III. They may have frequent bolus impactions requiring manual dislodgement.
IV. They frequently have odynophagia associated with dysphagia.

A. I and III
B. II and IV
C. I, II, and III
D. All of the above

462. A 47-year-old man presents with a six-month history of gradually worsening solid food dysphagia without weight loss. He has a long-standing history of mild pyrosis and does not smoke tobacco or drink alcohol. A barium swallow reveals a benign-appearing stricture in the midesophagus. Of the following, the MOST likely diagnosis would be:
A. Schatzki's ring
B. Squamous cell carcinoma of the esophagus
C. Barrett's esophagus with stricture
D. Infectious esophagitis

463. Which one of the following about patients with diffuse esophageal spasm is TRUE?
A. The primary disorder is muscular in origin.
B. The primary disorder is neural in origin.
C. The response to cholinergic stimulation is blunted.
D. The response to central nervous system stimulation is blunted.

464. An organism responsible for a disease with clinical features very similar to achalasia is:
A. *Helicobacter pylori*
B. *Clostridium tetani*
C. *Treponema pallidum*
D. *Trypanosoma cruzi*

465. Which of the following statements regarding the muscular layers of the esophagus are TRUE?
I. The proximal esophagus contains only striated muscle.
II. The distal esophagus contains only smooth muscle.
III. The middle esophagus contains both smooth and striated muscle.
IV. The upper esophageal sphincter has both smooth and striated muscle.

A. I and III
B. II and IV
C. I, II, and III
D. All of the above

466. Match the type of esophageal motor function with its description.
1. Secondary peristalsis
2. Tertiary contractions
3. Primary peristalsis
4. Tertiary peristalsis

A. The coordinated motor pattern of the esophagus initiated by a swallow
B. Progressive contractions in the esophageal body induced by stimulation of sensory receptors—not by a swallow
C. Uncoordinated or simultaneous contractions in the esophageal body
D. Contractions in the smooth muscle portion of the esophagus induced by a local intramural mechanism

467. Each of the following is a potential cause of oropharyngeal dysphasia EXCEPT:
A. Chagas' disease
B. Myasthenia gravis
C. Polymyositis
D. Parkinson's disease
E. Diabetes mellitus

468. Manometric findings of aperistalsis in the smooth muscle portion of the esophageal body and hypotension of the lower esophageal sphincter are MOST compatible with:
A. Diffuse esophageal spasm
B. Achalasia
C. Scleroderma
D. Diabetes mellitus
E. Huntington's chorea

469. Which of the following statements regarding pneumatic dilation of the esophagus for achalasia are TRUE?
I. At least 60% of patients have significant improvement in symptoms.
II. Patients with a poor response to the first pneumatic dilation are likely to respond to subsequent dilations.

III. The majority of patients suffering perforation with pneumatic dilation will not require surgical repair.
IV. Pneumatic dilation and surgical myotomy are equally effective in reducing symptoms.

A. I and III
B. II and IV
C. I, II, and III
D. All of the above

470. Which of the following statements regarding omeprazole are TRUE?
   I. Omeprazole must be given twice daily for optimum results.
   II. Omeprazole inhibits the hepatic cytochrome P-450 system.
   III. Most patients successfully responding to six to eight weeks of treatment are free of esophagitis at six months.
   IV. Omeprazole is more effective than standard doses of H_2 blockers for treating esophagitis.

   A. I and III
   B. II and IV
   C. I, II, and III
   D. All of the above

471. A 61-year-old man presents with complaints of dysphagia and fits of coughing every time he tries to swallow. He relates a history of alcohol and tobacco abuse and has lost 14 kg. The MOST appropriate initial diagnostic test is:
   A. Endoscopy
   B. Computed tomography of the chest
   C. Ultrasonography
   D. Barium swallow

472. Referring to the case history in question 471, after the diagnosis has been made, the initial treatment of choice would be:
   A. Radiation therapy
   B. Chemotherapy
   C. Esophageal stent
   D. Laser ablation

473. Achalasia is characterized by which of the following?
   I. A reduction in the number of ganglion cells located within the esophageal wall
   II. Normal progression of peristaltic waves with elevated resting pressure of the lower esophageal sphincter
   III. Incomplete relaxation of the lower esophageal sphincter after swallows
   IV. Resting intragastric pressures higher than intraesophageal pressures

   A. I and III

B. II and IV
C. I, II, and III
D. All of the above

474. Each of the following statements regarding lymphatic drainage of the esophagus is true EXCEPT:
   A. The cervical esophagus drains into the cervical nodes
   B. The middle esophagus drains into the mediastinum
   C. The distal esophagus drains into the mediastinum and porta hepatis
   D. The entire lymphatic system is highly interconnected

475. After an episode of acid reflux, the MOST important factor involved in restoring the intraesophageal pH is:
   A. Primary peristaltic contractions
   B. The rate of spontaneous swallowing after an episode of gastroesophageal reflux
   C. The volume of swallowed saliva
   D. Mucus and bicarbonate secretion from the esophageal mucosa

476. Which of the following statements about transient lower esophageal relaxations (tLESRs) are TRUE:
   A. They occur in normal subjects.
   B. The tLESR persists longer than does a swallow-induced lower esophageal (LES) relaxation.
   C. The physiologic purpose of tLESRs is to allow venting of gas from the stomach (belching).
   D. They account for the overwhelming majority of reflux events both in normal subjects and in patients with gastroesophageal reflux disease.

477. Which of the following conditions are associated with esophagitis?
   I. Scleroderma
   II. Sjögren's syndrome
   III. Zollinger-Ellison syndrome
   IV. Pregnancy

   A. I and III
   B. II and IV
   C. I, II, and III
   D. All of the above

478. Which of the following are characteristics of the Plummer-Vinson syndrome?
   I. Iron-deficiency anemia
   II. Increased risk of squamous carcinoma of the esophagus
   III. Cervical esophageal web
   IV. Resolution of dysphagia with iron repletion

   A. I and III
   B. II and IV

C. I, II, and III
D. All of the above

479. Which of the following is the best single test for evaluating a patient with oropharyngeal dysphasia?
A. Double-contrast esophagography
B. Endoscopy
C. Chest computed tomography
D. Barium swallow with videofluoroscopy
E. Single-contrast esophagography

480. Which of the following hormones are known to DECREASE lower esophageal sphincter pressure?
I. Secretin
II. Progesterone
III. Cholecystokinin
IV. Somatostatin

A. I and III
B. II and IV
C. I, II, and III
D. All of the above

481. Which of the following statements regarding the lower esophageal sphincter (LES) are TRUE?
I. Average LES pressure at rest approximates 20 mm Hg.
II. Calcium channel blockers reduce LES pressure.
III. LES pressure typically falls 1.5 to 2.5 seconds after a swallow and stays low for 6 to 8 seconds.
IV. Truncal vagotomy increases LES pressure.

A. I and III
B. II and IV
C. I, II, and III
D. All of the above

482. Which of the following are associated with an increased risk of squamous cell cancer of the esophagus?
I. Achalasia
II. Tylosis
III. Alcohol and tobacco use
IV. Raw fish

A. I and III
B. II and IV
C. I, II, and III
D. All of the above

483. Pill esophagitis may be caused by which of the following?
I. Doxycycline
II. Clinitest tablet
III. Zidovudine
IV. Ciprofloxacin

A. I and III

B. II and IV
C. I, II, and III
D. All of the above

484. The treatment of choice for candidal esophagitis in a patient with the acquired immunodeficiency syndrome is:
A. Fluconazole
B. Clotrimazole troches
C. Nystatin suspension
D. Amphotericin

485. The MOST common symptom reported by patients with diffuse esophageal spasm is:
A. Dysphagia
B. Heartburn
C. Chest pain
D. Regurgitation
E. Odynophagia

486. Which of the following is the MOST common congenital anomaly of the esophagus?
A. A vascular ring
B. An esophageal duplication
C. A congenital stenosis of the esophagus
D. A tracheoesophageal fistula

487. Each of the following increases lower esophageal sphincter pressure EXCEPT:
A. Cholinergic agonists
B. β-Adrenergic agonists
C. β-Adrenergic antagonists
D. α-Adrenergic agonists

488. Manometric findings commonly found with diffuse esophageal spasm include which of the following?
I. Frequent nonperistaltic contractions after swallows
II. Abnormalities of wave amplitude or duration
III. Periods of intense or repetitive contractions associated with baseline pressure elevation
IV. Poor relaxation of the lower esophageal sphincter

A. I and III
B. II and IV
C. I, II, and III
D. All of the above

489. The MOST common histologic pattern in Barrett's epithelium is:
A. Junctional or cardia-type Barrett's mucosa with a predominant foveolar surface pattern

B. Dysplastic stratified squamous epithelium
C. Specialized columnar epithelium with a villous architecture
D. Fundic-type Barrett's mucosa

---

490. The MOST damaging agent in esophagitis is:
A. Hydrogen ion
B. Pepsin
C. Bile acids
D. Food hyperosmolarity

---

491. Which of the following statements about idiopathic achalasia are TRUE?
A. Sublingual isosorbide dinitrate before meals improves symptoms.

B. Calcium channel blockers have demonstrated consistent clinical benefits.
C. Manometry can distinguish idiopathic achalasia from distal esophageal malignancy.

---

492. Which of the following structures or anatomic abnormalities cause a posterior indentation of the esophagus as seen on a barium esophagram?
  I. Aortic arch
 II. Left atrium
III. Left main-stem bronchus
IV. Aberrant right subclavian artery

A. I and III
B. II and IV
C. I, II, and III
D. All of the above

(452–B)   **(S&F, p. 514)**

Inflammatory changes due to esophagitis can be difficult to discern from true dysplasia. The current recommendations would be to treat with an intensive medical regimen and repeat surveillance biopsy in 12 weeks.

(453–B)   **(S&F, p. 551)**

Leiomyomas constitute the most common benign tumor of the esophagus. The majority are asymptomatic with symptoms primarily proportional to size. Endoscopic ultrasonography is useful in establishing a muscular origin of the tumor, although it cannot distinguish leiomyoma from leiomyosarcoma, other than by inference based on size. Papillomas arise from the epithelial surface and thus would not have normal overlying mucosa, and inflammatory fibroid polyps are extremely rare lesions.

(454–A)   **(S&F, pp. 498, 513–514)**

Neither intensive medical therapy nor surgical treatment has consistently been shown to have any effect on regression of Barrett's metaplasia. Men are ten times more likely to have Barrett's esophagus, and several carefully documented cases of adenocarcinoma have occurred in short segments of columnar-lined esophagus. Indeed, among white men in western societies, the incidence of adenocarcinoma of the esophagus is increasing in epidemic proportions.

(455–C)   **(S&F, pp. 520–525)**

Patients with the acquired immunodeficiency syndrome who have persistent odynophagia after empirical antifungal therapy merit endoscopic evaluation to exclude cytomegalovirus, herpes simplex virus, other fungal diseases, and large esophageal ulcers.

(456–B)   **(S&F, pp. 470–471)**

Excitatory neural discharges to the upper esophageal sphincter (UES) increase with each inspiration with a subsequent increase in UES pressure. The increased pressure prevents air from entering the esophagus and affords more airway protection.

(457–D)   **(S&F, pp. 475–476)**

Esophageal motor disorders are defined by characteristic patterns of muscle contraction. Therefore, manometry is a very important diagnostic tool. Intraluminal manometers measure both the hydrodynamic pressure within the fluid bolus and the squeeze pressure of the esophageal wall.

Studies are usually performed in a fasting state in the supine position. Sedation is not employed because it may affect swallowing and influence manometric results. Many factors can alter measured waves in the esophageal body, including the presence or absence of a swallowed bolus, the size and temperature of the bolus, the interval between swallows, and the diameter of the recording probe.

(458–D)   **(S&F, p. 507)**

Spontaneous perforation secondary to esophagitis is quite rare. Strictures develop in 8% to 20% of patients with esophagitis, and Barrett's metaplasia is seen with a similar frequency. Significant gastrointestinal hemorrhage complicating esophagitis occurs in less than 2% of patients.

(459–C)   **(S&F, pp. 530–531)**

All of the complications mentioned are more frequent with sclerotherapy than variceal ligation except for an esophageal tear caused by trapping mucosa between the endoscope and overtube. This complication can be largely prevented by careful insertion of the overtube with a Maloney dilator.

■■■ Reference

Laine, L., El-Newihi, H.M., Migikovsky, B., et al. Endoscopic ligation compared with sclerotherapy for the treatment of bleeding esophageal varices. Ann. Intern. Med. *119*:1, 1993.

(460–A)   **(S&F, pp. 457–459)**

The diaphragmatic hiatus has a vertical orientation such that the esophagus enters through a tunnel that is 5 to 6 cm in vertical height. This anatomic relationship has a bearing on the function of the lower esophageal sphincter and the antireflux barrier.

(461–C)   **(S&F, pp. 476–477)**

Patients with oropharyngeal dysphagia truly have difficulty swallowing. The food bolus cannot be propelled successfully from the hypopharyngeal region through the upper sphincter and into the esophagus. Tracheal aspiration and nasopharyngeal regurgitation are potential outcomes. Some patients describe recurrent bolus impactions that require manual dislodgement. These disorders can be so severe that saliva cannot be swallowed and drooling results. Odynophagia is not a feature of these disorders.

(462–C)   **(S&F, pp. 513–514)**

The history and radiographic findings suggest a diagnosis of Barrett's esophagus with a stricture. Up to 50% of patients with strictures will be found to have Barrett's metaplasia, and the stricture characteristically occurs near the proximally displaced squamocolumnar junction; hence it is a midesophageal stricture. The chronicity of the patient's dysphagia and the absence of weight loss argue against carcinoma.

Reference

Sphechler, S. J., Sperber, H., Doos, W. G., et al. The prevalence of Barrett's esophagus in patients with chronic peptic esophageal strictures. Dig. Dis. Sci. *28*:769, 1983.

(463–B)   *(S&F, pp. 486–487)*

Physiologic studies of patients with diffuse esophageal spasm suggest a neural defect. The esophagus is particularly sensitive to cholinergic stimulation. Agents such as bethanechol or carbachol will produce an exaggeration of abnormal manometric findings in many patients. Cholinesterase inhibitors produce similar results. Central nervous system disorders may contribute to the manometric abnormalities. Psychologic stress produces repetitive waves in normal subjects that resemble those in diffuse esophageal spasm. These findings may have a relationship to observations that anxiety and affective disorders are unusually prevalent in patients with contraction abnormalities.

(464–D)   *(S&F, p. 526)*

Chagas' disease develops 10 to 30 years after acute infection with *Trypanosoma cruzi*. The endoscopic and radiographic features are identical to those of achalasia. Manometric studies in Chagas' disease, however, reveal below-normal lower esophageal sphincter pressures and a response to nitrates.

(465–C)   *(S&F, p. 467)*

The proximal esophagus, including the upper esophageal sphincter, is composed of striated muscle only. The distal esophagus is made up solely of smooth muscle, with the transition zone in between composed of both smooth and striated muscle.

(466–1-B, 2-C, 3-A, 4-D)   *(S&F, p. 470)*

Esophageal contractions may be peristaltic or aperistaltic. Peristaltic contractions may result from several stimuli: primary peristaltic waves that are initiated by a wet swallow (presence of a bolus) or dry swallow (absence of a bolus); secondary waves, which are contractions not induced by a swallow but rather by stimulation of receptors in the esophageal body; and tertiary waves, which are contractions resulting from a local intramural mechanism.

(467–A)   *(S&F, pp. 476–478)*

Rapid and sequential contractions of striated muscle in the pharynx and hypopharynx propel food boluses through the relaxed upper sphincter. Signals to the pharynx and proximal esophageal region travel via the cranial nerves (principally IX, X, and XII). A variety of disorders can cause oropharyngeal dysphasia. These include structural lesions such as carcinoma, central nervous system diseases such as Parkinson's disease, cranial nerve diseases such as polymyositis, and neuromuscular disorders such as myasthenia gravis. (For a complete list see S&F, Table 18–2, p. 346.) Chagas' disease is a result of an infection by the parasite *Trypanosoma cruzi* that causes damage to the neural plexuses of the esophagus and other tubular organs. Esophageal involvement results in signs and symptoms markedly resembling achalasia.

(468–C)   *(S&F, pp. 490–492)*

The described manometric findings are classic for scleroderma of the esophagus. However, less than 40% of patients with these findings will have scleroderma. Persons with achalasia have aperistalsis with a hypertensive esophageal sphincter. Diffuse esophageal spasm has either nonperistaltic contractions or abnormalities of the contraction waves. Diabetes mellitus can produce findings resembling spastic disorders. Huntington's chorea is a neurologic disorder affecting the brainstem that produces proximal dysphagia.

(469–A)   *(S&F, pp. 484–485)*

At least 60% of patients have a good response to pneumatic dilation. Good results from surgical myotomy are reported in 88% to 90% of patients. Myotomy reduces the lower sphincter pressure more dependably than pneumatic dilation. Efficacy of pneumatic dilation is reduced by half for each subsequent dilation. Thus, patients who have a poor initial response are less likely to respond to future dilation. Morbidity of pneumatic dilation is mostly related to esophageal perforation, which occurs in approximately 5% of patients. Of those with perforation, fewer than half require surgical repair.

(470–B)   *(S&F, pp. 510–511)*

Omeprazole inhibits the cytochrome P-450 system, thereby delaying the metabolism of certain other drugs such as phenytoin and warfarin. Unlike cimetidine, omeprazole does not inhibit the metabolism of theophylline and propranolol. Omeprazole is very effective at treating esophagitis, but the recurrence rate after the initial response to therapy is 80% at 6 months.

(471–D)   *(S&F, pp. 542–543)*

The clinical history strongly suggests an esophageal carcinoma complicated by a tracheoesophageal fistula. The initial study should be a barium swallow to confirm the diagnosis. Tracheoesophageal fistulas occur in 6% to 12% of patients with squamous cell carcinoma.

(472–C)   *(S&F, p. 548)*

Whereas the role of esophageal stents in tumors without a tracheoesophageal fistula is debatable, stent placement across the fistula is the initial treatment of choice for symptomatic fistulas because the pulmonary complications are reduced. A wide variety of prostheses are available, including conventional plastic prostheses, metal prostheses, and self-expanding mesh stents.

Reference

Wu, W. C., Katon, R. M., Saxon, R. R., et al. Silicone-covered self-expanding metallic stents for the palliation of malignant esophageal obstruction and esophagorespiratory fistulas: Experience in 32 patients and a review of the literature. Gastrointest. Endosc. *40*:22, 1994.

(473–A) ***(S&F, pp. 479–482)***

The etiology of achalasia is unknown. The disease affects both sexes equally with little genetic predisposition. A neural lesion is believed to be responsible. Examination of the intraluminal esophageal nerve plexus has demonstrated a reduction in the number of ganglion cells. Achalasia displays several features on manometry. Sequentially propagated waves traversing the distal esophageal body are absent. Elevated resting pressure in the lower esophageal sphincter is found in 55% to 90% of untreated patients. Intraesophageal resting pressure is higher than intragastric pressure, which is the reverse of normal. The most important manometric finding is the demonstration of incomplete lower esophageal sphincter relaxation after a swallow.

(474–C) ***(S&F, p. 457)***

The distal esophagus drains via lymphatics into the celiac and gastric nodes. Although roughly separated into thirds, the entire lymphatic system is richly interconnected. This, coupled with the absence of a serosa over most of the esophagus, complicates surgical treatment of esophageal cancers.

(475–C) ***(S&F, pp. 502–503)***

The two principal mechanisms of esophageal acid clearance are esophageal peristalsis and neutralization of acid by salivary bicarbonate. Of the two, swallowed saliva is the most important with regard to restoring intraesophageal pH.

(476–A, B, C, D) ***(S&F, pp. 500–501)***

Transient lower esophageal relaxations are a normal, physiologic response to gastric distention by food or gas and allow for belching. The spontaneous relaxation persists for ten or more seconds, twice as long as a swallow-induced relaxation. Patients with gastroesophageal reflux disease have more frequent and more prolonged tLESRs.

(477–C) ***(S&F, p. 508)***

Pregnant women typically suffer from gastroesophageal reflux disease (GERD) but rarely have histologic esophagitis. The two conditions are not the same. GERD encompasses all aspects of GERD, whereas esophagitis specifically indicates mucosal injury. Esophagitis complicates Sjögren's syndrome because of xerostomia and the resulting inability of saliva to neutralize normally refluxed acid. Patients with scleroderma have severe esophageal dysmotility with resulting poor acid clearance and consequent esophagitis; they may also be troubled with Sjögren's syndrome, compounding the problem. Hypersecretory states such as Zollinger-Ellison syndrome are often complicated by esophagitis.

(478–D) ***(S&F, p. 465)***

The Plummer-Vinson, or Patterson-Brown-Kelly, syndrome refers to the association of upper esophageal webs with iron deficiency, benign cervical esophageal webs, and an increased risk of squamous carcinoma. The benign webs may resolve with treatment of the iron deficiency.

(479–D) ***(S&F, pp. 480–481)***

The modified barium swallow with videofluoroscopy demonstrates more aspects of oropharyngeal swallowing than any other technique. Routine barium swallow without videofluoroscopy, endoscopy, and chest computed tomography cannot adequately evaluate the rapid sequence of motor events in the region.

(480–D) ***(S&F, p. 502)***

Secretin, progesterone, cholecystokinin, and somatostatin along with gastric inhibitory polypeptide and vasoactive intestinal polypeptide decrease lower esophageal pressure, whereas gastrin, motilin, and substance P have been reported to have the opposite effect.

(481–C) ***(S&F, p. 473)***

The resting lower esophageal sphincter (LES) pressure approximates 20 mm Hg and is influenced by a number of neural and humoral factors. The muscular elements of the LES are calcium dependent, hence the inhibitory effect of calcium channel blockade. As part of a reflex mechanism, the LES relaxes after almost every swallow to allow passage of a bolus. Neither truncal vagotomy nor selective vagotomy has any influence on LES tone, responsiveness, or degree of relaxation.

(482–C) ***(S&F, p. 540)***

Alcohol and tobacco in combination result in an increased risk of esophageal carcinoma. In the United States, alcohol alone is not an independent risk factor. Achalasia is associated with a 16-fold increased risk of carcinoma that is delayed for an average of 20 years. Tylosis, a rare hyperkeratotic condition affecting the palms and soles, carries a 95% risk of esophageal cancer by age 65.

(483–D) ***(S&F, pp. 529–530)***

A growing list of commonly used medications may cause pill esophagitis. A careful history will usually elicit the diagnosis.

(484–A) ***(S&F, pp. 521–522)***

Fluconazole is as effective as ketoconazole in patients with the acquired immunodeficiency syndrome (AIDS), but fluconazole has the added advantage of antifungal activity in the setting of achlorhydria, which is present in many patients with AIDS. Clotrimazole may also be useful if the immune system is not severely depressed. Amphotericin is most useful in granulocytopenic patients with esophageal candidiasis.

(485–C) **(S&F, p. 487)**

Chest pain is reported in 80% to 90% of patients with diffuse esophageal spasm. The second most common symptom is dysphagia, which is reported in 30% to 60% of patients. Heartburn is reported in approximately 20% of patients. Regurgitation and odynophagia are rarely reported.

(486–D) **(S&F, pp. 460–461)**

The respiratory tract and the gut begin as a single tube and separate at two months of gestation. Failure to separate completely results in abnormal communications between the gut and respiratory tract. The most common of these, accounting for 85% of tracheoesophageal fistulas, is one with the proximal esophagus ending in a blind pouch and a fistula connecting the trachea with the distal esophagus. Such infants present with drooling, aspiration, and air in the gastrointestinal tract on abdominal radiographs.

(487–B) **(S&F, p. 502)**

β-Adrenergic agonists inhibit sphincter tone through β_1 and β_2 receptors, resulting in decreased muscle contractility and decreased acetylcholine release.

(488–C) **(S&F, pp. 487–489)**

Several types of manometric findings are included under diffuse esophageal spasm. The most consistent finding is nonperistaltic (simultaneous) contractions after swallows. However, many patients with esophageal spasm have peristaltic waves that are abnormal in amplitude or duration. The term *nutcracker esophagus* has been applied to patients with esophageal spasm associated with a marked increase in contraction amplitudes. Most patients with diffuse esophageal spasm have an elevation in resting lower

sphincter pressure; however, poor relaxation of the lower esophageal sphincter is not a feature of this disorder.

(489–C) **(S&F, pp. 499–500)**

There are four predominant mucosal patterns seen with Barrett's esophagus. In order of decreasing frequency they are (1) specialized columnar epithelium, (2) junctional or cardia type, (3) fundic type, and (4) indeterminate.

(490–A) **(S&F, pp. 504–505)**

Although several components of refluxed gastric contents are believed to render the esophageal mucosa more susceptible to injury, it is the hydrogen ion that diffuses into esophageal mucosa, causing inflammation and necrosis.

(491–A) **(S&F, pp. 479–486)**

Sublingual isosorbide dinitrate improves symptoms and radionuclide transit in the majority of patients with achalasia. However, placebo-controlled trials of calcium channel blockers have not demonstrated any consistent clinical benefits. Manometry is not able to distinguish idiopathic achalasia from any of the disorders that mimic achalasia, such as malignancy, amyloidosis, sarcoidosis, and Chagas' disease. Esophageal carcinoma has been reported in association with achalasia with rates as high as 20%. More meticulous studies report rates ranging from 2% to 7%.

(492–D) **Normal anatomic relationships (S&F, p. 458)**
Dysphagia lusoria (S&F, p. 463)

The aberrant right subclavian artery arises from the aorta below the left subclavian and courses posterior to the esophagus to the right arm. When an aberrant right subclavian artery causes esophageal obstruction, the term *dysphagia lusoria* is used and can be presumptively diagnosed at endoscopy by noting a diminished right radial pulse when the indentation is compressed by the endoscope.

Biliary Tract

S&F Section VIII

493. Each of the following is a true statement about cholangiography during laparoscopic cholecystectomy EXCEPT:
A. Cholangiography may detect unsuspected common bile duct stones.
B. Cholangiography confirms the physician's impression of the bile duct anatomy.
C. Between 8% and 16% of patients with biliary colic harbor common duct stones.
D. Ductal abnormalities are present in about 12% of cases.
E. All are true.

494. Each of the following is a true statement about treatment of common bile duct stones EXCEPT:
A. They should always be treated, because complications are common.
B. Endoscopic sphincterotomy successfully clears stones in 90% of cases.
C. Cholecystectomy should be performed to prevent passage of more stones.
D. Common bile duct stones found at laparoscopic cholecystectomy require conversion to open cholecystectomy with bile duct exploration.
E. Endoscopic sphincterotomy without cholecystectomy is appropriate for elderly or debilitated patients.

495. Each of the following is a true statement about laparoscopic cholecystectomy EXCEPT:
A. Mean operating time is longer than open cholecystectomy.
B. Hospital stay is about one third that of open cholecystectomy.
C. Standard procedure requires three small laparotomy incisions in the abdomen.
D. No controlled data comparing laparoscopic and open cholecystectomy exist.
E. The most common complication is infection of the wound site.

496. Which of the following are TRUE statements about primary sclerosing cholangitis (PSC) associated with inflammatory bowel disease?
A. PSC occurs in 2% to 4% of patients with inflammatory bowel disease.
B. Patients with pancolitis are more likely to have PSC than patients with proctitis.
C. Two thirds of patients with PSC have inflammatory bowel disease.

D. PSC occurs less commonly in Crohn's disease than in ulcerative colitis.
E. Proctocolectomy can often arrest or retard the progression of PSC.

497. Which of the following patients with incidentally discovered, asymptomatic gallstones would be the LEAST acceptable candidate for a prophylactic laparoscopic cholecystectomy?
A. A 21-year-old woman with sickle cell anemia
B. A 21-year-old woman of Amerindian ancestry
C. A 48-year-old woman awaiting renal transplantation
D. A 58-year-old man with mildly symptomatic coronary artery disease
E. A 38-year-old female astronaut planning prolonged space travel

498. Which of the following are TRUE statements regarding the management of cholangiocarcinoma?
A. Preoperative biliary decompression lowers operative mortality.
B. Proximal tumors are managed with a Roux-en-Y hepaticojejunostomy.
C. Unresectable tumors may be palliated with biliary stents.
D. Adjuvant radiation therapy improves survival.
E. Adjuvant chemotherapy with 5-fluorouracil improves survival.
F. Liver transplantation offers a 5-year survival of more than 50%.

499. All of the following are acceptable selection criteria for consideration of oral bile acid dissolution therapy for gallstones EXCEPT:
A. Symptomatic stone without a history of complications such as acute cholecystitis
B. Opacification of the gallbladder on oral cholecystography
C. Radiolucency of the stone(s) on a plain abdominal film
D. Single stone, diameter 15 mm
E. Multiple stones, diameter of all less than 5 mm

500. Which of the following statements regarding extracorporeal shock wave lithotripsy are TRUE?
A. Stone fragments less than 3 mm in diameter can usually pass into the intestine without causing symptoms.

B. Lithotripsy may be used as an adjunct to bile acid dissolution therapy.

C. Unlike bile acid dissolution alone, extracorporeal lithotripsy does not require a functioning gallbladder before treatment.

D. Multiple small stones are easier to treat than a single larger stone.

E. In highly selected patients, efficacy may approach 70%.

501. Important factor(s) in determining survival after hepatic portoenterostomy for biliary atresia include:
  I. Operation performed within 90 days of birth
  II. Cirrhosis
  III. Racial background

  A. I only
  B. II only
  C. I and II
  D. II and III
  E. All of the above

502. Each of the following is a proven risk factor for bile duct carcinoma EXCEPT:
  A. Caroli's disease
  B. Infection with *Clonorchis sinensis*
  C. Primary sclerosing cholangitis
  D. Gallstones
  E. Environmental carcinogens

503. Biliary disease in cystic fibrosis may include:
  I. Features consistent with idiopathic giant cell hepatitis and extrahepatic biliary atresia
  II. Mild elevation of aminotransferases and marked elevation of alkaline phosphatase
  III. Strictures of the common bile duct
  IV. Agenesis of the gallbladder

  A. I and III
  B. II and IV
  C. I, II, and III
  D. All of the above

504. Which one of the following statements regarding gallstone formation is NOT true?
  A. Up to 20% of patients with biliary sludge go on to have gallstones or acute cholecystitis.
  B. Gallbladder mucus may help prevent gallstones.
  C. Aspirin may help prevent gallstones.
  D. After an overnight fast, 80% to 90% of bile water is removed by the gallbladder, resulting in a concentrated bile.
  E. In the absence of a gallbladder, cholesterol gallstones rarely form.

505. Which of the following are TRUE statements regarding type I choledochal cysts?
  A. They account for less than 10% of choledochal cysts.

B. They exhibit segmental or diffuse fusiform dilatation of the common bile ducts.

C. They are true choledochal diverticula.

D. They consist of multiple intrahepatic and extrahepatic cysts.

506. Match the following statements to the disease entity. Each selection may be used once, more than once, or not at all.
  1. Abdominal pain is common
  2. Higher incidence among women
  3. Younger patient population
  4. Courvoisier's sign may be present
  5. Often presents as cholangitis

  A. Carcinoma of the gallbladder
  B. Carcinoma of the bile duct
  C. Both
  D. Neither

507. Which of the following are TRUE statements about dissolution therapy of gallstones?
  A. Ursodeoxycholate is less toxic than chenodeoxycholate.
  B. A single large stone will dissolve more rapidly than multiple small stones.
  C. The diameter of the stone decreases linearly with time.
  D. Ursodeoxycholate may cause an increase in serum cholesterol.
  E. Chenodeoxycholate may cause diarrhea.
  F. Stones with a computed tomographic density of less than 100 Hounsfield units are less likely to dissolve.

508. The most common presentation of gallbladder carcinoma is:
  A. A palpable mass in the right upper quadrant
  B. Jaundice
  C. Abdominal pain
  D. Cholangitis

509. Each of the following statements regarding the embryologic development of the liver and biliary tract is true EXCEPT:
  A. Primitive hepatocytes give rise to intrahepatic bile ducts.
  B. The liver develops from two primordia: the liver diverticulum and the septum transversum.
  C. The septum transversum gives rise primarily to the gallbladder, cystic duct, and common bile duct.
  D. Hepatic sinusoids arise from vitelline veins and serve as templates for the growth of hepatocytes.

510. Which of the following statements regarding primary bile acids are TRUE?
  A. Chenodeoxycholic acid, deoxycholic acid, and cholic acid are primary bile acids.
  B. Primary bile acids are formed from cholesterol in the liver.

C. Primary bile acids are conjugated with taurine or glycine to form conjugated bile acids.

D. Biotransformation of cholesterol to a primary bile acid involves 7α-hydroxylation and an epimerization of the 3α-hydroxy group.

511. Which one of the following is the MOST important physiologic stimulant of gallbladder contraction?
A. Vagal efferent fibers (cholinergic)
B. Motilin
C. Cholecystokinin (CCK)
D. Parasympathetic stimulation
E. Endogenous opiate release

512. Match the type of gallstone with its usual gross or microscopic description.
1. Cholesterol	A. Small, crumble easily, abundant mucin glycoproteins
2. Mixed	
3. Black pigment	B. Multiple, generally faceted
4. Brown pigment	C. Contain bacterial skeletons
	D. Large, often solitary

513. Each of the following statements concerning endoscopic biliary manometry is true EXCEPT:
A. A triple-lumen catheter and a constant perfusion system are used.
B. Angulation of the cannula should be avoided at all times.
C. Pressure is recorded while the catheter is advanced into the desired duct.
D. Sedation is accomplished with benzodiazepines and meperidine.

514. Which of the following are TRUE statements regarding gallbladder carcinoma?
A. The incidence in the United States is increasing.
B. There is a male preponderance.
C. Most cases occur in patients older than the age of 50.
D. Major advances in treatment have been made recently.

515. Children receiving parenteral nutrition are at increased risk for:
A. Reye's syndrome
B. Acalculous cholecystitis
C. Duodenal atresia
D. Pyogenic liver abscess

516. Which of the following statements regarding treatment of sphincter of Oddi dysfunction are TRUE?
A. Endoscopic sphincterotomy may relieve symptoms in patients with elevated resting basal pressures.
B. Surgical sphincteroplasty and endoscopic sphincterotomy are equally effective for patients with sphincter of Oddi stenosis.

C. Medical therapy with nitrates or oral nifedipine has been found to reduce pain, especially in patients with the milder type III sphincter of Oddi dysfunction.
D. Pancreatic sphincterotomy may be warranted in patients with pancreatic sphincter dysfunction and recurrent pancreatitis who did not respond to biliary sphincterotomy.

517. Each of the following is a true statement regarding common duct stones EXCEPT:
A. Alkaline phosphatase levels correlate with the degree of obstruction.
B. About 95% of patients with common duct stones also have gallbladder stones.
C. About 15% of patients with gallbladder stones also have common duct stones.
D. Cirrhotics and those with intermittent obstruction may exhibit no ductal dilation.
E. Bilirubin levels are typically 2 to 5 mg/dL and rarely exceed 12 mg/dL.

518. Which of the following statements regarding adjunctive tests for diagnosing gallbladder disease is FALSE?
A. Endoscopic retrograde cholangiopancreatography with filling of the gallbladder often detects stones missed by ultrasonography.
B. Examination of bile for cholesterol crystals is both sensitive and specific for cholesterol gallstones.
C. Abdominal computed tomography is as good as ultrasonography for detecting gallstones.
D. A gallbladder ejection fraction of less than 35% after cholecystokinin administration suggests disease.

519. Which of the following are TRUE statements regarding the natural history of gallstones?
A. The risk of asymptomatic stones becoming symptomatic is about 2% per year initially, less thereafter.
B. After an initial attack of biliary colic, the lifetime risk of recurrent attacks is approximately 70%.
C. The risk of developing biliary tract complications (cholangitis or pancreatitis) in patients with symptomatic gallstones is 1% to 2% per year.
D. Sixty to 80 percent of all gallstones are asymptomatic.

520. A patient with suspected choledocholithiasis is considered for endoscopic sphincterotomy and stone removal. In discussing the risk of sphincterotomy with the patient, which of the following complications is LEAST likely to occur?
A. Perforation of the periampullary duodenum
B. Hemorrhage
C. Impaction of the basket in the bile duct

D. Ascending cholangitis
E. Acute pancreatitis

521. Which of the following are TRUE statements about gallstone disease in children?
A. Gallstones in infants formed during parenteral nutrition may resolve spontaneously.
B. Laparoscopic cholecystectomy is rarely feasible in children.
C. Cholecystectomy is indicated for asymptomatic gallstones.
D. Chronic hemolysis is the most common cause of gallstones.
E. Long-term parenteral nutrition is an increasingly important cause of gallstones.

522. Each of the following statements concerning the pain of biliary colic is true EXCEPT:
A. It typically comes on gradually and lasts for an hour or more.
B. It is more common in the epigastrium than in the right upper quadrant.
C. It is usually precipitated by eating a meal.
D. It radiates to the back or other areas in more than half of patients.
E. Most patients have associated vomiting and diaphoresis.

523. Regarding cholangiocarcinoma, each of the following contraindicates resection for possible cure EXCEPT:
A. Vascular invasion of the portal vein
B. Perihilar adenopathy
C. Tumor invading the underside of the liver
D. Tumor extending into the intrahepatic ducts

524. Which of the following are TRUE statements about the enterohepatic circulation of bile acids?
A. More than 90% of secreted bile acids are reabsorbed by the small intestine.
B. Hepatic uptake of bile acids from blood is sluggish compared with ileal uptake from the intestine.
C. During fasting, most bile acids are found in the gallbladder.
D. During fasting after cholecystectomy, most bile acids are found in the liver.

525. Each of the following statements regarding ursodeoxycholate treatment of gallstones is true EXCEPT:
A. Unlike chenodeoxycholate, ursodeoxycholate can dissolve stones irrespective of their composition.
B. Dissolution with ursodeoxycholate is achieved in up to 70% of selected patients.
C. Ursodeoxycholate is much more expensive than chenodeoxycholate.
D. Ursodeoxycholate, unlike chenodeoxycholate, causes neither diarrhea or hepatotoxicity.

E. Recurrence of gallstones after successful dissolution is a problem.

526. Match the following statements to the correct patient group classification. Each selection may be used once, more than once, or not at all.
1. Patients have biliary-type pain.
2. Sphincter of Oddi stenosis is the most likely diagnosis; therefore, biliary manometry is optional.
3. Sphincter of Oddi manometry is essential for diagnosis.
4. Sphincter of Oddi dysfunction is unlikely; therefore, biliary manometry is of little value.

A. Sphincter of Oddi dysfunction: biliary group I
B. Sphincter of Oddi dysfunction: biliary group II
C. Sphincter of Oddi dysfunction: biliary group III
D. All of the above

527. An autosomal dominant disorder characterized by a decreased number of interlobular bile ducts, chronic cholestasis, and dysmorphic facies is:
A. Primary biliary cirrhosis
B. Alagille's syndrome
C. Caroli's disease
D. Biliary atresia

528. Which of the following statements about cholesterol polyps of the gallbladder are TRUE?
A. They are the most common type of gallbladder polyp.
B. They are a form of cholesterolosis of the gallbladder.
C. They are typically sessile.
D. They are often greater than 20 mm in diameter.
E. They are usually solitary.

529. Which of the following statements regarding acquired immunodeficiency syndrome (AIDS) cholangiography (infectious sclerosing cholangitis) are TRUE?
A. Patients generally present with pain, elevated alkaline phosphatase level, and jaundice.
B. Endoscopic sphincterotomy is warranted if a bile duct stone is present.
C. Endoscopic sphincterotomy with placement of an endoprosthesis is warranted to relieve persistent right upper quadrant pain.
D. Cholangiographic findings resemble those of primary sclerosing cholangitis.

530. The endoscopic approach to biliary cholangiography is preferred over the percutaneous approach in each of the following EXCEPT:
A. Patients with suspected ampullary lesions
B. Patients with prior biliary-enteric surgery

C. Patients with need to minimize morbidity and recovery time

D. Patients with suspected pancreatic lesions

---

531. Each of the following statements regarding the anatomy of the biliary tract is true EXCEPT:

A. The common bile duct and common hepatic duct possess a mucosa, submucosa, and muscularis.

B. The arterial supply of the bile ducts comes mainly from the right hepatic artery.

C. The right and left hepatic ducts merge inside the liver in the majority of cases.

D. The cystic duct may run a variable course before joining the medial aspect of the common bile duct.

---

532. Regarding the placement of a biliary endoprosthesis for the treatment of bile duct obstruction (either benign or malignant), which of the following statements are TRUE?

A. Stent occlusion is to be expected, with the mean time to occlusion ranging from 1 to 12 months.

B. The most frequent early complications after stent placement are due to the accompanying sphincterotomy.

C. Proximal bile duct lesions are more effectively drained than periampullary lesions.

D. Occluded stents usually become manifest by mild signs and symptoms rather than by frank cholangitis.

---

533. At first presentation, biliary atresia is associated with:

I. Hepatomegaly

II. Ascites

III. Coagulopathy

IV. Edema

A. I and III

B. II and IV

C. I, II, and III

D. All of the above

---

534. Acquired immunodeficiency syndrome (AIDS) cholangiopathy is commonly associated with each of the following EXCEPT:

A. Right upper quadrant pain

B. Jaundice

C. Cholangiographic findings resembling sclerosing cholangitis

D. Relief of pain after endoscopic sphincterotomy

---

535. Sphincter of Oddi dysfunction may play a causal role in all of the following EXCEPT:

A. Postcholecystectomy pain

B. Irritable bowel syndrome

C. Recurrent acute pancreatitis

D. Cholestasis

---

536. Each of the following is a common complication of percutaneous transhepatic biliary drainage EXCEPT:

A. Cholangitis

B. Sepsis

C. Pancreatitis

D. Bleeding

---

537. A 62-year-old woman presents to the emergency department complaining of a one-day history of unrelenting right upper quadrant and epigastric pain, nausea, and one episode of vomiting. Her past history is remarkable for a remote duodenal ulcer seen on an upper gastrointestinal series that also incidentally showed a periampullary duodenal diverticulum. On physical examination she is febrile to 38.8° C and has right upper quadrant tenderness without rebound. Bowel sounds are diminished. Laboratory data are remarkable for a white blood cell count of 16,500 cells/mm^3, total bilirubin value of 2.4 mg/dL, alkaline phosphatase level of 324 IU/L, aspartate aminotransferase value of 74 IU/L, and amylase value of 85 IU/L. An emergent abdominal ultrasound evaluation shows gallstones and a common bile duct that is dilated to 13 mm. Based on the most likely diagnosis, which of the following would be the most appropriate treatment?

A. Endoscopic retrograde cholangiopancreatography with sphincterotomy

B. Emergent cholecystectomy and common bile duct exploration

C. Percutaneous transhepatic biliary drainage

D. Supportive measures including intravenous fluids and antibiotics

---

538. Each of the following is a true statement regarding benign tumors of the gallbladder EXCEPT:

A. The most common lesions are "pseudotumors" (cholesterol polyps).

B. Adenomyomas are more likely to occur in the fundus.

C. The imaging study should be repeated in three to six months to assess growth.

D. Adenomas may harbor small foci of adenocarcinoma.

---

539. Which of the following statements concerning acute cholecystitis are TRUE?

A. Nausea and vomiting precede the onset of pain.

B. Acute cholecystitis can be aborted with nonsteroidal anti-inflammatory drug (NSAID) treatments.

C. Cholecystitis is rare in the absence of gallstones.

D. Cholescintigraphy has no role in diagnosing acute cholecystitis.

E. Mirizzi's syndrome is obstruction of the common bile duct due to a stone in the cystic duct.

---

540. Each of the following is a risk factor for gallstones EXCEPT:

A. Elevated serum cholesterol

B. Amerindian ancestry
C. Obesity
D. Weight loss
E. Total parenteral nutrition

541. Which of the following is the MOST frequent result of a chronically obstructed cystic duct after inflammation of the gallbladder subsides?
A. Porcelain gallbladder
B. Small, scarred gallbladder with luminal obliteration
C. Cancer of the gallbladder
D. Hydrops of the gallbladder
E. Polypoid gallbladder

542. Which one of the following statements regarding cholecystectomy is FALSE?
A. It is indicated for most symptomatic patients.
B. It causes complete relief of symptoms in over 80% of patients.
C. It should be avoided in elderly patients unless symptoms are severe.
D. It is considerably more hazardous in patients with portal hypertension.
E. It produces no measurable alterations in digestion or absorption.

543. Which of the following are TRUE statements about the complications of primary sclerosing cholangitis (PSC)?
A. Malabsorption of vitamin B_{12} is common, and monthly injections are recommended.
B. The pancreatic duct is often scarred and beaded in patients with PSC.
C. Cholangiocarcinoma is present in 30% to 40% of patients dying with PSC.
D. Hepatocellular carcinoma is rare in PSC.
E. Most patients in whom cholangiocarcinoma is found incidentally at liver transplantation do not develop metastatic disease.

544. Regarding gallstone pathogenesis, which one of the following statements is NOT true?
A. Intermittent secretion of saturated bile is common.
B. Bile contains proteins that delay cholesterol nucleation and crystallization.
C. Gallbladder motility is important for preventing gallstones.
D. Excretion of more than 1 g of cholesterol per day carries an increased risk.
E. Cholesterol solubility depends on bile salts and phospholipids in bile.

545. Which of the following statements regarding porcelain gallbladder are TRUE?
A. Spontaneous opacification of the gallbladder lumen is seen on plain films owing to concentrated calcium salts in bile.

B. The diagnosis is made by demonstrating intramural calcifications within the gallbladder wall on either plain abdominal films or abdominal computed tomography.
C. When an asymptomatic porcelain gallbladder is incidentally diagnosed in an otherwise healthy subject, careful annual follow-up with ultrasonography is warranted to screen for mass lesions of the gallbladder.
D. The lifetime risk of gallbladder cancer in porcelain gallbladder is 20%.

546. Match the following ultrasound features with the type of cholecystitis with which they are associated.
1. "Sonographic Murphy's sign"
2. Thickened gallbladder wall (>4 mm)
3. Gallbladder contents cast a shadow
4. Pericholecystic fluid collection
5. Dilation of the common bile duct more than 14 mm

A. Acalculous cholecystitis
B. Calculous cholecystitis
C. Both
D. Neither

547. Transport mechanisms have been identified in the canalicular membrane for each of the following EXCEPT:
A. Trihydroxy bile acids
B. Water
C. Conjugated bilirubin
D. Organic cations
E. Bicarbonate

548. Each of the following is a proven risk factor for carcinoma of the gallbladder EXCEPT:
A. Cigarette smoking
B. Gallstones
C. Environmental carcinogens
D. Native American background

549. Which of the following are TRUE statements about the pathology of primary sclerosing cholangitis?
A. Granulomas are commonly seen in portal tracts.
B. The gross appearance of the bile ducts is that of a thickened, hardened cord.
C. Lymph node enlargement may be present.
D. Biopsy may show periductular concentric fibrosis around interlobular bile ducts.
E. Proliferation of smaller bile ducts is seen in early disease.

550. Each of the following is a known risk factor for cholesterol gallstone formation EXCEPT:
A. Female gender
B. Hypercholesterolemia
C. Obesity
D. Rapid weight loss
E. Pregnancy

551. Each of the following should be part of a preoperative evaluation before gallstone surgery EXCEPT:
   A. Chest radiography
   B. Serum alkaline phosphatase determination
   C. Ultrasonography of the biliary tree
   D. Screen for signs and symptoms of congestive heart failure
   E. Electrocardiography

552. Which of the following are TRUE statements regarding treatment of gallbladder carcinoma?
   A. Symptomatic gallbladder cancers have an extremely poor prognosis with fewer than 10% cured by resection.
   B. Eighty percent of tumors occur in patients with gallstones.
   C. For most patients, palliation with biliary stents is the only therapy.
   D. "Incidental" cancer discovered in a gallbladder resected for biliary colic portends a poor prognosis.

553. The average bile acid pool size and the average number of times that it circulates per day are:
   A. Pool size 12 to 15 g and circulation 1 to 2 times
   B. Pool size 2 to 4 g and circulation 1 to 2 times
   C. Pool size 2 to 4 g and circulation 3 to 12 times
   D. Pool size 12 to 15 g and circulation 3 to 12 times

554. Percutaneous cholecystostomy is indicated in each of the following situations EXCEPT:
   A. Acute calculous cholecystitis in high-risk operative candidates
   B. Acute calculous cholecystitis with suspected choledocholithiasis
   C. To access the bile duct when the transhepatic approach has failed
   D. Acute acalculous cholecystitis as definitive therapy

555. A 24-year-old woman presents to your office with intermittent right upper quadrant pain for one month. It is not related to meals or ingestion of fatty foods. On physical examination she is mildly icteric and has a palpable mass in the right upper quadrant. Laboratory tests show mildly elevated aminotransferase, alkaline phosphatase, and total bilirubin levels. An abdominal ultrasound evaluation reveals a cystic lesion adjacent to the common bile duct and is otherwise unremarkable. What is the MOST likely diagnosis?
   A. Recurrent cholangiohepatitis
   B. Caroli's disease
   C. Choledochal cyst
   D. Hepatocellular carcinoma

556. With reference to the patient in question 555, what would be your recommended treatment?
   A. Ursodiol therapy
   B. Surgical resection
   C. Symptomatic treatment for abdominal pain
   D. Antibiotic therapy

557. Regarding treatment for ampullary carcinoma, which of the following statements is TRUE?
   A. Resection for cure is possible in less than 25% of patients.
   B. The Whipple procedure is the surgical treatment of choice.
   C. Regardless of therapy, overall five-year survival is less than 10%.
   D. Stenting rarely offers effective palliation.

558. Which of the following are TRUE statements about the presenting features of primary sclerosing cholangitis?
   A. Most patient are between 25 and 45 years of age.
   B. Males are more commonly affected than females.
   C. The most common presentation is right upper quadrant pain with fever.
   D. The spleen is enlarged in one third of patients, sometimes massively.
   E. The alkaline phosphatase level is rarely elevated more than five times normal.

559. Each of the following statements regarding the clinical features of acute cholecystitis is true EXCEPT:
   A. Mild jaundice is present in 20% to 40% of patients.
   B. Murphy's sign is a palpable, tender mass in the right upper quadrant.
   C. The temperature rarely rises above 102° F.
   D. Pain is poorly localized at first, then shifts to the right upper quadrant.
   E. More than half of unoperated cases resolve spontaneously.

560. A bile leak after gallbladder or bile duct surgery is BEST managed by:
   A. Immediate surgery
   B. Placement of a nasobiliary catheter
   C. Supportive measures, including intravenous fluids and antibiotics
   D. Percutaneous drainage of the biloma

561. Which of the following are TRUE statements regarding the sphincter of Oddi?
   A. Normal baseline pressures are lower than common bile duct pressures.
   B. Most phasic contraction waves propagate in an antegrade fashion.
   C. It can pump bile into the duodenum.

D. The sphincter prevents reflux of duodenal contents.

562. Each of the following statements about open cholecystectomy is true EXCEPT:
    A. The mortality rate is directly related to age and is less than 0.1% for patients younger than age 65.
    B. Perioperative myocardial infarction is the most common cause of death.
    C. The rate of complications, including bile leaks, pancreatitis, and bile duct injury, is 4% to 5%.
    D. Acute cholecystitis has little effect on the perioperative mortality.

563. Match each of the following factors with the type of cholecystitis with which it is associated.
    1. Middle-aged patients
    2. Elderly patients
    3. Female gender
    4. Male gender
    5. Right upper quadrant symptoms common at presentation
    6. Right upper quadrant symptoms uncommon at presentation
    7. Mortality about 1%
    8. Mortality greater than 10%
    9. Otherwise healthy patient
    10. Chronically debilitated patient

    A. Acalculous cholecystitis
    B. Calculous cholecystitis
    C. Both
    D. Neither

564. Each of the following statements regarding oral cholecystography is true EXCEPT:
    A. It measures cystic duct obstruction and gallbladder function better than ultrasonography.
    B. About 25% of normal persons do not opacify after a single dose.
    C. The rate of false-negative results is greater than that for ultrasonography.
    D. It requires normal intestinal absorption and hepatic secretion of dye.
    E. It provides useful information about the degree of calcification of the stones.

565. A 45-year-old woman with three episodes of biliary colic and nausea over the past six months is found on ultrasonography to have several gallstones measuring 4 to 7 mm in diameter. The stones are radiolucent, and the gallbladder opacifies on oral cholecystography. She is frightened of surgery and wants to discuss her options with respect to oral dissolution therapy with ursodiol. Which of the following statements are TRUE and should be discussed with the patient?
    A. In her case, ursodiol therapy has approximately a 40% chance of success.
    B. If the ursodiol were to work, the average time required for complete dissolution would be 6 to 12 months.
    C. Side effects of ursodiol include pruritus and hypercholesterolemia.

D. As the stones dissolve, biliary colic may be expected to temporarily worsen.
E. Even before the stones dissolve, biliary colic and nausea may lessen.

566. In a patient with cholangitis and a hilar tumor involving both intrahepatic ducts, the preferred management involves:
    A. Supportive therapy with antibiotics
    B. Endoscopic retrograde cholangiopancreatography and stent placement
    C. Percutaneous drainage of both right and left systems
    D. Percutaneous drainage of either the right or the left biliary systems

567. Caroli's disease is associated with:
    A. Segmental saccular dilatation of the intrahepatic ducts
    B. Congenital hepatic fibrosis
    C. Male preponderance
    D. All of the above

568. Each of the following statements about the efficacy of bile acid dissolution therapy for gallstones is true EXCEPT:
    A. It is much lower for stones less than 5 to 10 mm in diameter.
    B. Pretreatment fragmentation of stones may increase efficacy.
    C. Symptoms often get worse during treatment as smaller stones are passed.
    D. In the best patients, complete dissolution is achieved in 20% to 70%.
    E. Floating stones are more likely to dissolve than nonfloating stones.

569. Each of the following is a true statement about acalculous cholecystitis EXCEPT:
    A. It accounts for less than 1% of all cholecystectomies.
    B. It should be treated similarly to calculous cholecystitis.
    C. Predisposing factors include fasting, immobility, and hemodynamic instability.
    D. It can be prevented by administering cholecystokinin or lipid emulsions to stimulate gallbladder emptying.
    E. It has a substantially worse prognosis than calculous cholecystitis.

570. Each of the following is a common radiologic feature of gallbladder carcinoma EXCEPT:
    A. Porcelain gallbladder
    B. Gallstones
    C. Stricture of the common hepatic duct
    D. Fluid around the gallbladder

571. With respect to formation of brown pigment gallstones, which one of the following statements is NOT true?
A. They are the most common stone in patients with hemolytic disorders.
B. Their formation is probably triggered by bacterial infection.
C. Their incidence increases with age.
D. Females are at greater risk than males.
E. They may develop *de novo* in bile ducts.

572. The most common type of biliary atresia, associated with atresia of the common bile, hepatic, and cystic ducts at or above the porta hepatis, is called:
A. Type I
B. Type IIa
C. Type IIb
D. Type III

573. Match the following agents with their effect on sphincter of Oddi activity. Each selection may be used once, more than once, or not at all.
1. Anticholinergics
2. Glucagon
3. Morphine
4. Nitroglycerin
5. Calcium channel blockers
A. Inhibition
B. Stimulation

574. Each of the following is a true statement regarding carcinoma of the ampulla of Vater EXCEPT:
A. Cholangitis is more frequent than in gallbladder carcinoma.
B. Abdominal pain is a common presenting feature.
C. Jaundice may be intermittent.
D. Patients may present with pancreatitis.

575. Each of the following statements regarding the incidence of gallstones is true EXCEPT:
A. Females are affected more often than males.
B. Whites are affected more often than blacks.
C. Women with multiple pregnancies are affected less often.
D. Native Americans are affected more often than the general population.
E. The incidence of gallstones increases with age.

576. Each of the following statements regarding gallbladder anatomy is true EXCEPT:
A. Gallstones are most likely to perforate into the right colic gutter.
B. The cystic artery is an end artery that puts the gallbladder at risk for ischemic injury.
C. Venous drainage is provided entirely by the cystic vein.
D. Rokitansky-Aschoff sinuses are a potential source of infection, owing to chronic bacterial stasis.

577. Which of the following are TRUE statements regarding sphincter of Oddi dysfunction?
A. Pain is caused by spasm.
B. The most reliable abnormality is an elevated resting basal pressure.
C. Medical therapy can relieve pain.
D. Choledochal dysfunction predicts dysfunction in the pancreatic sphincter.

578. Which of the following are TRUE statements about the cholangiographic appearance of primary sclerosing cholangitis (PSC)?
A. The cholangiographic impression of PSC should be confirmed by biopsy.
B. Adequate visualization may require balloon dilation of dominant strictures.
C. Most patients have both extrahepatic and intrahepatic ductal involvement.
D. The pruned appearance of the ducts in PSC is often confused with that caused by cirrhosis.
E. Saccular and diverticular outpouchings are commonly seen.

579. A 65-year-old man presents with right upper quadrant pain, chills, and confusion of two days' duration. On examination, his temperature is 39.5° C, blood pressure is 100/65 mm Hg, and tenderness without guarding is present over the liver. He is not jaundiced. Laboratory tests show a leukocyte count of 5100 cells/mm^3 with predominant immature forms and a total bilirubin value of 2.1 mg/dL. An emergency ultrasonogram shows multiple gallstones in the gallbladder and a 7-mm diameter common bile duct. Of the following, which is the most likely diagnosis?
A. Acute cholecystitis
B. Acute pancreatitis
C. Cholangitis
D. Liver abscess
E. Appendicitis

580. Which bile acid is rapidly lost from the enterohepatic circulation secondary to poor ileal absorption?
A. Cholic acid
B. Deoxycholic acid
C. Lithocholic acid
D. Chenodeoxycholic acid

581. Which of the following are included under the definition of primary sclerosing cholangitis?
A. Sclerosing cholangitis lacking any apparent etiology
B. Sclerosing cholangitis associated with inflammatory bowel disease
C. Sclerosing cholangitis associated with systemic fibrosing conditions
D. Sclerosing cholangitis associated with autoimmune disorders

E. Sclerosing cholangitis associated with opportunistic infections
F. Sclerosing cholangitis associated with congenital biliary anomalies
G. Sclerosing cholangitis due to vasculitis

582. Regarding ultrasonography of the gallbladder, all of the following are true EXCEPT:
A. Gallstones are most easily seen in a distended gallbladder.
B. Chronic cholecystitis is diagnosed by finding a thickened wall.
C. Diagnosis of gallstones requires echogenicity, mobility, and an acoustic shadow.
D. Stones as small as 1 to 2 mm may be detected.
E. Sludge does not produce an acoustic shadow.

583. Regarding gallstone ileus, which one of the following statements is FALSE?
A. The stone is almost always greater than 2.5 cm in diameter.
B. The most common cause is erosion of a gallstone into the duodenum.
C. The mortality rate is 15% to 20%.
D. Most patients are elderly women.
E. The most common site of obstruction is the mid-jejunum.

584. Which of the following are TRUE statements about phosphatidylcholine (lecithin) secreted in bile?
A. Biliary phosphatidylcholine is hydrolyzed to lysophosphatidylcholine in the gut lumen.
B. Lysophosphatidylcholine is re-esterified to form phosphatidylcholine in the enterocyte.
C. Phosphatidylcholine is absorbed in the form of chylomicrons.
D. Phosphatidylcholine molecules that enter the hepatocyte are re-secreted as biliary phospholipids.

585. Each of the following is a true statement regarding sphincter of Oddi dysfunction (SOD) EXCEPT:
A. Basal pressure is considered elevated if it exceeds 35 mm Hg.
B. Biliary manometry is unnecessary in SOD type I because the diagnosis can be established on the basis of history and appropriate laboratory and cholangiographic findings.
C. Sphincterotomy in the absence of biliary manometry can be recommended in SOD type III (symptoms alone without objective laboratory or cholangiographic abnormalities) because a substantial fraction of these patients will achieve pain relief.
D. Eighty-five percent of patients with SOD type I will have elevated basal sphincter pressure.
E. Twenty-five percent of patients with SOD type III will have elevated basal sphincter pressure.

586. Which of the following are TRUE statements regarding evaluation of a patient with suspected sphincter of Oddi dysfunction?
A. Cholangiography is required to rule out a structural lesion.
B. Patients with sphincter dysfunction consistently show a change in the diameter of the common bile duct with a lipid-rich meal or cholecystokinin ultrasonography.
C. Biliary manometry is the gold standard in the evaluation of sphincter of Oddi function.
D. Pain at the time of endoscopic retrograde cholangiopancreatography supports the diagnosis.

587. Each of the following is a true statement EXCEPT:
A. Bile acids are synthesized in the liver and kidney.
B. Bile flow can be divided into "bile acid–dependent" and "bile acid–independent" components.
C. Bile acids enter hepatocytes by means of a sodium-coupled, active transport mechanism.
D. Bile acids are secreted into the canaliculus by an adenosine triphosphate–dependent transport mechanism.
E. Bile acids act as detergents, causing membrane damage at high concentrations.

588. Biliary cholesterol is not efficiently reabsorbed from the small intestine.
A. True
B. False

589. Which of the following statements about gallbladder polyps are TRUE?
A. Most are not true neoplasms but are the results of lipid deposition or inflammation.
B. The most common form is cholesterol polyps, followed by adenomyomas.
C. Inflammatory polyps are small, sessile, and almost never cause problems.
D. Adenomas are benign neoplasms and are less common than gallbladder cancer.
E. The usual symptoms of gallbladder polyps include vague right upper quadrant discomfort.

590. Each of the following is a true statement regarding bile secretion EXCEPT:
A. Secretion begins at the level of the bile canaliculus.
B. Bile flows from zone 1 to zone 3 of the liver acinus.
C. Bile secretion starts at around the seventh month of gestation.
D. Bile is responsible for the color of meconium.

591. Which of the following is NOT a synonym for adenomyomatosis of the gallbladder?
A. Diverticulosis of the gallbladder

B. Rokitansky-Aschoff sinuses
C. Adenoma of the gallbladder
D. Cholecystitis glandularis proliferans
E. Adenomyomatous hyperplasia

---

592. Which of the following drugs is LEAST likely to increase the risk of gallstones?
A. 3-Hydroxy-3-methylglutaryl–coenzyme A (HMG CoA) reductase inhibitors (e.g., lovastatin)
B. Oral contraceptives
C. Octreotide
D. Clofibrate
E. Ceftriaxone

---

593. Each of the following statements regarding the ultrasonographic diagnosis of acute cholecystitis and choledocholithiasis is true EXCEPT:
A. The "ultrasonic Murphy's sign" is focal gallbladder tenderness under the transducer.
B. The sensitivity of ultrasonography for detecting gallstones (>2 mm in diameter) in the gallbladder exceeds 95%.
C. The sensitivity of ultrasonography for identifying gallstones in the common bile duct is 90%.
D. Thickening of the gallbladder wall (in the absence of hypoalbuminemia) is suggestive of acute cholecystitis.
E. Pericholecystic fluid (in the absence of hypoalbuminemia) is suggestive of acute cholecystitis.

---

594. Each of the following statements regarding cholesterolosis of the gallbladder is true EXCEPT:
A. It is a histologic condition in which the macrophages in the gallbladder wall acquire excess cholesterol esters.
B. It is found in about 4% of gallbladders at autopsy.
C. It includes cholesterol polyps, which may be mistaken for gallstones.
D. It usually does not cause symptoms.
E. It may predispose to recurrent pancreatitis.

Biliary Tract

■■■■■*Answers*

(493–E)   **(S&F, p. 975)**

Although the value of routine cholangiography during open cholecystectomy has been questioned, it has many advantages in the setting of laparoscopic cholecystectomy, in which palpation of the common bile duct is not possible and the two-dimensional video image may not reveal ductal anatomy as clearly as direct inspection.

(494–D)   **(S&F, p. 967)**

Common bile duct stones may lead to serious complications such as cholangitis and pancreatitis. When found at laparoscopic cholecystectomy, these stones may be treated by either open cholecystectomy with bile duct exploration or laparoscopic duct exploration with or without choledochoscopy. Endoscopic sphincterotomy is effective in removing obstructing stones in over 90% of cases, allowing recovery from cholangitis or pancreatitis before cholecystectomy. In patients who are very elderly or who have serious concurrent disease, sphincterotomy may be the only treatment indicated.

(495–D)   **(S&F, pp. 975–976)**

Laparoscopic cholecystectomy has been adopted by patient demand rather than as a result of controlled clinical trials comparing it with open cholecystectomy. It offers the advantages of decreased perioperative morbidity, shorter hospitalization (1.2 vs. 4.5 days in one study), more rapid return to work, and less abdominal scarring. Against these advantages is an apparent greater incidence of common bile duct injury, although some of these may occur less frequently as surgeons become more experienced with the technique. The operation requires four incision sites: one larger site near the umbilicus to pass the operating telescope and three smaller sites for insufflation and passage of operating instruments.

(496–A, B, C, D)   **(S&F, p. 1007)**

The widespread availability of endoscopic retrograde cholangiopancreatography has documented the strong association of primary sclerosing cholangitis (PSC) with inflammatory bowel disease. Up to 14% of patients with ulcerative colitis will have abnormal results of liver function tests, and a large fraction of these patients will have global involvement of the biliary tree on cholangiography. The reverse association is even stronger, with two thirds of patients with PSC having evidence for inflammatory bowel disease (often subclinical). The association with ulcerative colitis is stronger than with Crohn's disease, and pancolitis is more likely to lead to PSC than proctitis. Although it was once thought that proctocolectomy could retard the progression of PSC, controlled studies indicate that this is not the case.

(497–D)   **(S&F, p. 956)**

Patients with sickle cell anemia and incidental gallstones have a significant risk of subsequently developing a complication of their gallstones that is difficult to distinguish from a pain crisis, and thus a prophylactic cholecystectomy is warranted. Young women of Amerindian ancestry who harbor gallstones are at high risk of subsequent complications, including gallbladder cancer, and likewise warrant cholecystectomy. Possible indications for prophylactic cholecystectomy include patients awaiting organ transplantation and those living in extremely remote locations in whom urgent medical care would prove impossible should a complication arise. Coronary artery disease *per se* is not an indication for a prophylactic cholecystectomy in an otherwise asymptomatic patient.

■■■■■**Reference**

Camilleri, M., Thompson, W. G., Fleshman, J. W., Pemberton, J. H. Clinical management of intractable constipation. Ann. Intern. Med. *121*:520–535, 1994.

(498–B, C, D)   **(S&F, pp. 1030–1031)**

Cholangiocarcinoma remains a challenging management problem. Although earlier studies suggested a lower mortality in patients receiving preoperative biliary decompression, most surgeons now believe that decompression does not alter operative outcome. The only advantage of placing a stent preoperatively would be to help guide the surgeon during resection. Proximal common bile duct or common hepatic duct tumors are best managed by reconstruction of the biliary tree using a Roux-en-Y hepaticojejunostomy. Palliation with biliary stents to relieve the biliary obstruction is the most useful form of therapy for unresectable tumors, although adjuvant radiation therapy can give modest increases in survival. Chemotherapy offers no proven benefit. The results of liver transplantation for cholangiocarcinoma have been disappointing. Three-year survival is 20% or less.

(499–D)   **(S&F, p. 986)**

Asymptomatic stones do not warrant treatment at all because most will remain asymptomatic; uncomplicated, symptomatic stones (biliary colic only) may be considered for oral bile acid therapy. The stone should be radiolucent on plain films or should not contain calcifications on computed tomography. The cystic duct must be patent, and gallbladder function (concentrating ability) must be preserved, both of which are demonstrated by an opacified gallbladder on an oral cholecystogram. The likelihood of success decreases dramatically with stones greater than 5 mm in diameter so a 15-mm stone can be excluded. Multiple stones may still dissolve over time, as long as no more than half of the gallbladder volume is occupied by stones.

(500–A, B, E)   **(S&F, pp. 987–990)**

Shock wave lithotripsy uses focused sound waves to disrupt stones. The stones most likely to respond are single cholesterol stones with little or no calcification. A single stone up to 20 mm in diameter is more likely to respond than are multiple smaller stones; and, in fact, lithotripsy should not be recommended in patients with multiple stones. When used in combination with ursodeoxycholate, between 47% and 68% of patients are stone free at six months. A major predictor of success was a well-functioning gallbladder, meaning preserved gallbladder contraction with emptying of more than 60% after meal stimulation. Transient edema of the gallbladder wall occurs in some patients, but no direct damage to tissues is caused by the treatment. About one third of patients experience one or more episodes of biliary colic during passage of the stone fragments, 2% develop mild biliary pancreatitis, and 1% develop transient cholestasis. These symptoms disappear when all fragments have been passed.

(501–E)   **(S&F, p. 914)**

The prognosis of untreated biliary atresia is extremely poor, with death from liver failure usually occurring within 2 years. A number of factors have been identified that contribute to the variable outcome after hepatic portoenterostomy. First, the age at which the operation is performed has been found to be crucial. Bile flow has been reestablished in several recent series in 80% to 90% of infants who were referred for surgery within 60 days after birth. More than 70% of these patients survived for at least ten years. In contrast, a success rate of less than 20% was observed in infants who were 90 days of age or older at the time of surgery. In the United States, predictors of a bad outcome include white race, operative age of more than 60 days, presence of cirrhosis on initial biopsy, totally nonpatent extrahepatic ducts, and absence of ducts at the level of transection in the liver hilus.

(502–D)   **(S&F, pp. 1029–1030)**

Although gallstones predispose to gallbladder cancer, no association between gallstones and bile duct carcinoma has been demonstrated.

(503–C)   **(S&F, p. 921)**

Patients with cystic fibrosis may develop cholestatic jaundice in the neonatal period. Clinical features may mimic other disorders, including idiopathic giant cell hepatitis and extrahepatic biliary atresia. Affected children demonstrate a variable degree of hepatomegaly. The liver edge is often hard and may be nodular. Marked splenomegaly may develop with the evolution of portal hypertension.

Laboratory studies may initially be normal but more typically include mild to moderate elevations of serum aminotransferase levels and moderate to marked elevations of serum alkaline phosphatase. Stricture of the distal common bile duct can occur, with over 50% affected in one series.

(504–B)   **(S&F, pp. 954–955)**

In the absence of a gallbladder, cholesterol stones form only rarely in the common bile duct. The gallbladder is thought to promote gallstone formation by concentrating bile, by providing a site where small stones can persist long enough to grow to clinical significance, and by secreting mucus (a putative nucleating agent). During periods of prolonged stasis, as in fasting, the mucus layer entraps microcrystals and multilamellar vesicles, forming sludge that can be detected using ultrasound. Up to 20% of patients with documented sludge go on to have gallstones or acute cholecystitis within a few years, suggesting that sludge is a precursor of gallstones. Aspirin and other prostaglandin inhibitors reduce mucus secretion in the gallbladder and protect against gallstone formation in experimental animals.

(505–B)   **(S&F, pp. 916–917)**

Type I choledochal cysts, accounting for 80% to 90% of all cases, exhibit segmental or diffuse fusiform dilation of the common bile duct. Type II cysts consist of a true choledochal diverticulum. A dilatation of the intraduodenal portion of the common bile duct or a so-called choledochocele (type III) may be a variation of this condition. Type IV cysts may be subdivided into type IVa multiple intrahepatic and extrahepatic cysts and type IVb multiple extrahepatic cysts. Type V, or Caroli's disease, consisting of single or multiple dilatation of the intrahepatic ductal system, may be viewed as a form of a choledochal cyst.

(506–1-C, 2-A, 3-B, 4-C, 5-B)   **(S&F, pp. 1029–1030)**

Abdominal pain is common in patients with either gallbladder carcinoma or cholangiocarcinoma, commonly a dull ache in the right upper quadrant. Carcinoma of the gallbladder has a female preponderance, likely due to the greater incidence of gallstone disease among women. Patients with carcinoma of the bile ducts tend to be younger because of the association between cholangiocarcinoma and primary sclerosing cholangitis. A palpable gallbladder (Courvoisier's sign) may be found with both cholangiocarcinoma (in the setting of a distal common bile duct lesion) or gallbladder carcinoma (with an obstructed cystic duct). Cholangitis is common in cholangiocarcinoma because of the strong association with sclerosing cholangitis.

(507–A, C, E, F)   **(S&F, pp. 985–986)**

Bile acid therapy should be limited to patients with noncalcified stones who have functioning gallbladders and infrequent or mild symptoms. Because of their greater surface-to-volume ratio, multiple small stones will dissolve more rapidly than a solitary larger stone. Chenodeoxycholate can cause diarrhea and may elevate the serum cholesterol level. It also may cause liver toxicity through conversion to lithocholate. Ursodeoxycholate does not have these undesirable features and is currently favored.

(508–B)   **(S&F, pp. 1026–1028)**

Jaundice is the most common presenting complaint in gallbladder carcinoma, reflecting bile duct involvement by tumor. Many patients present with acute cholecystitis indistinguishable from that due to stones. Abdominal pain, profound weight loss, and a palpable mass may be seen in advanced cases.

(509–C)   **(S&F, p. 905)**

The gallbladder, cystic duct, and common bile duct arise from the caudal portion of the hepatic diverticulum. The septum transversum consists of mesenchymal cells, which give rise to the vitelline veins and subsequently the hepatic sinusoids.

(510–B, C, D)   **(S&F, p. 941)**

In humans, two primary bile acids are formed in the liver from cholesterol. Cholesterol starts with a 3-hydroxy group. The rate-limiting step in bile acid biosynthesis is 7-hydroxylation, and the simplest bile acid that can be formed is the 3,7-dihydroxy bile acid chenodeoxycholic acid. If the 12 position is also hydroxylated, the result is the 3,7,12-trihydroxy bile acid cholic acid. Secondary bile acids are formed from primary bile acids by the action of intestinal bacteria. Most secondary bile acids are absorbed and secreted into bile. Those bile acids not absorbed by the terminal ileum enter the anaerobic environment of the cecum where bacterial enzymes may oxidize the hydroxy group at the 7 position, producing either deoxycholate from cholate or lithocholate from chenodeoxycholate. If the 7α hydroxyl group of chenodeoxycholate is not completely cleaved but only epimerized to the 7β configuration, then the rare (but therapeutically important) bile acid ursodeoxycholate (ursodiol) is formed.

(511–E)   **(S&F, pp. 954–955)**

Gallbladder emptying is controlled by both neural and humoral factors. The most potent stimulatory hormone is cholecystokinin (CCK). CCK release is triggered by absorbed long-chain fatty acids and, to a lesser extent, amino acids. The failure of patients with cystic fibrosis and pancreatic insufficiency to produce a normal CCK response to feeding explains the greater risk of gallstones in these diseases. Motilin and both endogenous and exogenous opiates stimulate gallbladder contraction, as does parasympathetic stimulation. In contrast, sympathetic stimulation, pancreatic polypeptide, pregnancy, and oral contraceptives inhibit emptying.

(512–1-D, 2-B, 3-A, 4-C)   **(S&F, p. 949)**

The type of gallstone can generally be identified by inspection. Large, pale, yellow-white stones are often referred to as pure cholesterol stones because they contain more than 90% cholesterol. The core of these stones is

usually dark and composed of the calcium salt of unconjugated bilirubin. Mixed cholesterol stones, containing more than 50% cholesterol, are more common and tend to be smaller and multiple. Their contiguous surfaces are usually faceted. Pigment stones are either black or brown. Black stones are composed mostly of the calcium salt of unconjugated bilirubin, are small, and crumble easily. Brown pigment stones are larger and firmer than black stones and contain a mixture of unconjugated bilirubin, cholesterol, and calcium soaps of fatty acids. They often contain bacterial cytoskeletons, suggesting that their formation is triggered by infection.

(513–C)   **(S&F, pp. 931–932)**

When performing biliary manometry, the cannula should be positioned deep into the desired duct and then slowly withdrawn until all side holes are positioned within the sphincter. Pressures are recorded during slow withdrawal of the catheter. Meperidine at a dose less than 1 mg/kg may be used for analgesia if basal sphincter pressures are used as the end point.

(514–C)   **(S&F, pp. 1026–1027)**

The incidence of gallbladder carcinoma on autopsy series is approximately 0.5% and appears to be steady. There is a female preponderance, which likely reflects a greater incidence of gallstone disease. Most cases occur after age 50. Despite recent advances in diagnostic imaging, survival after diagnosis has not improved significantly.

(515–B)   **(S&F, p. 925)**

Acalculous cholecystitis is acute inflammation of the gallbladder in the absence of gallstones. The disorder is uncommon in normal children but has been reported in infants receiving prolonged parenteral nutrition. Predisposing factors also include prolonged fasting and the use of narcotic analgesics. Acalculous cholecystitis may also follow abdominal trauma and has been observed with systemic vasculitis, periarteritis nodosa, and Kawasaki's disease.

(516–A, B, C, D)   **(S&F, pp. 933–934)**

Endoscopic sphincterotomy and surgical sphincteroplasty both relieve pain in the patients with type I sphincter of Oddi dysfunction (SOD) with elevated sphincter pressures. Medical therapy with nitrates or nifedipine will reduce mild pain in as many as 75% and should be considered as the first line of therapy in patients with the milder type III SOD. The role of sphincter of Oddi dysfunction in pancreatitis remains controversial. Pancreatic sphincterotomy is a procedure with a high complication rate and should be considered only when there is strong evidence that the pancreatitis was caused by sphincter of Oddi dysfunction. Some authors argue that a temporary trial with a pancreatic stent may identify those who might benefit from sphincterotomy. Pancreatic sphincterotomy or stenting in this setting should be performed only as part of clinical trials.

(517–A) **(S&F, pp. 966–967)**

Gallstones may pass from the gallbladder to the common duct, where they produce complications by obstructing bile flow. Alkaline phosphatase levels rise because of increased synthesis by canalicular epithelium, but the level bears no relationship to either the degree of obstruction or its cause. Ultrasonography or computed tomography commonly shows dilatation of the common and intrahepatic bile ducts, but this may not occur if the ducts are scarred from previous episodes of cholangitis or if cirrhosis is present. Dilatation may also be absent if the obstruction is low grade or intermittent.

(518–C) **(S&F, pp. 956–961)**

Endoscopic retrograde cholangiopancreatography (ERCP) with filling of the gallbladder causes many small stones to float at the bile-contrast interface where they can be detected easily. In one study, ERCP demonstrated stones in 78% of patients with pain and transient liver function abnormalities who had normal sonograms but was positive in only 2.5% of controls. In another study, cholesterol crystals were found in the bile of 88% of patients with cholesterol gallstones but not in the bile of patients without stones. Bile, which is obtained by either duodenal intubation or direct sampling at the time of ERCP, can also be used to detect calcium bilirubinate granules that indicate pigment stones. Computed tomography is less accurate than ultrasonography in detecting gallstones and is not routinely used. Several studies suggest that a low gallbladder ejection fraction after administration of cholecystokinin correlates with disease, but the sensitivity and specificity of this test remain controversial.

(519–A, B, D) **(S&F, p. 956)**

Prospective trials indicate that the risk of asymptomatic stones becoming symptomatic is about 2% per year for the initial five years and declines thereafter. Most patients who have biliary pain will have a repeat attack within two years, and the risk of acute cholecystitis in this group is about 3% per year. However, about 30% of patients who suffer a single attack of biliary pain never have a recurrence. Between 60% and 80% of all gallstones found by cross-sectional studies of adults are asymptomatic.

(520–C) **(S&F, p. 1039)**

In a study of more than 11,500 endoscopic sphincterotomies, the most common early complications were hemorrhage, pancreatitis, cholangitis, and perforation in 2.5%, 2.0%, 1.3%, and 1.1%, respectively. The risk of having the basket impacted in the bile duct was significantly lower at 0.2%.

(521–A, C, E) **(S&F, pp. 976–977)**

Gallstones in children are a common complication of parenteral nutrition and are also seen in hemolytic states. Unlike in the adult case, many experts recommend that asymptomatic stones should be removed to prevent compli-

cations during the life of the child. Because cholesterol gallstones may sometimes resolve spontaneously, surgery is not usually recommended unless stones persist for more than 6 to 12 months.

(522–C) **(S&F, pp. 961–962)**

Typical biliary colic is not colicky pain but comes on gradually over 15 to 60 minutes, with peak intensity lasting an hour or more and then gradually resolving. Pain may be precipitated by eating, but more commonly there is no inciting event. In order of decreasing frequency, the pain is felt in the epigastrium, right upper quadrant, left upper quadrant, and various parts of the precordium or lower abdomen. Radiation to other parts of the abdomen or back occurs in more than 50% of patients. Vomiting and diaphoresis occur in most patients. The interval between attacks may be weeks, months, or years and cannot be predicted. Diagnosis is made by confirming the presence of gallstones and excluding other disorders that could produce a similar clinical picture.

(523–B) **(S&F, p. 1030)**

Perihilar adenopathy is not considered a contraindication for surgical resection of cholangiocarcinoma.

(524–A, C) **(S&F, pp. 937–939)**

Most bile acids are found in the gallbladder during fasting and in the small intestinal lumen during digestion. When a meal is eaten, the gallbladder contracts and the bile acid pool is slowly discharged into the small intestine. Some passive absorption of the more lipophilic conjugated bile acids occurs in the proximal small intestine. The majority of bile acids reach the terminal ileum where an active transport process efficiently absorbs them from the lumen. More than 90% of secreted bile acids are reabsorbed and carried back to the liver, where they are efficiently cleared and promptly secreted once again into bile.

(525–A) **(S&F, p. 986)**

Ursodeoxycholate has greater safety and efficacy than chenodeoxycholate and is now the preferred agent for clinical use, though neither of the oral bile acids has any effect on pigment stones. Unlike chenodeoxycholate, it does not inhibit the synthesis of normal bile salts. Because normal cholesterol catabolism and excretion are maintained, serum cholesterol and low-density lipoproteins do not rise while the patient is under treatment, as is true for chenodeoxycholate. Side effects such as diarrhea and elevated aminotransferase levels are uncommon. The rate of stone dissolution is 20% to 40% at two years, with the best results in patients with small (<20 mm), radiolucent, floating stones made mostly of cholesterol. Patients whose gallbladders are diseased (e.g., unable to concentrate dye as assessed by an oral cholecystogram) should receive cholecystectomy instead. Recurrence of stones occurs in 50% of responding patients within five years. With the low morbidity and expense of laparoscopic cholecystectomy, the final role of bile salts in the treatment of gallstones is uncertain.

(526–1-D, 2-A, 3-B, 4-C) **(S&F, pp. 929–930)**

Hogan and Geenen developed a classification of patients with biliary-type pain and presumed sphincter of Oddi dysfunction. This classification attempts to interpret symptoms, biochemical abnormalities, and cholangiographic findings in terms of sphincter dysfunction. Group I patients have biliary-type pain, liver enzyme abnormalities, delayed drainage of contrast after cholangiography, and a dilated common bile duct. Sphincter of Oddi stenosis is very likely in this group, and manometry is therefore optional. Group II patients have less diagnostic symptoms than group I patients. Biliary manometry is therefore essential for diagnosis of sphincter dysfunction. Group III patients have only biliary-type pain. These patients are less likely to have sphincter of Oddi dysfunction as a cause of their complaints than are patients in the other two groups. All attempts should be made to rule out other causes of pain before resorting to biliary manometry.

(527–B) **(S&F, pp. 918–920)**

Syndromic paucity of intralobular bile ducts (Alagille's syndrome, or arteriohepatic dysplasia) is probably the most common form of familial intrahepatic cholestasis. This disorder is characterized by chronic cholestasis, a decreased number of interlobular bile ducts, and a variety of other congenital malformations. An autosomal dominant mode of transmission with reduced penetrance and variable expressivity has been suggested from familial pedigrees.

(528–A, B) **(S&F, p. 1002)**

Cholesterol polyps (also known as papillomas of the gallbladder) account for 60% of gallbladder polyps. They are typically small (<1 mm), multiple (with a mean of eight polyps per gallbladder in one study), and pedunculated. They are not a true neoplasm but are a variety of cholesterolosis caused by infiltration of the lamina propria with lipid-laden "foamy" macrophages. They rarely produce symptoms and are typically detected incidentally after cholecystectomy.

(529–B, D) **(S&F, p. 1047)**

Acquired immunodeficiency syndrome cholangiography (infectious sclerosing cholangitis) typically presents as pain and an elevated alkaline phosphatase level but not with jaundice. The cholangiographic appearance is similar to that seen in primary sclerosing cholangitis, namely beading and ulceration along the intrahepatic and extrahepatic bile ducts. These immunocompromised patients are extremely susceptible to bacterial cholangitis as a complication of an indwelling stent; therefore, stents should be placed across high-grade strictures only to relieve severe pruritus or acute bacterial infection, not just to relieve pain.

(530–B) **(S&F, p. 1033)**

The percutaneous approach to cholangiography is associated with more morbidity and a longer recovery time. Prior biliary-enteric surgery, such as a Roux-en-Y choledochojejunostomy, may preclude cholangiography by an endoscopic approach.

(531–C) **(S&F, pp. 906–908)**

The right and left hepatic ducts join outside the liver in most cases. It is uncommon for the ducts to merge inside the liver or for the cystic duct to join the right hepatic duct proximal to the hilum.

(532–A, B, D) **(S&F, pp. 1040–1041)**

Early complications from stent placement are indeed most likely due to the sphincterotomy and include hemorrhage, pancreatitis, perforation, and cholangitis. Stent patency averages 6 months, but occlusion may occur immediately or be delayed for up to 12 months. Therefore, when stenting a malignant obstruction, many investigators will not routinely replace stents but rather will wait until signs or symptoms suggest an occlusion. These include alkaline phosphatase level elevation and low-grade fever or chills. It is uncommon for an occluded stent to present as fullblown cholangitis and sepsis. Distal bile duct lesions are more effectively stented than are lesions occurring proximally at the hilum.

(533–A) **(S&F, p. 913)**

Most infants with biliary atresia are born at term after a normal pregnancy and have normal birth weight. Female infants are more commonly affected than males. Jaundice is usually observed by parents after the period of physiologic hyperbilirubinemia (after 14 days of age). The liver is typically enlarged with a firm edge palpable 2 to 6 cm below the right costal margin. Ascites and edema are not present initially, but coagulopathy due to vitamin K deficiency may occur.

(534–B) **(S&F, p. 1047)**

Patients with acquired immunodeficiency syndrome cholangiopathy may present with pain and a markedly elevated alkaline phosphatase level. However, the bilirubin value is normal in the vast majority of cases. Sphincterotomy may help those with pain, papillary stenosis, and a dilated extrahepatic duct system.

(535–D) **(S&F, p. 930)**

The existence of sphincter of Oddi dysfunction and its role in specific clinical conditions have been the cause of considerable controversy. Nevertheless, available evidence suggests that sphincter dysfunction may play a causative role in patients with postcholecystectomy pain, cholestasis, pancreatic-type pain, and idiopathic recurrent pancreatitis. The pain of sphincter of Oddi dysfunction is not relieved by either acid suppression therapy or treatment for the irritable bowel syndrome.

(536–C) **(S&F, p. 1035)**

Unlike endoscopic retrograde cholangiopancreatography, pancreatitis is unlikely after percutaneous biliary drainage because there is no direct injection of contrast into the pancreatic duct.

(537–A) *(S&F, p. 1038)*

This patient has cholangitis caused by choledocholithiasis. The unrelenting nature of the pain and the extrahepatic duct dilatation suggest an impacted stone. Even though she is known to have a duodenal diverticulum, the endoscopic approach is still favored. There does not appear to be a higher risk of complications from endoscopic retrograde cholangiopancreatography with sphincterotomy and stone removal in patients with a duodenal diverticulum.

(538–C) *(S&F, pp. 1028–1029)*

The distinction of gallbladder adenomas from early carcinoma is very difficult and cannot be made by ultrasound evaluation. Given the current availability of laparoscopic cholecystectomy, most experts no longer advise observing adenomas for growth but recommend immediate cholecystectomy.

(539–B, E) *(S&F, pp. 961–966)*

The first sign of cholecystitis is diffuse abdominal pain, which is generally followed by nausea and vomiting. Inflammation of the gallbladder is thought to be caused by activation of inflammatory mediators rather than by infection. In one study of patients with biliary colic, progression to overt cholecystitis was completely prevented by treatment with diclofenac sodium, a nonsteroidal anti-inflammatory drug (NSAID). Cholecystitis occurs in the absence of gallstones about 10% of the time, mostly in the setting of starvation, rapid weight loss, or total parenteral nutrition. The primary value of cholescintigraphy in acute cholecystitis is its ability to demonstrate obstruction of the cystic duct in patients when the diagnosis remains in doubt. Newer agents (e.g., DISIDA) can be used even in jaundiced patients. Mirizzi's syndrome is obstruction of the common hepatic or bile duct by extrinsic compression caused by the cystic duct stone itself or surrounding inflammation.

(540–A) *(S&F, p. 950)*

Serum cholesterol level has not been found to be a direct risk factor for gallstones, and in several studies there has actually been an inverse relationship. Obesity, particularly morbid obesity, is a strong risk factor, although many people with gallstones are not overweight. A positive family history is also a risk factor, although it is not known whether genetic or socioeconomic factors are responsible. Patients with Amerindian ancestry (some Mexican Americans and all Native Americans) have a higher risk. Women with lower socioeconomic status are at greater risk, as are those who have rapid weight loss due to dieting. Patients on total parenteral nutrition tend to develop biliary sludge and stones as well as acalculous cholecystitis. This risk can be reduced by periodic stimulation of gallbladder emptying using lipid emulsions.

(541–D) *(S&F, p. 963)*

Early changes in acute cholecystitis consist principally of hyperemia and edema, and the gallbladder becomes distended with bile, inflammatory exudate, or, rarely, pus. With time, bile salts and pigments are absorbed and replaced with thin mucoid material, pus, or blood. After the attack subsides, the mucosal surface heals and the wall becomes scarred and nonfunctional. If the cystic duct remains obstructed, the lumen may become distended with clear mucoid fluid, termed *hydrops of the gallbladder.*

(542–C) *(S&F, pp. 974–975)*

Cholecystectomy is the definitive treatment of gallstone disease and is indicated for most symptomatic patients. Between 88% and 95% of patients with presumed biliary colic have complete relief of their symptoms with cholecystectomy. Age by itself is not a contraindication to elective cholecystectomy. Elective cholecystectomy is considerably more hazardous in patients with cirrhosis and portal hypertension. The concentration of bile acids in intestinal contents does not appear to be altered by cholecystectomy.

(543–B, C, D) *(S&F, pp. 1012–1013)*

Malabsorption of fat-soluble vitamins (A, D, E, and K) is common in primary sclerosing cholangitis (PSC) due to cholestasis and may produce night blindness, clotting abnormalities, and osteoporosis unless supplements are given. Abnormal pancreatograms have been found at endoscopic retrograde cholangiopancreatography in 8% to 77% of patients but rarely lead to pancreatitis or pancreatic insufficiency. Cholangiocarcinoma is a common and deadly complication of PSC and is reported in 30% to 40% of patients dying with PSC and 9% to 33% of patients undergoing liver transplantation for PSC. The survival after liver transplantation is good, with recurrent PSC uncommon. However, 60% of patients transplanted who are incidentally found to have cholangiocarcinoma in their explant die of metastases within two years.

(544–D) *(S&F, pp. 952–955)*

Cholesterol gallstones tend to form when bile is frequently supersaturated. The solubility of cholesterol in bile depends on its ratio to bile acids and phospholipids, with which it forms biliary particles called micelles. Factors that decrease bile acid secretion (e.g., interruption of the enterohepatic circulation of bile salts) or increase cholesterol secretion (high-fat diets) increase the risk of gallstones. Complete emptying of the gallbladder can prevent stone formation by excreting stones before they can grow large enough to produce disease. Thus, stone disease is more common in patients with reduced gallbladder motility (including fasting during hospitalization). Bile contains proteins that can both accelerate and delay cholesterol nucleation and crystallization. Normal bile contains several grams of cholesterol per day.

(545–B, D) *(S&F, p. 969)*

Porcelain gallbladder is defined as intramural calcifications and has a high risk of gallbladder cancer. When detected, whether asymptomatic or not, a prophylactic cholecystectomy is warranted, not observation over time.

(546–1-C, 2-C, 3-B, 4-C, 5-D)   **(S&F, p. 996)**

The features of acalculous cholecystitis are similar to those of calculous disease and include thickening of the gallbladder wall, tenderness when the transducer is pressed over the gallbladder (the "sonographic Murphy's sign"), and pericholecystic fluid collections. Fluid collections indicate severe inflammation, necrosis, and/or perforation and are more common in acalculous than in calculous disease. The presence or absence of stones, detected as echogenic foci that cast sonographic shadows, determines whether the disease is termed *calculous* or *acalculous* cholecystitis. Treatment of both forms is cholecystectomy. In patients who are too sick to undergo surgery, percutaneous tube decompression of the gallbladder is an option.

(547–B)   **(S&F, pp. 937–943)**

Specific transport mechanisms have been identified for multiple molecules in bile. Many of these are adenosine triphosphate–dependent, although the energetics have not been well established. There is no specific transporter for water. As in most epithelia, its movement is governed by the movement of osmotically active solutes such as bile acids, organic anions, cations, and inorganic electrolytes.

(548–A)   **(S&F, p. 1026)**

Cigarette smoking has never been associated with a higher incidence of carcinoma of the gallbladder. Workers in the rubber and automotive industries appear to be at an increased risk (likely due to environmental carcinogens), as are Native Americans by virtue of the high incidence of gallstone disease.

(549–B, C, D)   **(S&F, p. 1008)**

The gross appearance of the bile ducts in primary sclerosing cholangitis (PSC) is that of a thickened, hardened cord, likened by some surgeons to a thrombosed vessel. Inflammatory adhesions may be present around the duct, and lymph nodes in the hilum may be enlarged. The duct wall is thickened by a mixed inflammatory infiltrate, and a characteristic "onion skin" fibrosis around interlobular and septal bile ducts is present in around one half of cases. The finding of concentric fibrosis obliterating the small ducts is virtually diagnostic but occurs in only 10% of cases. Granulomas and bile duct proliferation on liver biopsy suggest primary biliary cirrhosis, not PSC.

(550–B)   **(S&F, pp. 950–951)**

Hypercholesterolemia by itself is not a risk factor for cholesterol gallstone formation, although hypertriglyceridemia is positively associated with gallstone disease. Being female, obese, or pregnant or having a history of rapid weight loss are all independent risk factors.

(551–A)   **(S&F, p. 974)**

Serum alkaline phosphatase level, if elevated, suggests choledocholithiasis. The abdominal ultrasonogram confirms the diagnosis of biliary disease and may detect evidence of common duct stones of obstruction. Any evidence

of congestive heart failure greatly increases the risk of surgery. An electrocardiogram should be done in older patients or patients for whom the diagnosis of biliary colic is not secure. In the absence of other evidence of cardiopulmonary disease, a chest radiograph is not required.

(552–A, C)   **(S&F, p. 1026)**

Eighty percent of gallbladder cancers occur in the setting of cholelithiasis. The only potentially curative treatment for gallbladder carcinoma is surgery. Unfortunately, less than 10% of tumors are resectable for cure at exploration and the five-year survival is less than 5%. Whether high-risk populations such as Native Americans should undergo prophylactic cholecystectomy remains controversial. With the advent of laparoscopic cholecystectomy, the indications for cholecystectomy may broaden. For the majority of patients who are unresectable at presentation, stenting of the biliary obstruction offers the only form of therapy available. Incidental cancers are discovered in 1% to 2% of gallbladders resected for biliary colic and have a much more favorable prognosis than does symptomatic gallbladder cancer.

(553–C)   **(S&F, pp. 937–939)**

When a meal is ingested, bile acids are secreted into the intestine. Bile acid secretion can be measured by duodenal perfusion techniques and is 12 to 24 g/day, depending on dietary intake. The bile acid pool averages 2 to 4 g, so that the pool circulates on average 3 to 12 times a day. Pool size and cycling frequency are inversely related so that the secretion rate is relatively constant over a wide range of pool sizes.

(554–B)   **(S&F, p. 1038)**

Percutaneous cholecystostomy can be performed successfully in almost all patients and is often the definitive therapy in those with acute acalculous cholecystitis. In high-risk patients with gallstone-induced acute cholecystitis, percutaneous cholecystostomy can "buy time" until definitive surgical therapy can be undertaken. Patients with suspected choledocholithiasis in addition to acute cholecystitis need clearance of the bile duct so a cholecystectomy followed by endoscopic retrograde cholangiopancreatography (or vice versa) would be preferable to a percutaneous cholecystostomy.

(555–C)   **(S&F, pp. 916–917)**

The diagnosis in this case is a choledochal cyst. This congenital lesion is more common in females and is symptomatic in approximately 25% of cases. The symptom triad is abdominal pain, jaundice, and an abdominal mass.

(556–B)   **(S&F, p. 917)**

The treatment of choice for choledochal cysts is surgical resection. Potential complications if not resected include stones, cholangitis, carcinoma, and perforation.

(557–B)   **(S&F, p. 1031)**

Ampullary carcinoma has a much better prognosis than gallbladder or bile duct carcinoma. Surgical resection is possible in as many as 75% of patients. The Whipple procedure is the surgery of choice. With surgery, the overall five-year survival is 40%. Stenting provides effective palliation for those patients whose carcinoma is unresectable.

(558–A, B, D)   **(S&F, pp. 1011–1012)**

Most patients presenting with primary sclerosing cholangitis are between 25 and 45 years of age, and males are one and one-half to two times more commonly affected than females. The most common presenting symptoms are jaundice, pruritus, mild to moderate right upper quadrant pain, and fatigue. Febrile episodes may occur, but acute septic cholangitis is rare at presentation. The liver and spleen are often enlarged, and splenomegaly may be marked in some cases. Alkaline phosphatase levels are usually increased, with elevations up to 20 times normal not uncommon. Serum aminotransferase levels are often increased, as are those of immunoglobulins (particularly IgM).

(559–B)   **(S&F, p. 963)**

Acute cholecystitis usually begins with biliary colic due to obstruction of the cystic duct with a stone. As inflammation progresses, the pain becomes localized to the right upper quadrant and systemic signs of inflammation develop. These may include a temperature of 102° F, leukocyte counts of 12,000 to 15,000 cells/mm^3, and an increase in serum aminotransferase and alkaline phosphatase levels. Mild jaundice (bilirubin <4 mg/dL) is common, particularly in older patients. Marked elevation of the serum bilirubin, amylase, or aminotransferase values suggests a common duct stone. Murphy's sign is pain and inspiratory arrest when the patient takes a deep breath during palpation of the right subcostal region. It is caused by contact of the inflamed gallbladder with the examiner's hand. The gallbladder is palpable in about one third of cases, often lateral to its normal location. Because acute cholecystitis is primarily a chemical inflammation, more than half of unoperated cases resolve spontaneously without complications, though about 10% will develop a localized perforation and 1% a free perforation. Most attacks last seven to ten days, but they may resolve completely within 24 hours in some cases.

(560–B)   **(S&F, p. 1043)**

A bile leak can be managed nonoperatively by placement of a nasobiliary catheter or a pigtail stent or by performing endoscopic sphincterotomy. All of these measures reduce further leakage, allowing time for the leak to heal. Supportive measures and percutaneous drainage of the biloma can improve the patient's overall well-being but will not help in sealing the leak.

(561–B, D)   **(S&F, pp. 929–933)**

Baseline sphincter of Oddi pressures are 10 to 30 mm Hg higher than duodenal pressures and 5 to 15 mm Hg higher than common bile duct pressures. The majority of phasic waves propagate antegrade toward the duodenal lumen. Although a pumping action has been demonstrated in the opossum, it is unclear whether phasic wave activity translates into a pumping action in humans. The sphincter serves an important role as an antireflux barrier, especially during phase III of the migrating motor complex (MMC).

(562–D)   **(S&F, pp. 974–975)**

Overall, open cholecystectomy is a safe procedure with low rates of postoperative death and serious morbidity. Most deaths occur in elderly patients or in those with serious complications of gallstone disease, such as cholangitis or acute cholecystitis. Whereas the overall mortality rate is 0.5% to 1.5% for elective surgery in most series, surgery for acute cholecystitis or common bile duct obstruction has a mortality rate about three times larger.

(563–1-B, 2-A, 3-B, 4-A, 5-B, 6-A,   **(S&F, p. 995)**
7-B, 8-A, 9-B, 10-A)

Unlike the more commonly seen calculous cholecystitis, acalculous cholecystitis occurs primarily in elderly persons who are postsurgical, require total parenteral nutrition, or are otherwise at chronic bed rest with poor oral intake. It may also be seen in the setting of trauma, vasculitis, or vascular instability. Males are affected more often than females. Diagnosis is often delayed, because initial symptoms are localized to the right upper quadrant in only 25% and other reasons for pain or fever usually exist. The disease is much more fulminant than calculous cholecystitis, with half of all patients developing gangrene or perforation and a mortality of 10% to 50%.

(564–C)   **(S&F, p. 960)**

Although ultrasonography is the first test ordered in most cases, the oral cholecystogram (OCG) is still useful. Both tests have a similar sensitivity (90% to 95%) and specificity (95% to 100%). The OCG is most commonly used to evaluate patients with high index of suspicion for gallstones who have a negative ultrasonogram. About 25% of patients require two doses of contrast dye to opacify their gallbladders. It is also useful in patients for whom dissolution therapy is being considered, because cholesterol stones can often be differentiated from other stone types by their radiolucency, lack of extensive calcifications, and tendency to float. OCG should not be used in patients with significant intestinal or hepatic disease, because false-positive results may occur, owing to failure to absorb or secrete the dye.

(565–A, B, E)   **(S&F, pp. 986–988)**

This patient, with small, radiolucent stones and a functioning gallbladder, is a reasonable candidate for an attempt at oral dissolution therapy, and the success rate could be expected to be about 40%. If all stones were less than 5 mm and "floated" on an oral cholecystogram, she would be an ideal candidate, with a 70% chance of success. Stones dissolve (if at all) at a rate of approximately 0.7 mm/month; thus, her stones would take about seven months to dissolve. Ursodiol has virtually no side effects, and, surprisingly, symptoms often abate within the first few weeks of therapy, perhaps because microscopic cholesterol has dissolved.

(566–C)   **(S&F, p. 1045)**

In the setting of cholangitis, both systems must be drained to avoid risk of persistent infection. Endoscopic retrograde cholangiopancreatography can be technically difficult when dealing with hilar or intrahepatic lesions; therefore, the percutaneous approach is favored.

(567–D)   **(S&F, pp. 917–918)**

Segmental, saccular dilatation of the intrahepatic bile ducts is referred to as Caroli's disease. This rare disorder is congenital. It may consist solely of ectasia of the hepatic bile ducts or may be associated with features of congenital hepatic fibrosis. About 75% of patients are male.

(568–C)   **(S&F, pp. 986–987)**

The best candidates for dissolution therapy have small, floating, radiolucent stones. Efficacy rates range from 20% to 70% depending on how rigidly selection criteria are applied. Although there is a theoretical risk that smaller stones would obstruct the cystic or common ducts, most patients actually notice a decrease in symptoms before complete dissolution is achieved. Approximately 50% of successfully treated patients redevelop gallstones within five years.

(569–A)   **(S&F, pp. 995, 997)**

Acalculous cholecystitis, also called necrotizing chole-cystitis, has a distinct etiology, pathology, and prognosis. It accounts for up to 10% of cholecystectomies in the general population and up to 50% of cholecystectomies in patients hospitalized for other problems. The triad of prolonged fasting, immobility, and hemodynamic instabil-ity appears to predispose to a breakdown of the gall-bladder's resistance to the damaging effects of bile. Be-cause many patients are already ill with other diseases, it can be difficult to diagnose early. Clinical features include fever, leukocytosis, and hyperamylasemia. Tenderness in the right upper quadrant is very helpful if present but is seen in only 25% of cases at presentation. The prognosis is relatively poor, with a mortality rate of 10% to 50% and a complication rate of about 50%.

(570–D)   **(S&F, p. 1026)**

Fluid around the gallbladder is rare in gallbladder carci-noma. When seen, it suggests perforation.

(571–A)   **(S&F, p. 955)**

Black pigment stones occur more commonly in patients with hemolysis. In contrast, brown pigment stones are most often seen in patients with infections of the biliary tree. Bacteria release enzymes that deconjugate bile acids (bile salt deconjugase) and bilirubin (β-glucosidase), causing the aqueous concentration of unconjugated bilirubin (which is highly insoluble) to rise. They also release phospholipase A, which liberates long-chain fatty acids that form insolu-ble soaps with calcium. Asian populations have a particu-larly high incidence of brown pigment stones, although this incidence is falling as the risk of infection with *Clonorchis sinensis* and other biliary infections is reduced.

(572–D)   **(S&F, p. 913)**

Three main types of biliary atresia have been defined on the basis of the site of the lesion. Type I is atresia of the common bile duct with patent proximal ducts. Type II atresia involves the hepatic duct with cystic dilatation of the bile ducts at the porta hepatis. In type IIa, the cystic and common ducts are patent, whereas in type IIb, these structures are obliterated. These forms of biliary atresia are usually surgically correctable but unfortunately comprise less than 10% of all cases. The remaining patients have type III atresia involving obstruction of ducts at or above the porta hepatis.

(573–1-A, 2-A, 3-B, 4-A, 5-A)   **(S&F, pp. 931–932)**

Anticholinergics, glucagon, and nitrates all inhibit sphincter of Oddi activity, whereas morphine and choliner-gic drugs stimulate it. Meperidine (at a dose of 1 mg/kg) and benzodiazepines do not affect basal sphincter pressure and thus can be used for analgesia during sphincter of Oddi manometry.

(574–B)   **(S&F, p. 1031)**

Painless jaundice, which may be intermittent, is the most common manifestation of carcinoma of the ampulla of Vater. Patients may also present with pancreatitis or gastro-intestinal bleeding. Pain is usually a late manifestation.

(575–C)   **Ethnic (S&F, p. 949)**
                                       Age, gender, parity
                                       (S&F, pp. 950–951)

Gallstones are two to three times more common in women than in men. The incidence of gallstones rises with age and is 5% to 20% in white females between age 30 and 50 and 25% to 30% thereafter. Similar rates have been reported for Hispanic and Mexican American women. The rate approaches 70% in female Pima Indians and is gener-ally high in other Native American groups. Blacks seem to have a lower prevalence than whites in both the United States and Africa. Multiple pregnancies appear to increase the risk of gallstones slightly, perhaps because gestational hormones predispose to sludge formation in the gallbladder.

(576–A)   **(S&F, pp. 908–909)**

The posterior aspects of the fundus and body of the gallbladder lie in proximity with the transverse colon and duodenum. Thus, perforation of gallstones occurs most often into these structures.

(577–B, D) **(S&F, pp. 929–935)**

The cause of pain in sphincter of Oddi dysfunction is unclear. Although some have postulated that pain comes from sphincter spasm, others believe it is due to distention of the proximal biliary tree. An elevated resting basal pressure (>40 mm Hg) is the most accepted abnormality. Medical therapy with nitroglycerin and calcium channel blockers can reduce resting pressures, but it is unclear whether symptoms are improved. When one portion of the sphincter has an elevated resting pressure, the other portion is abnormal in 33% to 65% of cases.

(578–B, C, E) **(S&F, p. 1009)**

The typical cholangiographic abnormalities in primary sclerosing cholangitis (PSC) consist of multifocal strictures, diffusely distributed, and usually short (0.2 to 2 cm) with intervening segments of normal dilated ducts, producing a highly characteristic beaded appearance. When seen in a compatible clinical setting, these findings are diagnostic of PSC. Small branches may fill poorly, giving rise to a "pruned" appearance. This picture is usually readily distinguished from that produced by cirrhosis. Major localized areas (dominant strictures) may occur and are most common near the bifurcation of the common bile duct. These findings are in contrast to secondary sclerosing cholangitis due to infection or toxins, in which the area of stricturing is often quite localized with marked dilation of the biliary tree distal to the obstruction.

(579–C) **(S&F, p. 958)**

The classic Chacot triad of right upper quadrant pain, fever, and jaundice is highly suggestive of cholangitis, usually due to choledocholithiasis. Unfortunately, the complete triad is present in only 70% of patients. In this case the chills, confusion, and hypotension point to bacteremia, which is present in the majority of patients with cholangitis. Leukocytosis and jaundice are missing in 20% of patients with cholangitis, making the diagnosis more subtle. Against acute cholecystitis is the presence of a high fever, and a liver abscess would have been seen on the ultrasonogram. The finding of a dilated common bile duct on ultrasonography is lacking in 25% of patients with a common duct stone, so a normal ultrasonogram cannot exclude choledocholithiasis. The patient needs resuscitation, antibiotics, and urgent endoscopic retrograde cholangiopancreatography.

(580–C) **(S&F, p. 941)**

Most cholic acid and chenodeoxycholic acid conjugates are absorbed from the ileum without undergoing bacterial modification. However, small amounts of these acids are converted by intestinal bacteria to deoxycholic acid (DCA) and lithocholic acid (LCA). These secondary bile acids are absorbed, conjugated with glycine or taurine in the liver, and secreted into bile. Absorption of DCA conjugates by the ileal transport system is actually more efficient than that of the primary bile acid conjugates. As a result, DCA

may comprise 20% to 40% of the biliary bile acids in most adults. In contrast, LCA conjugates are poorly absorbed by the terminal ileum, so that they are rapidly lost from the enterohepatic circulation into the feces.

(581–A, B, C, D) **(S&F, pp. 1006–1007)**

The biliary tree has a limited repertoire of responses to disease. In most cases, sclerosing cholangitis is the result. The current definition of primary sclerosing cholangitis has been broadened to include a spectrum of disorders characterized by diffuse biliary stricturing and associated with apparent autoimmunity and includes options A through D. Specifically excluded are sclerosing cholangitis due to tumors, recurring pyogenic cholangitis (as in congenital anomalies), opportunistic infections (as in the acquired immunodeficiency syndrome), vasculitis, allograft rejection, or graft-versus-host disease. However, management is similar regardless of cause.

(582–B) **(S&F, pp. 957–960)**

Because gallstones are most easily seen in a distended gallbladder, patients are fasted for at least eight hours before ultrasound examination. Although thickening of the wall suggests chronic cholecystitis, this is a nonspecific finding. Criteria for diagnosing gallstones include echogenic foci in the gallbladder that are mobile and produce an acoustic shadow. Sludge is mobile and echogenic but does not produce a shadow.

(583–E) **(S&F, pp. 968–969)**

Gallstone ileus is caused when a stone, usually greater than a 2.5 cm in diameter, passes though a cholecystenteric fistula into the bowel and becomes impacted. Most patients are elderly women, and most have no history of cholecystitis. The most common level of obstruction is the ileocecal area. Plain films often show air in the biliary tree, ileus, and a calcified stone outside the normal distribution of the gallbladder. This diagnosis should be considered in elderly persons presenting with bowel obstruction, particularly when no history of prior surgery is present. Mortality is high and is mostly due to delay in diagnosis and coexistent medical problems. Treatment is emergency laparotomy.

(584–A, B, C) **(S&F, pp. 943–944)**

Of all the organic constituents of bile, only the bile acids participate in a true enterohepatic circulation. Biliary phosphatidylcholine (PC) is hydrolyzed to lyso-PC, which is then re-esterified to form PC in the enterocyte. It is absorbed in the form of chylomicrons but rapidly exchanges with other PC molecules in lipoproteins and cell membranes. PC molecules that enter the hepatocyte are extensively metabolized and do not contribute significantly to biliary phospholipids.

(585–C) **(S&F, p. 930)**

The sphincter of Oddi has received considerable recent attention because of evidence that sphincter dysfunction can produce symptoms or accentuate disease processes in some patients. The sphincter has a basal resting pressure 5 to 10 mm Hg greater than in the common bile duct, and pressures exceeding 35 mm Hg are clearly abnormal. Sphincter of Oddi dysfunction (SOD) type I patients have typical biliary pain and liver enzyme elevations at least twice normal on two occasions and delayed drainage on endoscopic retrograde cholangiopancreatography and a dilated common bile duct. Such patients have an 85% probability of having elevated sphincter pressures; thus, manometric study adds little. Those with SOD type III have biliary pain only without objective abnormalities; thus, manometry is mandatory before sphincterotomy because patients with SOD type III with normal pressures have only a 10% chance of benefiting from the sphincterotomy.

(586–A, C)   **(S&F, p. 931)**

Biliary manometry is the most physiologic test of sphincter of Oddi activity available and has become the gold standard for evaluating sphincter dysfunction. Although endoscopic biliary manometry is technically difficult, findings appear to be reproducible. Cholangiography should always be performed before manometry to rule out anatomical lesions and stone disease. Administration of a lipid-rich meal or intravenous cholecystokinin results in dilatation of the common bile duct (measured ultrasonographically) in the setting of common bile duct obstruction. However, similar studies have been inconsistent in patients with sphincter of Oddi dysfunction. Pain at the time of contrast agent injection has a very low predictive value for sphincter of Oddi dysfunction.

(587–A)   **(S&F, pp. 937–943)**

Bile acids are synthesized exclusively by the liver and recycle through the liver, bile, and intestine through the enterohepatic circulation. The transport proteins on the sinusoidal and canalicular surface have been characterized. Both appear to be energy-dependent transporters that can be competitively inhibited by a variety of agents. Total bile flow is driven by the osmotic activity of secreted bile acids plus that due to other solutes.

(588–A)   **(S&F, pp. 943–945)**

In contrast to most dietary lipids, biliary cholesterol is not efficiently absorbed from the small intestine. The majority (50% to 70%) passes into the large intestine and is eliminated in feces. This process accounts for nearly all cholesterol excretion from the body. When biliary cholesterol secretion is interrupted by cholestasis, accumulation of cholesterol may result in xanthoma formation.

(589–A, B, C, D)   **(S&F, pp. 1001–1004)**

The vast majority of gallbladder polyps are either cholesterol polyps (localized accumulation of cholesterol esters in foamy macrophages in the gallbladder wall) or adenomyomas (non-neoplastic proliferation of the surface mucosa). Only about 4% are neoplastic. Unlike other gastrointestinal mucosas, adenomas are actually less common than adenocarcinoma; and no clear progression from adenomas to carcinomas has been demonstrated. Except in the case of invasive carcinomas, gallbladder polyps rarely produce any symptoms. Surgery in symptomatic patients is usually indicated only if stones are also present, or if the polyp is large enough to be worrisome for cancer (>10 mm).

(590–B, C)   **(S&F, pp. 906–907)**

The bile canaliculus corresponds to the smallest branch of the biliary tree and is where bile secretion begins. Canalicular bile flows from the central lobular cells (zone 3) to the portal triads (zone 1) before joining larger ductules. Bile secretion starts at the beginning of the fourth month of gestation. The secreted bile pigments color the contents of the gut (meconium) a dark green.

(591–C)   **(S&F, p. 999)**

Adenomyomatosis of the gallbladder is an acquired, hyperplastic lesion of the gallbladder characterized by excessive proliferation of the surface epithelium with invaginations into the muscularis or beyond. Despite the prefix "adeno," it is a benign condition with no malignant potential. It is found in about 1% of autopsies and is three times more common in women. Because the gallbladder has no muscularis mucosa, the epithelial layer may deepen and penetrate into the muscular layer, forming Rokitansky-Aschoff sinuses. These sinuses are present in about 90% of gallbladders resected for stone disease. The disorder is commonly localized to the fundus of the gallbladder and causes thickening of the gallbladder wall. Like cholesterolosis, it rarely causes symptoms and is not usually an indication for surgery.

(592–A)   **(S&F, p. 951)**

Lovastatin reduces serum cholesterol by blocking hepatic synthesis of cholesterol and may actually reduce the risk of cholesterol gallstones. Oral contraceptive users have a greater risk of gallstones, particularly if they are younger than 40 years old. This appears to be largely due to the estrogen content and is less of a problem with current formulations. Clofibrate and other fibrate drugs strikingly increase gallstones. Octreotide inhibits gallbladder emptying and leads to gallstones whereas ceftriaxone is extremely concentrated in bile and may precipitate with calcium to form stones.

(593–C)   **(S&F, p. 959)**

The sensitivity of ultrasonography for detecting stones is the gallbladder is 95%, but less than 50% of stones in the common bile duct are actually visualized by ultrasonography. The presence of common duct stones can be inferred by the finding of a dilated bile duct, which has a sensitivity of 75%. The presence of tenderness under the transducer as it passes over the gallbladder (ultrasonographic Murphy's sign) is highly suggestive of acute cholecystitis. Other less specific findings include wall thickening (>4 mm) and pericholecystic fluid. Thickening of the gallbladder wall may also be seen with congestive heart failure, hypoalbuminemia, the acquired immunodeficiency syndrome, and renal failure.

(594–B)   *(S&F, pp. 997–998)*

Cholesterolosis of the gallbladder is generally a benign condition in which epithelial macrophages become laden with excess cholesterol esters. The gallbladder may be diffusely involved, or the infiltrated tissue may be localized, causing cholesterol polyps. These small (2 to 10 mm) polyps do not usually cause symptoms, but they are important because they may be mistaken for gallstones on cholecystography. Some authors believe that pieces of cholesterol polyps may break free and cause common duct obstruction, leading to recurrent pancreatitis. Autopsy studies have found cholesterolosis of the gallbladder in 5% to 40% of cases.

595. A 23-year-old woman is referred with elevated aminotransferase levels and pruritus. She is at week 35 of gestation with her second child. Her previous pregnancy was uncomplicated. Physical examination reveals excoriations but is otherwise unremarkable without jaundice or stigmata of liver disease. No evidence of fetal distress is present. Repeat serum alanine aminotransferase level is 520 IU/L, with an alkaline phosphatase value of 500 IU/L and a normal gamma glutamyl transpeptidase. Tests for viral hepatitis are negative. Regarding the most likely diagnosis, which of the following statements are TRUE?
A. Serum bile acid levels are elevated.
B. The fetus is at minimal risk.
C. Symptoms will resolve promptly after parturition.
D. Treatment with ursodeoxycholate is indicated.
E. The risk of recurrence with subsequent pregnancies is small.

596. A 62-year-old man is referred by his primary care physician for evaluation of hepatomegaly. On questioning he admits to fatigue for the past year, a 10-kg weight loss, and dependent edema. He is not obese, does not drink alcohol, and was previously well. Physical examination shows a 16-cm liver span and evidence of congestive heart failure. He is anicteric and no stigmata of liver disease are present. Routine liver test results are normal. Regarding the most likely diagnosis, which of the following statements about this patient are TRUE?
A. Urinalysis would probably be abnormal.
B. Liver biopsy is not usually needed to make the diagnosis.
C. The prognosis is poor.
D. Death is usually not related to liver disease.

597. Overall patient survival after orthotopic liver transplantation in adults is:
A. 70% at one year and 55% at five years
B. 80% at one year and 68% at five years
C. 90% at one year and 78% at five years
D. 85% at one year and 50% at five years

598. Absolute contraindications to liver transplantation include each of the following EXCEPT:
A. Human immunodeficiency virus seropositivity
B. Extrahepatic malignancy
C. Advanced cardiac or pulmonary disease
D. Hepatitis B with viremia
E. Uncontrolled extrahepatic infection

599. Which of the following statements about liver transplantation are TRUE?
A. Survival is better with cholestatic forms of liver disease.
B. Renal insufficiency is a relative contraindication.
C. Primary hepatocellular carcinoma is an absolute contraindication.
D. More patients in poorer United Network Organ Sharing (UNOS) functional categories are undergoing transplants than previously.

600. Which of the following statements about recurrent hepatitis B after liver transplantation are TRUE?
A. Immunosuppression tends to reduce viral damage to the graft.
B. Viral titers after recurrence are extremely high.
C. Recurrence rates are higher with chronic than acute hepatitis B.
D. The presence of HBeAg predicts a higher risk of recurrence.
E. Hepatitis B immune globulin (HBIG) may be stopped after one year if the patient remains HBsAg negative.

601. Which of the following is MOST likely to explain hepatic allograft dysfunction occurring more than 30 days after transplantation?
A. Hepatic artery thrombosis
B. Preservation injury
C. Cytomegaloviral hepatitis
D. Azathioprine toxicity
E. Hyperacute rejection

602. Which of the following statements about biliary complications of liver transplantation are TRUE?
A. Bile leaks occur in up to 25% of patients.
B. The bile duct anastomosis is the most common site for strictures.
C. Hilar strictures suggest hepatic artery thrombosis.
D. Strictures are more common with ABO-incompatible transplants.
E. Strictures are more common after prolonged cold ischemia.

603. Which one of the following statements about hepatitis C after liver transplantation is FALSE?
A. Hepatitis C virus is the major cause of post-transplant hepatitis.

B. Interferon-α clears viral RNA in approximately 20% of patients treated.

C. The most common histologic lesion is mild inflammation.

D. Patients infected with genotype 1b have a worse outcome.

E. Hepatitis C viral titers increase markedly after liver transplantation.

---

604. Which one of the following statements regarding nonhepatic complications of liver transplantation is FALSE?

A. The average gain in body weight after transplantation is 10% at 10 months.

B. Hyperlipidemia occurs in up to 40% of patients.

C. Hemolytic anemia is more common after transplantation from an ABO-incompatible donor.

D. Graft-versus-host disease after transplantation may produce diarrhea.

E. Pleural effusions are usually clinically insignificant.

---

605. Regarding the controversial issue of orthotopic liver transplantation (OLT) in patients with alcoholic liver disease (ALD), which of the following statements are TRUE?

A. Survival of patients with ALD undergoing OLT is less than that in non-ALD recipients.

B. Recidivism to alcoholism after OLT is approximately 50%.

C. Post-transplant compliance with medical therapy is less in ALD patients than in non-ALD patients.

D. The percentage of ALD patients who return to work after OLT is less than that seen in non-ALD patients.

---

606. Each of the following statements regarding treatment of hepatitis C with interferon-α is true EXCEPT:

A. Liver disease may be exacerbated in patients with autoimmune features.

B. Patients with advanced disease are less likely to respond.

C. Interferon is contraindicated in transplant patients.

D. High titers of hepatitis C viral RNA predict a greater likelihood of a sustained response.

E. Viral genotype is a determinant of clinical response.

---

607. A 40-year-old man presents with fulminant hepatic failure. Each of the following are important criteria in determining the need for liver transplantation EXCEPT:

A. Variceal hemorrhage

B. Underlying cause

C. Prothrombin time greater than 100 seconds

D. Degree of hyperbilirubinemia

---

608. Which statements regarding treatment of chronic hepatitis B with interferon-α are TRUE?

A. Interferon produces a lasting improvement in 33% to 37% of patients.

B. Patients with decompensated liver disease should be treated to forestall the need for transplantation.

C. The standard regimen for hepatitis B is 3 million units thrice weekly.

D. Re-treatment or use of higher doses is recommended if the patient relapses or fails to respond.

---

609. A 34-year-old Mexican American man presents with a one-week history of fatigue, nausea, vomiting, dark urine, acholic stools, and jaundice. He denies ethanol ingestion or history of exposure to other toxins. An ultrasonogram performed at an outside hospital was normal. His physical examination on June 3 was notable for icterus, a liver span of 10 cm, no palpable spleen tip, and a normal neurologic examination. Laboratory values included the following:

	6/3	6/8	6/20	8/17	10/19
Asparatate aminotransferase	1010	2715	305	45	39
Alanine aminotransferase	1832	4246	695	73	51
Alkaline phosphatase	181	202	216	109	110
Gamma glutamyl transpeptidase	277	184	192	81	58
Total bilirubin	14.6	20.5	3.2	1.3	1.0
Prothrombin time	15.0	19.0	12.5		

HBsAg reactive, anti-HBc IgM reactive, anti-HBc reactive, anti-HAV IgM nonreactive

Which statements are TRUE?

A. He should have been hospitalized for observation before his second visit.

B. Had he developed fulminant liver failure, he would have been a poor candidate for liver transplantation.

C. Spouse and any sexual partners of the patient should be tested for hepatitis B and if negative should receive hepatitis B vaccine and hepatitis B immune globulin.

D. His probability of developing chronic hepatitis B is reduced by the presence of antibodies to HBcAg.

---

610. Which of the following groups of findings in a patient with alcoholic cirrhosis is most likely to indicate bleeding from esophageal varices?

A. Hepatic vein gradient 24 mm Hg, no varices, Child's A

B. Hepatic vein gradient 16 mm Hg, small varices, Child's A

C. Hepatic vein gradient 12 mm Hg, large varices, Child's A

D. Hepatic vein gradient 6 mm Hg, small varices, Child's B

611. Rank in declining order of frequency these indications for liver transplantation in pediatric patients:
   A. Viral liver disease
   B. Biliary atresia
   C. α_1-Antitrypsin deficiency
   D. Drug toxicity

612. "Quality of life" indications for liver transplantation include all of the following EXCEPT:
   A. Intractable pruritus
   B. Intractable encephalopathy
   C. Intractable ascites
   D. Intractable fatigue
   E. Intractable bleeding

613. Common complications of treatment with cyclosporine and tacrolimus include all of the following EXCEPT:
   A. Renal failure
   B. Hypotension
   C. Gingival hyperplasia
   D. Hyperlipidemia
   E. Central nervous system toxicity

614. Which one of the following statements about primary biliary cirrhosis (PBC) is FALSE?
   A. Most patients have aberrant expression of class II HLA antigens on bile duct surfaces.
   B. Lesions are confined to small intrahepatic bile ducts.
   C. Up to 25% of patients are diagnosed with asymptomatic disease.
   D. Pruritus steadily worsens with histologic progression.
   E. The typical patient is a woman in her early 50s.

615. Match the stages of primary biliary cirrhosis with their descriptions.
   1. Stage I   A. Ductular proliferation
   2. Stage II   B. Scarring and fibrosis
   3. Stage III   C. Florid duct lesion
   4. Stage IV   D. Fibrous septa with regenerative nodules

616. Which one of the following statements about the differential diagnosis of primary biliary cirrhosis (PBC) is FALSE?
   A. Liver biopsy does not reliably differentiate PBC from primary sclerosing cholangitis.
   B. Hepatitis B can occasionally produce granulomatous inflammation about bile ducts.
   C. Sarcoidosis can produce cholestasis and similar histology on a biopsy specimen.
   D. Inflammatory bowel disease is rarely associated with PBC.
   E. Antimitochondrial antibodies are present in up to 25% of patients with autoimmune hepatitis.

617. Which of the following treatments of primary biliary cirrhosis are of proven efficacy?
   A. Azathioprine
   B. Colchicine
   C. Corticosteroids
   D. Methotrexate
   E. Penicillamine
   F. Ursodeoxycholic acid

618. A 54-year-old man is referred for an incidental finding of high iron transferrin saturation (55%) on routine screening. Serum ferritin is 350 ng/mL (normal, 20–200 ng/mL) and alanine aminotransferase level is normal. He takes no medications and is clinically well. Family history is negative for liver problems, and social history reveals daily consumption of 100 mL of ethanol, mostly as wine. The next diagnostic test should be:
   A. Repeat iron studies
   B. Human leukocyte antigen typing
   C. Genetic screen for hemochromatosis
   D. Liver biopsy
   E. Iron studies on family members

619. A 44-year-old man presents with constant right upper quadrant abdominal pain. Review of systems is positive for fatigue, arthralgias, and impotence over the past year. He does not drink alcohol. Examination shows mild epigastric tenderness and a 14-cm liver span without other evidence of liver disease. Initial laboratory testing shows an alanine aminotransferase level of 120 IU/L, normal alkaline phosphatase value, negative serologic tests for hepatitis B and C, and a positive antibody to *Helicobacter pylori*. This clinical picture is MOST compatible with:
   A. Peptic ulcer disease
   B. Hemochromatosis
   C. α_1-Antitrypsin deficiency
   D. Wilson's disease
   E. Gallstones

620. The MOST appropriate treatment for hemochromatosis is:
   A. Deferoxamine until ferritin is less than 50 ng/mL
   B. Phlebotomy, 1 unit per week, until ferritin is less than 50 ng/mL
   C. Phlebotomy, 1 unit per month, until ferritin is less than 50 ng/mL
   D. Both A and B
   E. Both A and C

621. Which of the following statements about nonalcoholic steatohepatitis are TRUE?
   A. Liver biopsy is required to differentiate it from alcoholic liver disease.
   B. It almost never progresses to cirrhosis.
   C. It is equally common in males and females.

D. Patients are typically aged 25 to 40.

E. The physical examination is typically normal.

622. Match each liver test with the basis for the abnormality. Each option may be used once, more than once, or not at all.

1. Aminotransferases
2. Prothrombin time
3. Albumin
4. Alkaline phosphatase
5. Bilirubin

    A. Decreased clearance from blood
    B. Overproduction
    C. Decreased synthesis
    D. Leakage from damaged tissue

623. A 36-year-old man with chronic hepatitis C presents with new-onset ascites. He is otherwise asymptomatic. A diagnostic paracentesis is performed, showing a neutrophil count of 75 cells/mm^3 and gram-negative rods and gram-positive cocci on Gram's stain. What is the MOST likely diagnosis?

A. Spontaneous bacterial peritonitis

B. Intra-abdominal abscess

C. Fitz-Hugh–Curtis syndrome

D. Traumatic paracentesis

624. A 45-year-old man with long-standing alcoholic liver disease characterized by jaundice, spider telangiectasia, palmar erythema, and moderate ascites presents with confusion, disorientation, somnolence, and amnesia. On examination, he has hypoactive reflexes, nystagmus, clonus, and muscular rigidity. What is the correct staging of his hepatic encephalopathy?

A. Subclinical

B. Stage 1

C. Stage 2

D. Stage 3

E. Stage 4

F. He likely does not have hepatic encephalopathy.

625. What is the pathophysiologic cause of hepatitis B virus–associated polyarteritis nodosa and membranous glomerulonephritis?

A. HBeAg and anti-HBe immune complexes

B. Anti-HBV DNA antibodies

C. HBsAg and anti-HBs immune complexes

D. HBcAG and anti-HBc immune complexes

626. Which of the following are TRUE statements regarding solitary cysts of the liver?

A. They are usually associated with cysts in other organs.

B. They involve the left lobe more often than the right.

C. They are hereditary.

D. They occur at all ages.

627. Regarding the use of corticosteroids in the treatment of acute alcoholic hepatitis, which of the following statements are TRUE?

A. Corticosteroids given orally are as effective as when given intravenously.

B. Hepatic encephalopathy is a relative contraindication for the use of corticosteroids.

C. Unfortunately, only milder cases of alcoholic hepatitis (discriminant function <32) show a response to corticosteroids.

D. Serum creatinine value greater than 2.5 mg/dL is a relative contraindication to the use of corticosteroids.

628. A diagnostic paracentesis is an extremely useful test in evaluating patients with ascites, but each assay ordered on the ascitic fluid costs money. Which TWO of the following tests are virtually useless measurements in testing for ascitic fluid?

A. Blood cell count

B. Triglycerides

C. Albumin

D. Cholesterol

E. pH

F. Amylase

G. Bilirubin

629. Regarding the proper technique of diagnostic paracentesis, all of the following statements are true EXCEPT:

A. Patients with a prothrombin time greater than 17 seconds should receive frozen plasma before the paracentesis to prevent intra-abdominal hemorrhage.

B. With a midline insertion site, the risk of bleeding is greater for supraumbilical taps compared with infraumbilical taps.

C. A midline abdominal scar is a contraindication to a midline insertion site.

D. Either right or left lower quadrant insertion sites (4 cm superior and 4 cm medial to the anterior superior iliac spine) are safe alternative sites if the midline is scarred.

630. Which of the following is a specific physical finding in alcoholic cirrhosis?

A. Dupuytren's contracture

B. Parotid gland enlargement

C. Muercke's lines

D. None of the above

631. Hepatic histology showing an intact limiting plate, occasionally isolated foci of intralobular necrosis, but no evidence of significant periportal inflammation, bridging necrosis, or fibrosis has been associated with each of the following diseases EXCEPT:

A. Primary biliary cirrhosis

B. Hepatitis B
C. Hepatitis C
D. Untreated autoimmune hepatitis
E. Portal inflammation secondary to an extrahepatic disorder such as pancreatitis

---

632. A 20-year-old female presents with fatigue, headache, and nausea. She is despondent over the breakup of a recent relationship and has been drinking more alcohol than usual. A chemistry panel is obtained and reveals aspartate aminotransferase level of 1523 IU/L, alanine aminotransferase level of 2000 IU/L, alkaline phosphatase value of 235 IU/L, total bilirubin level of 5.0 mg/dL, and prothrombin time of 15 seconds (control, 11 to 13 seconds). What additional history would be most helpful in treating this patient?
A. The amount of alcohol she has been drinking
B. Whether she takes oral contraceptives
C. Whether she has taken any acetaminophen
D. Whether she has had a recent viral illness

---

633. Each of the following statements regarding hepatitis D virus (HDV) is true EXCEPT:
A. The diagnosis of HDV infection relies mainly on assays for antibody to viral antigen.
B. Patients with hepatitis D progress to cirrhosis and hepatic failure in a high proportion of cases.
C. Hepatitis D virus requires hepatitis B virus for its replication.
D. Twenty-five to 30 percent of patients with hepatitis D have sustained remissions after therapy with interferon-α.
E. Vaccination can prevent infection by hepatitis D.

---

634. True statements regarding hepatitis B include all of the following EXCEPT:
A. Most HBsAg carriers can recall an acute episode of jaundice associated with hepatitis B.
B. Between 2% and 10% of adult patients with acute hepatitis B develop chronic infection.
C. Hepatocytes containing HBsAg may have a ground-glass appearance.
D. In acute hepatitis B, cells expressing HBcAg and human leukocyte antigen class I antigens are destroyed by cytotoxic T cells.

---

635. Which one of the following statements about spontaneous bacterial peritonitis is FALSE?
A. Gram-negative rods are more common than gram-positive cocci.
B. The Gram stain is usually positive.
C. Low-protein ascites is a major risk factor for its development.
D. About half of patients are bacteremic at the time of diagnosis.

---

636. Each of the following statements about secondary bacterial peritonitis is true EXCEPT:
A. A low ascitic fluid glucose concentration is a clue to diagnosis.
B. Empirical antibiotic coverage should include an agent effective against anaerobes.
C. Peritoneal fluid cultures remain positive after 48 hours of antibiotics.
D. A high serum ascites/albumin gradient argues against the diagnosis.

---

637. A 30-year-old woman with no prior medical problems presents with biliary colic. She denies any risk factors for chronic liver disease, and her only medication has been an oral contraceptive for many years. Her laboratory test results are as follows: aspartate aminotransferase, 27 IU/L; alanine aminotransferase, 36 IU/L; alkaline phosphatase, 150 IU/L; total bilirubin, 0.7 mg/dL; and a normal prothrombin time. All viral serologic studies are negative, and she has normal ceruloplasmin and α-fetoprotein levels. An ultrasonogram reveals cholelithiasis and a 5 × 6-cm subcapsular, multilobulated mass in the right lobe of the liver. A radionuclide scintigraphy ("liver scan") is normal. What is the MOST likely cause of the liver lesion?
A. Fibrolamellar hepatocellular carcinoma
B. Cirrhosis with a regenerative nodule
C. Focal nodular hyperplasia
D. Splenic vein thrombosis
E. Gallbladder carcinoma

---

638. In developed countries, the causes of ascites in order from the most to least frequent are:
A. Tuberculosis
B. Malignancy
C. Cirrhosis
D. Pancreatitis

---

639. Which antibody confers the greatest resistance to reinfection by hepatitis B?
A. Anti-HBc IgM
B. Anti-HBc IgG
C. Anti-HBs
D. Anti-HBe

---

640. A 45-year-old Chinese man with chronic hepatitis B and cirrhosis presents with hepatomegaly. An abdominal ultrasonogram shows a mass in the right lobe of the liver without evidence of cirrhosis. An α-fetoprotein value is normal. What is the MOST likely diagnosis?
A. Hepatic adenoma
B. Hepatocellular carcinoma
C. Cystadenocarcinoma
D. Hemangioma

641. A 56-year-old woman with a history of chronic hepatitis B presents with increased abdominal girth. On physical examination, the patient is afebrile and anicteric and moderate ascites is present. Ascites is confirmed on abdominal ultrasonography, and no hepatic masses are identified. Laboratory data show the following: white blood cell count (WBC), 4200 cells/mm³; hematocrit, 39%; platelet count, 105,000 cells/mm³; sodium, 143 mEq/L; potassium, 4.1 mEq/L; blood urea nitrogen, 16 mg/dL; creatinine, 0.7 mg/dL; bilirubin, 1.7 mg/dL; albumin, 3.1 g/dL; prothrombin time (INR), 1.2 seconds; α-fetoprotein, normal. Diagnostic paracentesis shows a total WBC of 140 cells/mm³ and an albumin level of 1.1 g/dL. A decision to treat the ascites is made. Each of the following measures is likely to be helpful EXCEPT:
A. Salt restriction
B. Fluid restriction
C. Dietary education
D. Diuretics

642. Although medical management was initially successful, ascites has now worsened and the patient in question 641 requires therapeutic paracentesis every two weeks. She has been evaluated for liver transplantation but was rejected owing to an unstable social situation. Placement of a peritoneovenous shunt is considered. With regard to peritoneovenous shunting, which of the following is FALSE?
A. It will permit discontinuation of diuretics in most patients.
B. It does not reduce the incidence of infections.
C. It does not improve survival.
D. It will prolong the interval between hospitalizations.

643. Which of the following causes of chronic liver disease also pose an increased risk of hepatocellular carcinoma? (More than one answer may be correct.)
A. Wilson's disease
B. Chronic hepatitis C
C. Chronic hepatitis B
D. Genetic hemachromatosis

644. Each of the following hormones or neurotransmitters has been postulated to contribute to ascites in the setting of cirrhosis EXCEPT:
A. Nitric oxide
B. Norepinephrine
C. Acetylcholine
D. Aldosterone
E. Renin

645. Which of the following are TRUE statements about pyogenic hepatic abscesses?
A. The most common cause is biliary tract infection.
B. Radiologic differentiation from amebic abscess is difficult.

C. Right upper quadrant tenderness is common.
D. Treatment with percutaneous drainage plus antibiotics is usually effective.

646. A patient presents with a history of drinking a fifth of vodka daily for the past six months. Physical examination reveals marked jaundice, tender hepatomegaly, ascites. and multiple angiomas. The serum bilirubin level is 25 mg/dL, the prothrombin time is 17 seconds (control, 11 to 13 seconds), and the serum albumin level is 2.1 g/dL (3.5 to 4.8 g/dL). This patient's one-month mortality is:
A. Approximately 15%
B. Approximately 50%
C. Not able to be estimated because a liver biopsy is needed to determine the patient's prognosis
D. Not able to be estimated because the patient's five-year mortality is independent of his underlying liver disease

647. A 42-year-old man with a long-standing history of ethanol dependence presents with new-onset ascites. A diagnostic paracentesis reveals a polymorphonuclear leukocyte count of 75 cells/mm³. The following day an ascitic fluid culture is growing gram-negative rods. Under which conditions should empirical antibiotic treatment be started?
A. If abdominal pain or fever is present
B. If the organism is identified as *Pseudomonas*
C. If the ascitic fluid protein concentration is low
D. Under all circumstances

648. Assuming the primary tumor is resectable, for which of the following malignancies does surgical resection of liver metastases have the BEST survival?
A. Melanoma
B. Renal cell carcinoma
C. Wilms' tumor
D. Ovarian cancer
E. Colon cancer

649. A 20-year-old man presents with malaise, jaundice, and fatigue. His parents report that he has recently been acting strangely and has become very combative. On careful questioning, he denies any licit or illicit drug use, tattoos, blood transfusions, or sexual contacts. Laboratory tests reveal the following: aspartate aminotransferase, 1500 IU/L; alanine aminotransferase, 2000 IU/L; alkaline phosphatase, 125 IU/L; total bilirubin, 26 mg/dL (direct 10 mg/dL); prothrombin time, 14 seconds (control, 11 to 13 seconds); hemoglobin, 9 g/dL. Viral serologic studies are negative. Which of the following tests would be MOST likely to establish a diagnosis?
A. Head computed tomography
B. 24-Hour urinary copper
C. Slit-lamp examination

D. Serum ceruloplasmin
E. Acetaminophen level

650. The patient in question 649 is admitted to the hospital for observation. What therapy should be initiated?
A. D-Penicillamine
B. Orthotopic liver transplantation
C. Trientine
D. Deferoxamine

651. Which of the following tests of peritoneal fluid has the greatest sensitivity for detecting spontaneous bacterial peritonitis?
A. White blood cell count
B. Gram's stain
C. pH
D. Lactate

652. The primary toxic metabolite of ethanol is:
A. Ethyl aldehyde
B. Acetaldehyde
C. Formaldehyde
D. None of the above

653. A 32-year-old woman presents because of right upper quadrant discomfort. She denies any fatigue, weight loss, fever, chills, nausea, or vomiting. She has been taking oral contraceptives for many years. On examination she has a 14-cm liver span with mild tenderness over the right upper quadrant. Laboratory tests reveal an aspartate aminotransferase level of 45 IU/L, alanine aminotransferase level of 59 IU/L, alkaline phosphatase level of 150 IU/L, and a total bilirubin level of 1 mg/dL. All other laboratory test results are normal except for a mild anemia. Hepatitis serologic studies are negative. An abdominal ultrasonogram is obtained and reveals an 8-cm solid mass in the right lobe of the liver with a normal biliary system. Which one or more of the following are appropriate for managing this patient?
A. Recommend she stop taking oral contraceptives.
B. Repeat the ultrasonogram in six months.
C. Obtain an immediate surgical consultation.
D. Obtain a tagged red blood cell scan.

654. Which of the following represents a contraindication to abdominal paracentesis?
A. Obesity
B. Extensive prior abdominal surgery
C. Abdominal aortic aneurysm
D. Disseminated intravascular coagulation

655. Each of the following is a true statement concerning routine culture of neutrocytic ascites EXCEPT:
A. It has a sensitivity similar to that of bedside inoculation of blood culture bottles.

B. The median bacterial concentration in ascitic fluid is one organism per milliliter.
C. Approximately half of cultures are negative.
D. Both aerobic and anaerobic cultures should be done.

656. Which of the following countries has the lowest incidence of hepatocellular carcinoma?
A. China
B. Japan
C. Mexico
D. Italy
E. South Africa

657. A 25-year-old homosexual man is admitted to your service with fatigue, arthralgias, abdominal pain, and dark urine. He was well until 3 days ago but now has difficulty staying awake during the evaluation. Physical examination reveals mild scleral icterus, mild right upper quadrant abdominal tenderness on palpation, and asterixis. Initial laboratory studies reveal an alanine aminotransferase level of more than 2000 IU/L and negative HBsAg determination. A screen for toxins and urine copper is normal, and there is no history of mushroom ingestion. His clinical status continues to deteriorate and he requires mechanical ventilation. Which of the following is MOST likely to cause the death of this patient?
A. Acute renal failure
B. Sepsis
C. Gastrointestinal hemorrhage
D. Cerebral edema

658. Each of the following laboratory abnormalities is suggestive of alcoholic liver disease EXCEPT:
A. Hypoalbuminemia
B. Parallel elevation of the aspartate and alanine aminotransferases
C. Erythrocyte macrocytosis
D. Leukocytosis

659. Acute infection with the hepatotropic viruses HAV, HBV, or HCV may rarely result in fulminant hepatic failure. In western countries, the rank order for the probability of acute infection progressing to fulminant hepatic failure is:
A. HCV→HBV→HAV
B. HAV→HBV→HCV
C. HBV→HAV→HCV
D. HBV→HCV→HAV

660. Regarding the decision of whether to treat autoimmune hepatitis, all of the following are considered to be absolute indications for treatment EXCEPT:
A. Incapacitating symptoms
B. Severe cytopenia
C. Aspartate aminotransferase greater than ten times normal

D. Aspartate aminotransferase greater than five times normal and gamma globulin greater than two times normal

E. Bridging necrosis on liver biopsy

---

661. Each of the following hepatobiliary disorders is associated with a renal lesion EXCEPT:
A. Choledochal cyst
B. Congenital hepatic fibrosis
C. Caroli's disease
D. Adult polycystic disease

---

662. Which physical sign has the highest diagnostic accuracy for detection of ascites?
A. Bulging flanks
B. Shifting dullness
C. Fluid wave
D. Puddle sign

---

663. Which of the following is the MOST effective long-term therapy for hepatic hydrothorax?
A. Chest tube drainage
B. Salt restriction and diuretics
C. Liver transplantation
D. Peritoneovenous shunting

---

664. Regarding the serologic diagnosis of hereditary hemochromatosis (HHC), which of the following statements are TRUE?
A. The combination of a transferrin saturation of more than 55% and a serum ferritin level greater than 300 ng/mL has a positive predictive value of 93% for HHC.
B. The combination of a transferrin saturation of less than 50% and a serum ferritin level less than 250 ng/mL has a negative predictive value of 97% that the patient does not have HHC.
C. Most patients with HHC present with fatigue, arthralgias, pruritus, or impotence.
D. Rapid absorption of dietary iron after a meal may give a falsely elevated transferrin saturation; hence, blood should be obtained in a fasting state for testing.

---

665. The single best imaging test in evaluating a hepatic cyst is:
A. Abdominal ultrasonography
B. Abdominal computed tomography
C. Radionuclide scanning
D. Abdominal magnetic resonance imaging

---

666. In acetaminophen-related fulminant hepatic failure, which of the following findings portends the WORST prognosis?
A. Metabolic acidosis, pH less than 7.3
B. Cerebral edema

C. Renal failure
D. Hyperbilirubinemia

---

667. The rate of metabolism of acetaldehyde in alcoholics versus nonalcoholics is:
A. Accelerated due to induction of hepatic aldehyde dehydrogenase by ethanol
B. Delayed due to reduced levels of aldehyde dehydrogenase in the liver
C. The same in alcoholics and nonalcoholics

---

668. Each of the following may cause fulminant hepatic failure EXCEPT:
A. Lassa fever
B. Yellow fever
C. Cytomegalovirus infection
D. Hepatitis D

---

669. Which of the following is MOST common in spontaneous bacterial peritonitis?
A. Encephalopathy
B. Abdominal pain
C. Rebound tenderness
D. Fever

---

670. Each of the following factors is an important risk factor for alcoholic liver disease EXCEPT:
A. Ethnic background
B. Coexisting hepatitis C
C. Gender
D. Nutritional status
E. All of the above are risk factors

---

671. Each of the following conditions can decrease the diagnostic accuracy of the serum ascites/albumin gradient EXCEPT:
A. Hyperglobulinemia
B. Chylous ascites
C. Hypotension
D. Diuretics

---

672. Each of the following agents has been shown to be cholestatic EXCEPT:
A. Estrogens
B. Flucloxacillin
C. Chlorpromazine
D. Ursodeoxycholic acid
E. Anabolic steroids

---

673. Which of the following is the most objective way to follow the response of ascites to diuretics?
A. 24-Hour urine volume
B. Abdominal girth
C. Serum ascites/albumin gradient
D. Daily weight

674. Each of the following statements regarding autoimmune hepatitis is true EXCEPT:
   A. Fatigue is the most common presenting complaint.
   B. All patients have an elevated aspartate aminotransferase level.
   C. Smooth muscle antibody, antinuclear antibody, or anti-LKM1 markers are present in approximately 50% of cases.
   D. Hepatomegaly or jaundice is present in approximately two thirds of cases.

675. Ingestion of ethanol has all the following effects EXCEPT:
   A. Reduction of nicotinamide-adenine dinucleotide to the reduced form
   B. Inhibition of fatty acid oxidation in the liver
   C. Formation of acetaldehyde-protein adducts (attachment of acetaldehyde to cellular proteins)
   D. Stimulation of gastrin release

676. A 62-year-old woman with Alzheimer's disease presents to the emergency department with complaints of nausea and vomiting for three days. Her physical examination is normal except for memory loss. Laboratory tests reveal a normal complete blood cell count with differential and a normal serum amylase value, and liver function tests are normal except for an alanine aminotransferase value of 177 IU/L. Which of the following diagnostic steps would be the MOST appropriate?
   A. Ultrasonography of the upper abdomen, with special attention to search for cholesterolosis of the gallbladder
   B. Hepatitis A virus IgM, HBsAg, and hepatitis C virus serologic tests
   C. Inquiry as to tacrine use, and, if present, then discontinue and discharge patient
   D. Lumbar puncture with cerebrospinal fluid examination for rapid plasma reagin (PRP)

677. Each of the following causes of ascites is associated with a high serum ascites/albumin gradient EXCEPT:
   A. Nephrotic syndrome
   B. Fatty liver of pregnancy
   C. Constrictive pericarditis
   D. Hepatic vein thrombosis

678. Which of the following liver lesions is associated with the use of anabolic steroids?
   I. Hepatic adenoma
   II. Hemangioma
   III. Peliosis hepatis
   IV. Cystadenoma

   A. I and III
   B. II and IV

   C. I, II, and III
   D. All of the above

679. Which of the following laboratory findings in an alcoholic with fulminant hepatic failure would MOST suggest acetaminophen overdosage?
   A. Disproportionately elevated prothrombin time in comparison to aminotransferase levels
   B. Markedly elevated alanine aminotransferase level of 8000 IU/L
   C. Hyperammonemia
   D. Hyperbilirubinemia

680. A 35-year-old Chinese woman presents for evaluation of jaundice and pruritus. She is in the United States visiting a relative. She has a long history of recurrent fevers, right upper quadrant abdominal pain, and jaundice. Recently she has noted some weight loss. What is the MOST likely cause of this patient's problem?
   A. *Ascaris* infection
   B. *Clonorchis sinensis* infection
   C. *Escherichia coli* cholangitis
   D. Schistosomiasis

681. Survival may be improved by abstaining from alcohol in patients with alcoholic liver disease. Which of the following statements regarding the effect of abstinence on prognosis are TRUE and supported by objective evidence?
   A. The prognosis of cirrhosis without accompanying complications (portal hypertension, encephalopathy) is favorably affected by abstinence.
   B. The prognosis of cirrhosis with accompanying complications (portal hypertension or encephalopathy) is not significantly affected by abstinence.
   C. Hepatic inflammation on biopsy is as equally an ominous finding as cirrhosis in terms of survival.
   D. Women, in particular, may show progressive liver disease despite abstinence.

682. All of the following statements regarding portal hypertensive gastropathy are true EXCEPT:
   A. Endoscopic findings of mild cases of portal hypertensive gastropathy include a mosaic (snakeskin) pattern of erythema.
   B. Endoscopic findings of severe cases of portal hypertensive gastropathy include bright red punctate erythema and brown or black submucosal macules indicative of mucosal hemorrhages.
   C. Despite its name, the lesion is often seen in patients without portal hypertension, especially in elderly women.
   D. Although spontaneous remission is seen, the lesion usually progresses slowly.
   E. It accounts for up to 20% of acute or chronic bleeding in patients with portal hypertension.

683. As a rule, alcohol is not good for the liver, but it specifically worsens hepatotoxicity from all of the following drugs EXCEPT:
A. Chlorpromazine
B. Acetaminophen
C. Methotrexate
D. Isoniazid

684. Which of the following complications of fulminant hepatic failure is LEAST common?
A. Pulmonary edema
B. Pancreatitis
C. Infection
D. Cerebrovascular accidents

685. When given as a single agent, which antibiotic has the greatest efficacy in treatment of spontaneous bacterial peritonitis?
A. Ampicillin
B. Aztreonam
C. Cefotaxime
D. Chloramphenicol

686. Nonalcoholic steatohepatitis (NASH) shares many biochemical and histologic features with alcoholic liver disease. Which of the following findings favors the diagnosis of NASH over alcoholic liver disease?
A. Fatty liver
B. Mallory bodies
C. Neutrophilic infiltration of the liver
D. Fibrosis
E. None of the above

687. Which of the following are TRUE statements regarding acute viral hepatitis?
A. Fever, arthralgia, arthritis, and rash may develop two to three weeks before jaundice.
B. Coryza, headache, and pharyngitis are not associated with viral hepatitis.
C. Splenomegaly strongly suggests a chronic process.
D. With the onset of jaundice, the fever usually declines and the constitutional symptoms begin to subside.
E. The stool may be acholic during the preicteric phase.

688. A 28-year-old woman presents with nausea and vomiting, fatigue, and right upper quadrant pain. She is 35 weeks pregnant and has had no complications during her pregnancy. On physical examination, she is mildly hypertensive with jaundice and mild right upper quadrant tenderness but no hepatomegaly. She is hospitalized and found to have an aspartate aminotransferase level of 550 IU/L, alanine aminotransferase level of 300 IU/L, alkaline phosphatase value of 250 IU/L, total bilirubin level of 10 mg/dL, prothrombin time of 15 seconds (control, 11 to 13 seconds), and moderate proteinuria. One week into the hospitalization, her bilirubin level continues to rise, as does her prothrombin time. What would be the BEST therapy for this patient?
A. Acetylcysteine
B. Supportive care
C. Induction of labor
D. Magnesium sulfate

689. Which one of the following is likely to be the LEAST reliable predictor of clinical outcome in patients with fulminant hepatic failure?
A. Degree of encephalopathy
B. Duration of jaundice
C. Prothrombin time
D. History of acetaminophen ingestion
E. Liver histology

690. Chylous ascites is associated with each of the following conditions EXCEPT:
A. Cirrhosis
B. Lymphoma
C. Pancreatitis
D. Lymphatic trauma

691. Which of the following are TRUE statements regarding autoimmune liver disease?
A. Treatment includes prednisone alone or in combination with azathioprine.
B. Approximately 20% of patients will suffer a relapse after successful medical treatment.
C. Initial (two week) response to medical therapy has little prognostic value in predicting long-term outcome.
D. Follow-up liver biopsies are helpful in assessing the long-term course.

692. Which of the following are TRUE statements regarding chronic hepatitis B?
A. Females are more likely to progress to chronic infection.
B. More than 90% of neonates born to HBeAg-positive mothers become chronically infected.
C. Vertically transmitted hepatitis B infrequently progresses to cirrhosis.
D. Patients receiving cancer chemotherapy are more likely to progress to chronic hepatitis B.

693. Which of the following statements regarding hepatitis C and hepatocellular carcinoma are TRUE?
A. Hepatitis C is present in approximately 40% of patients with hepatocellular carcinoma in the United States.
B. Hepatocellular carcinoma occurs on average 20 to 30 years after initial infection with hepatitis C virus.

C. Although the onset of chronic hepatitis C may be insidious, patients observed for 20 years often develop cirrhosis or hepatocellular carcinoma.

D. Specific hepatitis C virus genotypes (type 1b > type 2) predict viral load and correlate with disease progression.

694. Which of the following are TRUE statements regarding treatment of hepatitis B with interferon-α?
A. Interferon enhances expression of human leukocyte antigen class I antigens on the hepatocyte surface.
B. Approximately 60% of HBeAg-positive patients receiving interferon-α lose markers of active replication.
C. Less than 10% of infected patients lose HBsAg.
D. Interferon is particularly useful in decompensated liver disease.

695. What is the usual time sequence of the serologies seen in self-limited acute hepatitis B?
A. HBsAg, anti-HBc IgM, HBeAg, anti-HBs
B. HBsAg, HBeAg, anti-HBc IgM, anti-HBs
C. anti-HBs, HBeAg, anti-HBc IgM, HBsAg
D. anti-HBs, anti-HBc IgM, HBsAg, HBeAg
E. anti-HBc IgM, HBsAg, HBeAg, anti-HBs

696. The only potentially curative treatment for primary hepatocellular carcinoma is surgical resection.
A. True
B. False

697. Each of the following statements regarding umbilical hernias in cirrhotic patients with ascites is true EXCEPT:
A. Incarceration is the most common complication.
B. Rupture is associated with a mortality of 10% to 45%.
C. Preoperative removal of ascites reduces the rate of hernia recurrence.
D. Skin ulceration is an indication for surgery.

698. Which of the following are TRUE statements regarding acute viral hepatitis?
A. Enzyme elevations always precede jaundice.
B. Alanine aminotransferase levels are usually higher than aspartate aminotransferase levels in both early and late phases.
C. Aminotransferase levels are greater in icteric than in anicteric hepatitis.
D. Hepatitis B leads to a more gradual rise in enzyme values than does hepatitis A.

699. A 47-year-old patient presents for evaluation of abnormal liver function tests. The patient reports he is a moderate drinker, consuming 8 to 12 beers per day on weekends only, and has a remote history of intravenous drug use. He is asymptomatic. Laboratory tests reveal an aspartate aminotransferase level of 75 IU/L, alanine aminotransferase level of 26 IU/L, alkaline phosphatase level of 130 IU/L, total bilirubin value of 0.9 mg/dL, prothrombin time of 13 seconds (control, 11 to 13 seconds), white blood cell count of 5000/mm³, hemoglobin of 14 g/dL, and platelet count of 100,000/mm³. On examination, the liver is large but no nodularity is appreciated. The MOST likely diagnosis in this patient is:
A. Chronic hepatitis caused by hepatitis C virus
B. Fatty infiltration
C. Acute hepatitis
D. Alcoholic cirrhosis

700. Which of the following statements regarding alcohol consumption and alcoholic liver disease are TRUE?
A. As a national policy, prohibition of alcohol from 1919 to 1932 in the United States had little effect on the rate of death from cirrhosis.
B. For men, an average cumulative dose of ethanol of 600 kg (2.8 L beer/day × 20 years) is required before chronic liver disease is seen.
C. A majority of alcoholics will eventually develop evidence of liver disease.
D. When adjusted for differences in weight, men and women have approximately equal tolerances for ethanol.

701. Which of the following are TRUE statements regarding hepatitis A?
A. Most viral shedding occurs before the onset of symptoms.
B. Patients may develop persistent jaundice and chemical evidence of intrahepatic cholestasis.
C. Onset of symptoms is often insidious.
D. Infectivity persists for approximately 60 days after the onset of jaundice.

702. In what disease setting is ascites MOST likely to respond to diuretics?
A. Peritoneal carcinomatosis
B. Primary biliary cirrhosis
C. Miliary tuberculosis
D. Lupus erythematosus

703. Each of the following is a benign cystic disease of the liver EXCEPT:
A. Caroli's disease
B. Adult polycystic disease
C. Congenital hepatic fibrosis
D. All are benign cystic diseases

704. A 40-year-old Japanese man presents with confusion, fatigue, weight loss, and mild right upper quadrant pain. He is found to have mildly abnormal liver function tests as follows: aspartate aminotransferase,

50 IU/L; alanine aminotransferase, 73 IU/L; alkaline phosphatase, 271 IU/L; and total bilirubin, 0.8 mg/dL. He is found to be HBsAg positive, HBeAg positive, anti-HBc positive (IgM negative), and anti-HCV negative. Which of the following would be the BEST serologic test to perform next in this patient?
A. Carcinoembryonic antigen level
B. α-Fetoprotein level
C. CA 19-9 level
D. CA 125 level

---

705. The patient in question 704 is found to have a 3 × 6-cm mass in the right lobe of the liver by abdominal ultrasonography. Shortly after admission, he is found in his bed, mumbling unintelligibly and inappropriately. His vital signs are stable and he has not received any medications. What is the MOST likely cause of his altered mental status?
A. Hepatic encephalopathy
B. Hypoglycemia
C. Brain metastases
D. Intracerebral hemorrhage
E. Rupture with bleeding into the peritoneum

---

706. A patient presents with jaundice, weakness, and right upper quadrant abdominal pain for the past week. He has been drinking more than 12 cans of beer per day. On physical examination his sclerae are icteric, his liver is markedly enlarged and tender to palpation, and he has moderate ascites. In addition, he is found to have dark stools positive for occult blood. Laboratory test results are as follows: total bilirubin, 20 mg/dL; aspartate aminotransferase, 146 IU/L; alanine aminotransferase, 44 IU/L; alkaline phosphatase, 240 IU/L; white blood cell count, 10,000 /mm^3; hemoglobin, 7 g/dL (mean corpuscular volume of 94); platelet count, 100,000/mm^3; and prothrombin time, 20 seconds (control, 11 to 13 seconds). What would be the best next step in this patient?
A. Start intravenous methylprednisolone.
B. Start intravenous vasopressin infusion.
C. Provide supportive care and observation.
D. Perform upper endoscopy.

---

707. The MOST important factors predicting a favorable response to interferon-α therapy in chronic hepatitis B are:
A. Low alanine aminotransferase and low serum hepatitis B viral DNA level
B. Elevated alanine aminotransferase and low serum hepatitis B viral DNA levels
C. Low alanine aminotransferase and high serum hepatitis B viral DNA levels
D. Elevated alanine aminotransferase and high serum hepatitis B viral DNA levels

---

708. Which of the following is the MOST important determinant of survival in patients with bleeding from esophageal varices?
A. Severity of the underlying liver disease

B. Hepatic vein gradient
C. Size of the varices
D. Presence of red wale marks

---

709. Which of the following is NOT a true statement about the use of octreotide for treating variceal bleeding?
A. It must be given parenterally.
B. It reduces azygous blood flow.
C. Its use should be limited to 48 hours or less.
D. It has fewer complications than vasopressin.
E. It is as effective as sclerotherapy for controlling acute variceal bleeding.

---

710. Each of the following causes of ascites is associated with a low serum ascites/albumin gradient EXCEPT:
A. Pancreatitis
B. Biliary duct perforation
C. Tuberculosis with cirrhosis
D. Mesothelioma

---

711. Each of the following statements regarding hepatitis C is true EXCEPT:
A. About 1% of the adult population in the United States, Japan, and Europe is infected with hepatitis C.
B. Hepatitis C viral RNA is detectable in liver when aminotransferase levels are elevated.
C. Currently available assays for hepatitis C virus antibody detect over 95% of cases of acute hepatitis C.
D. Currently available assays for hepatitis C virus antibody detect over 95% of cases of chronic hepatitis C.

---

712. Diagnostic laparoscopy is MOST likely to be helpful in identifying which of the following causes of ascites?
A. Pancreatic
B. Tuberculous
C. Chylous
D. Myxedematous

---

713. Each of the following is believed to play a specific role in the pathogenesis of spontaneous bacterial peritonitis EXCEPT:
A. Increased gut permeability
B. Low ascites/albumin concentration
C. Bacterial seeding of mesenteric lymph
D. Reticuloendothelial cell dysfunction

---

714. Which of the following laboratory findings is MOST suggestive of alcoholic liver disease?
A. Elevation of gamma glutamyl transpeptidase
B. Elevation of aspartate aminotransferase
C. A normal alanine aminotransferase

D. Elevation of the aspartate aminotransferase:alanine aminotransferase ratio greater than 2

---

715. Approximately 75% of patients who present with grade IV hepatic encephalopathy die within 48 hours of admission to the hospital unless liver transplantation is done.
A. True
B. False

---

716. A 50-year-old woman presents with jaundice and mild right upper quadrant tenderness that has been present for two weeks. History reveals that she is married to a business executive and spends many nights alone. She admits to drinking up to three glasses of wine per day. On physical examination, you would expect to find:
A. Hepatomegaly
B. Evidence of intravenous drug use
C. A small liver
D. Sclerodactyly

---

717. Laboratory test results for the patient in question 716 are as follows: aspartate aminotransferase, 154 IU/L; alanine aminotransferase, 25 IU/L; alkaline phosphatase, 127 IU/L; total bilirubin, 15 mg/dL; prothrombin time, 18 (control, 11 to 13 seconds); white blood cell count, 15,000/mm³; hemoglobin, 11 g/dL; hematocrit, 33%; and platelet count, 150,000/mm³. Which of the following would be the MOST appropriate next step?
A. Institute corticosteroid therapy.
B. Start her on antibiotics.
C. Obtain blood, urine, and sputum cultures.
D. Observe her and administer vitamin K, folate, and thiamine.

---

718. Each of the following is associated with diffusely infiltrating disease of the liver EXCEPT:
A. Colon cancer
B. Lung cancer
C. Breast cancer
D. Lymphomas

---

719. A 65-year-old Mexican American man in generally good health is found to have hepatomegaly on a routine examination. He uses tobacco but not alcohol and lives with his family, none of whom are ill. He moved to the United States from rural northern Mexico 12 years ago. A sonogram reveals a 12-cm cyst occupying the right lobe of the liver with daughter cyst enclosed. Laboratory test results are normal except for eosinophilia. Which of the following steps should be undertaken next?
A. Repeat the sonogram in three months and aspirate cystic fluid if lesion is larger.
B. Aspirate the fluid for culture (acid-fast bacilli—fungal and bacterial) and cytology.

C. Obtain serologic test for hydatidosis with surgical resection if positive and aspiration if negative.
D. Offer patient surgical resection of the lesion.
E. Obtain serologic test for hydatidosis; if test is positive, treat with mebendazole or albendazole.

---

720. Alcoholic cirrhosis is characterized by:
A. Micronodules
B. Macronodules
C. Mixed pattern (micronodules and macronodules)
D. All of the above may be seen.

---

721. Each of the following metabolic changes is commonly seen in fulminant hepatic failure EXCEPT:
A. Hyperglycemia
B. Hypoglycemia
C. Respiratory alkalosis
D. Hyponatremia

---

722. A 25-year-old woman presents for evaluation of right upper quadrant discomfort with bloating. She also complains of alternating constipation and diarrhea. Physical examination is normal. To further evaluate the right upper quadrant pain, you send the patient for an abdominal ultrasonogram, which reveals a 4 × 6-cm mass in the right lobe of the liver. The only laboratory abnormality is mild thrombocytopenia. What would be the BEST test to do next?
A. Hepatic arteriography
B. Bolus-contrast computed tomography with sequential scans
C. Technetium scan
D. Colonoscopy
E. Computed tomographic–guided liver biopsy

---

723. What is the probable cause of the thrombocytopenia in the patient in question 722?
A. Idiopathic thrombocytopenic purpura
B. Kasabach-Merritt syndrome
C. Hypersplenism
D. Wiskott-Aldrich syndrome

---

724. A young woman presents to the emergency department with severe mental confusion. She is not icteric and was well enough to hike 20 miles three days earlier. She had several episodes of nausea and vomiting the previous day. What is the suspected cause of this patient's illness?
A. Herbal teas
B. Acute intermittent porphyria
C. *Amanita phalloides* toxicity
D. Viral hepatitis
E. Giardiasis

---

725. Each of the following is a common symptom of chronic hepatitis EXCEPT:
A. Depression with difficulty sleeping

B. Increased abdominal pain after exercise
C. Right upper quadrant abdominal pain
D. Relief of pain by sitting with the knees raised
E. Severe fatigue

---

726. Congenital hepatic fibrosis is associated with each of the following EXCEPT:
A. Berry aneurysms
B. Deformity of the gallbladder
C. Pancreatic insufficiency
D. Congenital heart disease

---

727. Common paraneoplastic findings in hepatocellular carcinoma include each of the following EXCEPT:
A. Hypercalcemia
B. Erythrocytosis
C. Dermatomyositis
D. Hypoglycemia

---

728. The liver's production of certain serum proteins may rise or fall during acute systemic inflammatory conditions (acute phase response). All of the following serum proteins produced by the liver increase during an acute phase response EXCEPT:
A. Fibrinogen
B. Ferritin
C. Haptoglobin
D. Transferrin
E. Ceruloplasmin

---

729. Each of the following biopsy findings is consistent with alcoholic hepatitis EXCEPT:
A. Councilman bodies
B. Mallory bodies
C. Microvesicular and macrovesicular fat
D. Hepatocyte degeneration

---

730. A 45-year-old woman presents with right upper quadrant fullness. She is otherwise asymptomatic. Abdominal examination reveals a poorly defined mass in the right upper quadrant. Her physical examination is otherwise unremarkable. Laboratory test results are normal. An abdominal ultrasound evaluation reveals a 3 × 4-cm simple cyst in the right lobe of the liver. With this finding, what would be your recommendation?
A. Aspiration of the cyst
B. No further treatment or evaluation
C. Surgical resection
D. Injection of a sclerosant

---

731. Conditions other than cystic fibrosis that may be associated with transiently elevated sweat electrolyte concentrations include:
  I. Acute respiratory disorders
 II. Chronic respiratory disorders

III. Adrenal insufficiency
IV. Hyperthyroidism

A. I and III
B. II and IV
C. I, II, and III
D. All of the above

---

732. Which of the following is LEAST likely to be the cause of ascites formation?
A. Spontaneous bacterial peritonitis
B. Peritoneal carcinomatosis
C. Nephrotic syndrome
D. Congestive heart failure
E. Peritoneal tuberculosis

---

733. Which of the following statements regarding transjugular intrahepatic portosystemic shunts is FALSE?
A. The goal is to lower portal pressure below 12 mm Hg.
B. Technical success can be achieved in 95% of patients.
C. Encephalopathy is uncommon and develops in 5% of patients.
D. Shunt stenosis occurs in about 50% of patients within one year.
E. Shunt stenosis is associated with a 30% chance of recurrent variceal bleeding within two years.

---

734. Which of the following methods can be used for the prenatal diagnosis of cystic fibrosis?
A. Monoclonal antibodies to measure microvillous enzyme levels in amniotic fluid
B. DNA probes linked to the cystic fibrosis gene
C. Direct mutation analysis
D. All of the above

---

735. A young woman is brought to the emergency department 48 hours after an overdose of acetaminophen. She is admitted and started on acetylcysteine therapy. Despite treatment, her mental status deteriorates and by hospital day four she sleeps most of the time and is markedly confused. How would you grade her encephalopathy?
A. Grade I
B. Grade II
C. Grade III
D. Grade IV

---

736. A 45-year-old woman with four children presents with vague, right upper quadrant discomfort of two months' duration and nausea. Her physical examination is normal. Liver function tests are normal, and an ultrasonogram, looking for gallstones, instead identifies a 5-cm solitary, solid lesion in the right lobe of the liver. A test for α-fetoprotein is normal as are serologic studies for hepatitis C and B viruses.

Of the following tests, which would be the BEST in terms of cost, safety, and specificity of diagnosis?
A. Colonoscopy and upper endoscopy
B. Fine-needle aspiration of the liver lesion under ultrasonographic guidance
C. Bolus-enhanced computed tomography with rapid phase sequential scans of the liver
D. Hepatic arteriography
E. Laparoscopic biopsy of the liver lesion

---

737. The woman in question 736 has a spiral computed tomogram that shows peripheral enhancement of the liver lesion consistent with a cavernous hemangioma. Of the following, which is the BEST course of action?
A. Perform laparoscopic biopsy of the lesion for tissue confirmation.
B. Perform arteriographic embolization of the lesion.
C. Offer patient resection of the lesion for symptom relief.
D. Offer patient resection of the lesion if rupture occurs.
E. Prescribe oral contraceptives to reduce likelihood of hemangioma enlargement.

---

738. The absorption of which of the following vitamins is LEAST dependent on intact hepatic function?
A. Vitamin A
B. Cobalamin
C. Vitamin K
D. Tocopherol (vitamin E)
E. Vitamin D

---

739. A 30-year-old white man with a history of intravenous drug abuse presents with the following hepatitis serologies: HBsAg-positive, anti-HBc-positive, anti-HBc IgM-negative, anti-HCV-negative. He has no evidence of cirrhosis on physical examination, and his aminotransferase values are two to three times normal. He is treated with interferon-α 5 million units/day for 16 weeks. During the course of treatment, HBeAg and hepatitis B viral DNA are cleared from the serum. During clearance of these serologic markers, the serum aminotransferase levels will characteristically:
A. Decrease to normal
B. Increase and then decrease to normal
C. Decrease but remain abnormal
D. Remain unchanged
E. Show a sustained increase

---

740. Which of the following are believed to contribute to the pathogenesis of hepatic encephalopathy?
 I. Colonic absorption of ammonia and mercaptans (produced by bacterial action on proteins and urea in the lumen) and subsequent impaired hepatic clearance
 II. Gamma-aminobutyric acid (GABA)

 III. Production of false neurotransmitters
 IV. Norepinephrine

A. I and III
B. II and IV
C. I, II, and III
D. All of the above

---

741. Each of the following is a neurologic manifestation of alcoholism EXCEPT:
A. Wernicke-Korsakoff encephalopathy
B. Cerebellar degeneration
C. Dementia
D. Peripheral neuropathy

---

742. A 37-year-old man who has been being treated for ulcerative colitis presents with jaundice and pruritus. He reports a 4-kg weight loss but attributes this to recent stress. He was first diagnosed with ulcerative colitis at age 15, and at that time colonoscopy revealed pancolitis. He had a mildly elevated alkaline phosphatase level but normal aminotransferase values at that time, and liver function tests have been performed periodically since. Over the years, the test results progressively worsened; and at age 22 he underwent endoscopic retrograde cholangiopancreatography because of an elevated alkaline phosphatase value (435 IU/L). Findings were consistent with sclerosing cholangitis. The patient has remained asymptomatic until now. His colitis has been under control on oral prednisone 5 mg/day. Azathioprine, 75 mg/day, was recently added as a corticosteroid-sparing agent. Which of the following is the MOST likely cause of his new symptoms?
A. Choledocholithiasis
B. Drug hepatotoxicity
C. Cholangiocarcinoma
D. Metastatic colon cancer

---

743. Match the following (potential) hepatotoxins with the mechanism of liver injury:
1. Acetaminophen	A. Granulomatous hepatitis
2. Isoniazid	B. Cholestasis without hepatitis
3. Oral contraceptives	C. Acute hepatitis
4. Carbamazepine	D. Dose-dependent hepatotoxicity

---

744. Which of the following laboratory findings are likely to be present in acute viral hepatitis?
A. Leukocytosis
B. Thrombocytopenia
C. Anemia
D. Elevated α-fetoprotein level
E. Elevated serum iron level

---

745. The risk of acquiring viral infection from a single needlestick accident when the blood is known to be infective is:
A. HCV < HBV < HIV

B. HBV < HCV < HIV
C. HIV < HBV < HCV
D. HIV < HCV < HBV
E. HCV < HIV < HBV

---

746. Match the following conditions with the associated characteristics of peritoneal fluid:

1. Hepatocellular carcinoma
2. Lymphatic obstruction
3. Peritoneal carcinomatosis
4. Bile duct laceration

A. Abnormal cytology
B. High serum ascites/albumin gradient
C. High bilirubin concentration
D. High triglyceride concentration

---

747. A 40-year-old businessman presents because on a routine examination he was found to have abnormal liver test results (aspartate aminotransferase, 45 IU/L; alanine aminotransferase, 59 IU/L; alkaline phosphatase, 185 IU/L; total bilirubin, 0.3 mg/dL). All other laboratory tests including a complete blood cell count (CBC), platelets, and urinalysis are normal. The patient has no complaints and has no previous medical history. He is a social drinker, consuming three to four drinks per night. If a liver biopsy were performed, what would be the MOST likely finding?
A. Steatohepatitis
B. Fatty liver
C. Cirrhosis
D. Acute hepatitis

---

748. Specify which viruses are associated with each finding.
1. Virus may be found in blood
2. Mortality in acute infection of 0.5% to 1.0%
3. Chronic infection may occur
4. Fecal-oral transmission
5. Incubation period 28 to 160 days
6. Sexual transmission prominent in the United States
7. Requires helper virus for infection
8. Vertical transmission efficient
9. Clinical diagnosis detects viral component in blood
10. Up to 70% of cases progress to chronic infection
11. Produces little or no disease

A. Hepatitis A
B. Hepatitis B
C. Hepatitis C
D. Hepatitis D
E. Hepatitis E
F. Hepatitis B, C, D, and G
G. Hepatitis G
H. Hepatitis A and E
I. All viruses

---

749. After post-transfusion hepatitis C, what percentage of the patients are likely to develop chronic hepatitis?
A. Less than 10%

B. 20%
C. 40%
D. More than 60%

---

750. Regarding the natural history of untreated autoimmune hepatitis, all of the following statements are true EXCEPT:
A. A patient with an aspartate aminotransferase level greater than ten times normal has a 10% survival after ten years.
B. A patient with an aspartate aminotransferase level greater than five times normal and a gammaglobulin level greater than two times normal has a 10% survival after ten years.
C. A patient with an aspartate aminotransferase level less than five times normal and a gammaglobulin level less than two times normal has a 90% survival after ten years.
D. Histologic findings of both periportal hepatitis and bridging necrosis have similar five year survival rates of 50%.

---

751. In which malignancy is the ascitic fluid cytology LEAST likely to be positive?
A. Hepatocellular carcinoma
B. Ovarian carcinoma
C. Pancreatic carcinoma
D. Breast carcinoma

---

752. A 35-year-old woman with a history of intravenous drug abuse 15 years earlier presents with a purpuric rash on her lower extremities, renal insufficiency, and abnormal liver tests. Hepatitis B serologic studies include negative HBsAg, positive anti-HBc, and a negative anti-HBc IgM. Which of the following statements are TRUE?
A. The patient likely has acute hepatitis D superimposed on chronic hepatitis B.
B. The patient likely has type II essential mixed cryoglobulinemia and hepatitis C.
C. During interferon therapy, purpura may improve but will often rebound after the interferon is discontinued.
D. The patient likely has porphyria cutanea tarda complicating hepatitis C.
E. The patient likely has active hepatitis on liver biopsy.

---

753. Each of the following statements regarding annular pancreas is true EXCEPT:
A. It is the most common anomaly obstructing the duodenum in infancy.
B. Most cases involve the first portion of the duodenum.
C. It may be asymptomatic.
D. Pancreatic tissue extends into the duodenal wall.

754. A 30-year-old woman presents with right upper quadrant discomfort. Abdominal examination reveals hepatomegaly with no cutaneous stigmata of chronic liver disease. She has been taking oral contraceptives since age 16. An abdominal ultrasound evaluation reveals a solid 3 × 4-cm mass in the right lobe of the liver. Liver function tests, viral serologic studies, and α-fetoprotein are normal. Of the following the MOST likely diagnosis is:
A. Metastatic colon cancer
B. Hepatocellular adenoma
C. Metastatic ovarian cancer
D. Fibrolamellar hepatocellular carcinoma

755. Which of the following portosystemic shunts would be MOST appropriate for a patient with recurrent variceal bleeding (despite ligation therapy) who is a candidate for a liver transplant in the future?
A. Transjugular intrahepatic portosystemic stent shunt
B. End-to-side portacaval shunt
C. Distal splenorenal shunt
D. Side-to-side portacaval shunt

756. Which of the following are TRUE statements regarding arthritis associated with hepatitis B?
A. It is a symmetric, polyarticular arthritis.
B. Synovial thickening is common.
C. An associated rash is common.

D. Joint fluid leukocyte count is less than 5000 cells/mm³.
E. Inflammatory cells within the joint fluid are predominantly mononuclear.

757. A 60-year-old patient with chronic hepatitis C presents with worsening ascites. He contracted hepatitis C from a blood transfusion he received during the Vietnam War. He is compliant and takes his diuretics as instructed and also follows a strict low-sodium diet. He denies any fever, chills, nausea, or vomiting. Which of the following is the BEST next step in managing this patient?
A. Check an α-fetoprotein level.
B. Admit the patient to the hospital for bed rest and a strict low-sodium diet.
C. Admit the patient to the hospital and perform a large-volume paracentesis.
D. Perform an abdominal ultrasound evaluation to rule out hepatic vein thrombosis.

758. The patient in question 757 is found to have an elevated α-fetoprotein level. Abdominal computed tomography is performed that reveals two liver masses. Which of the following computed tomographic findings would make the patient's masses surgically nonresectable?
A. Both masses greater than 6 cm in diameter in the right lobe
B. Right lobe mass 1 cm, left lobe mass 1 cm
C. Splenomegaly
D. Intra-abdominal venous collaterals

(595–A, C, D) **(S&F, pp. 1253–1254)**

This woman has cholestasis of pregnancy, a common form of intrahepatic cholestasis that typically occurs during the third trimester of pregnancy. The principal symptom is pruritus, which may be severe, typically involves the soles and palms, and is worse at night. In addition to an elevated alkaline phosphatase level, aminotransferase values may be elevated to as high at 1000 IU/L, making differentiation from hepatitis difficult. Resolution after delivery is prompt and complete. Risk to the fetus is significant but can be reduced by early delivery if fetal distress develops. Treatment with cholestyramine may help symptoms but may aggravate associated malabsorption of fat-soluble vitamins. Ursodeoxycholate treatment provides symptomatic improvement at minimal risk to the fetus. Up to 70% of patients affected during their initial pregnancies have recurrence with subsequent pregnancies.

(596–A, B, C, D) **(S&F, pp. 1391–1395)**

This patient has systemic amyloidosis with cardiac, hepatic, and renal involvement. No specific laboratory tests are available, and the diagnosis requires biopsy. Because early data suggested an increased risk of bleeding from liver biopsies in this condition, it is prudent to sample other potentially affected tissues (e.g., rectum) first. Hepatic function is usually well preserved, and death typically ensues from cardiac or renal failure or from the underlying malignant (e.g., multiple myeloma) or inflammatory condition. If chronic inflammation is present, effective treatment of that condition will sometimes arrest the amyloidosis.

(597–B) **(S&F, p. 1404)**

Survival rates after orthotopic liver transplantation have improved dramatically. In 1996, most leading programs achieved a one-year survival rate of more than 85% and a five-year survival rate of more than 75%. Overall figures for the same period in the United States were 79% and 68%, respectively, reflecting the lower survival in programs that do fewer transplants.

(598–D) **(S&F, p. 1405)**

Although active hepatitis B infection was once viewed as an absolute contraindication to liver transplantation in many centers, the ability to prevent overt viral recurrence by regular lifelong administration of hepatitis B immune globulin (HBIG) has eliminated this barrier. Additional absolute contraindications not listed include multisystem organ failure and inability to comply with an immunosuppression protocol.

(599–A, B) **(S&F, pp. 1404–1406)**

Because the course of cholestatic liver diseases such as primary biliary cirrhosis and primary sclerosing cholangitis is easy to predict, more patients are transplanted with optimum timing, resulting in better survival rates. Relative contraindications include renal insufficiency, hepatitis B infection with viremia, primary hepatocellular carcinoma, hemochromatosis, and fulminant hepatic failure. Improved survival rates after liver transplantation have led to a higher percentage of patients undergoing transplantation before other organs begin to fail.

(600–B, C, D) **(S&F, pp. 1407–1408)**

Although it often takes 10 to 20 years for immunocompetent patients with chronic hepatitis B to develop advanced liver disease, progression to cirrhosis is much more rapid after recurrence in the graft. Viral titers are often very high, posing a substantial risk to family and health care workers. Because the intense immune response may clear the virus during fulminant acute hepatitis B infection, recurrence rates tend to be lower. Patients with active replication at the time of transplantation (positive serum tests for HBeAg or hepatitis B viral DNA) are more likely to experience a recurrence. Administration of hepatitis B immune globulin is effective at preventing recurrent infection but is costly and appears to be required for life.

(601-C) **(S&F, pp. 1408–1410)**

Immediate dysfunction (1–5 days after transplantation) is most likely due to hepatic artery thrombosis, preservation injury, or hyperacute rejection. Dysfunction after 5 to 30 days is usually due to acute cellular rejection, bile leaks, azathioprine toxicity, or preservation injury. Delayed dysfunction (>30 days) is typically due to rejection, viral infection (cytomegalovirus, hepatitis B and C viruses), biliary strictures, or recurrence of the underlying primary biliary cirrhosis or primary sclerosing cholangitis.

(602–A, B, C, D, E) **(S&F, pp. 1410–1411)**

The biliary tree has been described as the "Achilles heel" of liver transplantation. Complications include leaks, stricture, obstruction due to stones or sludge, and infection. Bile leaks are most common early and occur in as many as 25% of recipients. The choledochocholedochostomy is the most common site for strictures, followed by hilar and diffuse strictures. Ischemia such as that occurring after hepatic vein thrombosis commonly presents as a hilar stricture but may present as anastomotic or diffuse strictures. Strictures are more common with ABO-incompatible donors and prolonged cold ischemia time. Treatment with balloons or stents may be useful, but many patients with strictures ultimately require retransplantation.

(603–B)   **(S&F, p. 1411)**

Hepatitis C is the major cause of hepatitis after orthotopic liver transplantation. Infection may reflect recurrent disease or new infection from the donor or from exposure to blood products. No effective prophylaxis is available. Interferon-α rarely produces complete responses, does not improve histology, and may precipitate rejection. Patients with hepatitic C virus genotype 1b tend to have a worse outcome. As with most other viral titers, hepatitic C virus titers increase dramatically with immunosuppression after transplantation.

(604–A)   **(S&F, pp. 1414–1415)**

Obesity is common after liver transplantation in adults. The average gain in body weight is approximately 30% within the first 10 months after orthotopic liver transplantation (OLT). A common cause of diarrhea after OLT is hospital-acquired infection with *Clostridium difficile*. However, diarrhea may occur due to graft-versus-host disease caused by immunocompetent cells co-transplanted with the graft. The most common findings of graft-versus-host disease in this setting are fever and leukopenia, followed by diarrhea, often with rash. Pleural effusions are extremely common after OLT but are usually clinically insignificant. They typically occur on the right side and resolve spontaneously within one month of surgery.

(605–None are true)   **(S&F, p. 1407)**

Concern about limited organ availability notwithstanding, it is difficult to objectively state that the clinical outcome of orthotopic liver transplantation (OLT) in alcoholic patients is any worse than non–alcoholic liver disease transplant recipients. Recidivism rates are 10% to 20%, and survival is good or better than for nonalcoholic liver diseases. The primary issue is the acceptable period of sobriety required before consideration of OLT. Many transplant centers currently require six months of sobriety before transplantation.

(606–D)   **(S&F, pp. 1153–1155)**

Selection of patients with chronic hepatitis C for interferon therapy requires care. In patients with features of autoimmunity, liver disease may be exacerbated by interferon-α. Host and viral factors that predict a greater likelihood of sustained response include early and less advanced disease and lower titers of hepatitis C viral RNA. Patients with hepatitis C genotype 1 (common in the United States) have higher viral titers and lower complete response rates than do patients with other strains more common in Japan and Europe.

■■■■**Reference**

Cuthbert, J. A. Hepatitis C: Progress and problems. Clin. Microbiol. Rev. 7:505, 1994.

(607–A)   **(S&F, pp. 1358–1359)**

In a study by O'Grady and associates, important prognostic indicators included the underlying cause of hepatic failure, the degree of prolongation of the prothrombin time, the level of hyperbilirubinemia, and the age of the patient. The presence or absence of variceal bleeding did not correlate with the need for transplantation in this setting.

■■■■**Reference**

O'Grady, J. G., Alexander, G. J. M., Hayllar, K. M., Williams, R. Early indicators of prognosis in fulminant hepatic failure. Gastroenterology 97:439, 1989

(608–A)   **(S&F, pp. 1141–1142)**

Treatment of chronic hepatitis B with interferon-α has several shortcomings. Although more than half of the patients show improvement while on interferon, only 33% to 37% have any lasting benefit from treatment. Patients with decompensated cirrhosis should generally not be treated for fear of precipitating a crisis. Platelets often decrease while on treatment, and the increased inflammation and the death of infected hepatocytes required for successful clearance of the virus may precipitate bleeding, coma, or death. The approved treatment for hepatitis B is 5 million units daily for four months, whereas a dose of 3 million units three times a week for six to twelve months is commonly used for hepatitis C. In nonresponders, repeat courses of treatment and use of higher doses are rarely beneficial.

■■■■**Reference**

Korenmann, J., Baker, B., Waggoner, J., et al. Long-term remission in chronic hepatitis B after alpha interferon therapy. Ann. Intern. Med. 114:629, 1991.

(609–A, C)   **(S&F, pp. 1135–1140)**

The patient has severe acute hepatitis B, as evidenced by the elevation of the prothrombin time, indicating markedly decreased synthetic capacity of the liver. Close observation is indicated in any liver patient with an elevated prothrombin time, whereas admission to the hospital is indicated in patients with acute hepatitis and elevations of the prothrombin time above about 17 seconds. Most cases of acute hepatitis B improve spontaneously. However, supportive care with adequate dietary intake and volume resuscitation is often necessary. Although hepatitis B infection typically recurs after liver transplantation, clinical infection can be prevented by administration of hepatitis B immune globulin (HBIG). Sexual partners of the patient should be tested for hepatitis B and, if negative, should receive hepatitis B vaccine. Any needlesticks among medical personnel should be treated with HBIG and hepatitis B vaccine. Antibodies to HBcAg are universal in hepatitis B and do not confer immunity or prevent chronic infection.

(610–C)   *(S&F, p. 1293)*

Studies performed in patients with alcoholic cirrhosis have shown that a hepatic vein gradient of more than 10 to 12 mm Hg is necessary to develop variceal hemorrhage. The degree of elevation above this level does not further increase the risk of bleeding. Patients with large varices, varices with red wale spots, and advanced liver disease are more likely to develop variceal bleeding.

(611–B, C, A, D)   *(S&F, p. 1404)*

The most common disease indications for orthotopic liver transplantation in pediatric patients are extrahepatic biliary atresia (55%) and α_1-antitrypsin deficiency (7%). Viral liver disease in infants is usually asymptomatic and almost never produces liver failure.

(612–D)   *(S&F, pp. 1405–1406)*

The most common quality-of-life indication for orthotopic liver transplantation is ascites that is refractory to diuretic therapy. Although transjugular intrahepatic portosystemic shunt is effective in relieving ascites in some patients, its long-term benefits are still under study. Encephalopathy refractory to medical therapy is the second most common indication, followed by bleeding and pruritus. Intractable fatigue is rarely an indication, because it can be very difficult to differentiate fatigue due to liver failure from that due to depression.

(613–B)   *(S&F, pp. 1412–1414)*

Cyclosporine and tacrolimus are immunosuppressive agents with similar toxic profiles that are often used in combination. The most important side effect of these agents is nephrotoxicity. Acute renal toxicity is reversible. Ten to 20 percent of patients develop acute renal failure requiring hemodialysis shortly after orthotopic liver transplantation. Chronic renal toxicity tends to be irreversible and is often associated with a type IV renal tubular acidosis with hyperkalemia. Dose-dependent hypertension requiring treatment occurs in 30% to 85% and is more common with cyclosporine than with tacrolimus. Central nervous system neurotoxicity occurs in 15% to 20% of those treated. Opportunistic infections and gingival hyperplasia are also common, whereas lymphoma is much more common than in untreated patients.

(614–D)   *(S&F, p. 1279)*

Primary biliary cirrhosis is an autoimmune disease associated with abnormalities in both the cellular and humoral immune systems. The antimitochondrial antibody (AMA) is a very sensitive test, although AMA-negative cases may occur and AMA is occasionally positive in autoimmune hepatitis, primary sclerosing cholangitis, or syphilis. Up to 25% of patients are diagnosed before symptoms occur, often when an elevated cholesterol or alkaline phosphatase level is found during routine screening. The most common symptom is fatigue (65%), followed by pruritus (55%) and

hepatomegaly (25%). Only 10% present with jaundice. Pruritus, when present, correlates poorly with histologic progression and may remit as the disease progresses or may develop later in the course of the disease. Ninety percent or more of patients are women, typically presenting in their early 50s.

(615–1-C, 2-A, 3-B, 4-D)   *(S&F, p. 1277)*

Primary biliary cirrhosis progresses through characteristic histologic stages. In stage I, there is focal inflammatory destruction around smaller intrahepatic bile ducts, often termed the *florid duct lesion*. The portal tracts are usually expanded by lymphocytes, and the parenchyma is typically normal. In stage II, inflammation extends from the portal tract into the hepatic parenchyma with ductular proliferation and piecemeal necrosis. In stage III, scarring and fibrosis ensue, leading to stage IV, cirrhosis.

(616–B)   *(S&F, pp. 1277–1278)*

Hepatitis C can occasionally be associated with granulomatous inflammation around the bile ducts, leading to a histologic picture that may be confused with primary biliary cirrhosis (PBC). The liver biopsy does not reliably differentiate PBC from primary sclerosing cholangitis (PSC). However, the presence of inflammatory bowel disease, which is rare in PBC, should raise the suspicion of PSC. Granulomatous liver disease due to sarcoidosis can be confirmed by chest radiography in over 90% of sarcoid cases. Elevated antimitochondrial antibodies may be seen in autoimmune hepatitis, PSC, syphilis, myocarditis, and drug-induced liver disease.

(617–F)   *(S&F, pp. 1280–1281)*

A large number of treatments have been tried for primary biliary cirrhosis, but only ursodeoxycholate (10–15 mg/kg/day) has definite efficacy. Ursodeoxycholate produced clinical and biochemical improvement in four large trials and improved long-term survival in one trial. Corticosteroids may improve biochemical parameters and symptoms, but the high risk of bone disease has prevented large scale trials. The other treatments listed are of little if any value. Liver transplantation remains the treatment of choice for patients with advanced disease.

(618–A)   *(S&F, pp. 1100–1101)*

Up to 80% of cases of hemochromatosis are detected by routine screening of serum iron and saturation while still asymptomatic. Serum iron studies should first be repeated while fasting, because most persons have transiently elevated serum iron levels after eating. If the abnormality is confirmed, liver biopsy is required to exclude (or confirm) the diagnosis of hemochromatosis. The current case could be early hemochromatosis or, more likely, iron overload associated with alcoholism. Liver biopsy with measurement of the hepatic iron index (liver iron content divided by the patient's age) is the best way to differentiate between these two possibilities. Human leukocyte antigen typing is of no value in this setting but could be used to identify affected siblings and children if the patient is found to have hemochromatosis. Specific genetic testing for hemochromatosis is becoming available but does not offer the additional information on iron loading and histology provided by a liver biopsy.

(619–B) **(S&F, pp. 1099–1100)**

Most patients with symptomatic hereditary hemochromatosis present between ages 40 and 50. Clinically affected males outnumber females by up to 8:1, although the gene frequency is the same for both. The most common presenting symptoms are weakness, lethargy, abdominal pain, loss of libido or potency, and arthralgias. Physical findings include hepatomegaly in the majority of patients. Hemochromatosis is a common disease, with approximately 1:400 persons homozygous. Other diagnoses are less likely. Peptic ulcer disease due to *Helicobacter pylori* may explain this patient's abdominal tenderness, but it is more likely that he is an asymptomatic carrier. The patient is too old for a hepatic presentation of Wilson's disease. α_1-Antitrypsin deficiency can produce cirrhosis in adults and cholelithiasis can produce constant abdominal pain, but they do not produce the nonhepatic manifestations reported here.

(620–B) **(S&F, pp. 1101–1102)**

Deferoxamine is an iron chelator that can be used to reduce total body iron stores in patients unable to tolerate phlebotomy; typically, these are transfusion-dependent persons. Most patients with hemochromatosis can be treated with weekly phlebotomy. Each unit contains about 250 mg of elemental iron, so about 100 units are required to remove the excess iron from someone with 25 g of total body iron.

(621–None are true) **(S&F, pp. 1215–1219)**

Nonalcoholic steatohepatitis (NASH) is a disease of unknown etiology. Because it can display all of the features of alcoholic hepatitis (including Mallory hyaline), liver biopsy is more useful for staging than for diagnosis. NASH may also be seen in diabetes, total parenteral nutrition, jejunoileal bypass, and with certain drugs and toxins. Progression to fibrosis and cirrhosis is well documented, although most patients have a more indolent course. It is typically seen in obese middle-aged women. Most patients are asymptomatic, although fatigue, malaise, and vague right upper quadrant discomfort may occur. Hepatomegaly is present in up to 75% of affected persons. The diagnosis should not be made until after excluding other possible causes. Treatment is nonspecific and consists of weight loss, withdrawal any drugs or toxins that could be responsible, and control of blood glucose and lipid levels.

(622–1-D, 2-C, 3-C, 4-B, 5-A) **(S&F, p. 1113)**

Common "liver function tests" such as aminotransferase and alkaline phosphatase levels are not actually function tests but are markers of injury. Aminotransferase levels are elevated when damaged liver cells either leak cytoplasm or shed vesicles into blood. Synthesis of alkaline phosphatase is elevated by cholestasis. Elevated alkaline phosphatase levels may be delayed for hours after biliary obstruction because of the time required for synthesis. Albumin and prothrombin levels are better markers of hepatic function because they depend on the rate of hepatic synthesis. However, albumin levels change too slowly to be of use in acute liver conditions, and both albumin and the prothrombin time are affected by nonhepatic factors, including the rate of consumption or excretion.

(623–D) **(S&F, p. 1321)**

The neutrophil count is usually greater than 250 cells/mm³ in spontaneous bacterial peritonitis, intra-abdominal abscess (a cause of secondary bacterial peritonitis), and Fitz-Hugh–Curtis syndrome (chlamydial or gonococcal peritonitis). Polymicrobial peritonitis is also uncommon. Thus, this is most likely a case of bacterial contamination, which is generally the result of gut perforation by the paracentesis needle. Treatment with a third-generation cephalosporin or serial paracentesis is indicated.

(624–D) **(S&F, p. 1335)**

The patient has all the features of stage 3 hepatic encephalopathy. If he were only drowsy or had only impaired computation or poor memory, he would be considered to have stage 2, whereas stupor or coma would obviously change this to stage 4.

(625–C) **(S&F, p. 1137)**

Anti-HBs/HBsAg complexes are regularly detected in the serum of patients with hepatitis B virus–associated polyarteritis nodosa and membranous glomerulonephritis. These complexes may also be found in the serum of a significant percentage of patients with chronic hepatitis B liver disease.

(626–D) **(S&F, pp. 1381–1383)**

Unlike polycystic disease, solitary cysts of the liver are not associated with cysts in other organs. They occur in the right lobe of the liver more often than in the left. They are not hereditary and occur at all stages of life.

(627–A, D) **(S&F, p. 1209)**

Corticosteroids are most effective in the subset of patients with more severe cases of acute alcoholic hepatitis. These include patients with hepatic encephalopathy or a discriminant function (= 4.6 × [PT − control] + bilirubin [mg/dL]) of more than 32. Corticosteroids are as effective when given orally, but patients with baseline renal impairment fare poorly, with a high rate of progression to renal failure and a mortality of 75% with or without corticosteroids.

(628–D, E) (S&F, p. 1315)

Neither ascitic fluid pH nor cholesterol is helpful in distinguishing infected fluid (pH) or malignant ascites (cholesterol) from other conditions that can cause ascites, and these two tests should rarely be ordered.

(629–A) (S&F, p. 1312)

Because the risk of bleeding is only approximately 1% in patients not receiving frozen plasma, its prophylactic use is not warranted. A midline site below the umbilicus is preferred if large ascites is present, but either the right or left lower quadrants may be used if the midline is scarred or if insufficient fluid is present. Whichever side is duller to percussion is used.

(630–D) (S&F, pp. 1199–1211)

There are no physical findings that are pathognomonic for alcoholic cirrhosis. Dupuytren's contracture is more commonly found in alcoholics but can be seen in other individuals, as is true for the other conditions listed.

(631–D) (S&F, p. 1265)

The most frequent causes for this histologic pattern are hepatitis B and hepatitis C. Other conditions include primary biliary cirrhosis, drug reactions from a variety of agents, the portal inflammatory lesion associated with inflammatory bowel disease (pericholangitis), and portal inflammation secondary to extrahepatic biliary tract disorders such as pancreatitis and choledocholithiasis. This histologic pattern is unusual in patients with idiopathic autoimmune chronic hepatitis who have not received corticosteroid therapy but can be seen in treated patients.

(632–C) (S&F, p. 1229)

Acetaminophen is a well-recognized cause of fulminant hepatic failure. The usual toxic dose of acetaminophen is 8 to 15 g, but it may be as little as 2 to 6 g in the setting of heavy ethanol use. Ethanol induces the P-450 system responsible for converting acetaminophen into its toxic metabolites. In addition, heavy drinkers may be malnourished, reducing the levels of protective glutathione in the liver. Treatment with acetylcysteine would help restore normal glutathione levels and prevent progression of her toxic hepatitis.

(633–D) (S&F, pp. 1156–1160)

Diagnosis of hepatitis D depends on antibody to hepatitis D virus antigen. Most patients with this infection have very active histologies with rapid progression to fibrosis and cirrhosis. The delta virus is "defective" in that it cannot code for its own coat protein. Instead, it borrows the coat protein from hepatitis B (HBsAg). Thus, hepatitis D occurs only in patients previously or simultaneously infected with hepatitis B, and vaccination against hepatitis B will also prevent hepatitis D. Patients co-infected with hepatitis B and hepatitis D exhibit a relatively poor response to treatment with interferon-α.

■■■■**Reference**

Di Bisceglie, A., Negro, F. Diagnosis of hepatitis delta virus infection. Hepatology *10*:1014, 1989.

(634–A) (S&F, pp. 1135–1139)

The majority of patients with chronic hepatitis B have an asymptomatic or relatively mild initial illness with persistent mild hepatomegaly. Most HBsAg carriers cannot recall an acute episode of hepatitis B. Up to 13% of adults who acquire hepatitis B have some evidence of long-term sequelae, with 1% to 3% developing active histology such as piecemeal necrosis. Chronic hepatitis B ensues when an ineffective immune response is mounted against hepatocytes containing hepatitis B virus. Cells containing the virus are normally destroyed by cytotoxic T lymphocytes directed against cells expressing both hepatitis B core antigen and human leukocyte antigens (HLAs) class I. Liver cells normally express low levels of HLA class I, which is the major reason that liver transplantation does not require a tissue match. Interferon therapy for chronic viral hepatitis works in part by inducing the liver cells to express more HLAs class I.

(635–B) (S&F, pp. 1322–1325)

Gram-negative rods, in particular *Escherichia coli* and *Klebsiella,* account for the majority of organisms responsible for spontaneous bacterial peritonitis. A positive Gram stain is rare and suggests the diagnosis of secondary bacterial peritonitis (e.g., perforation). The opsonic activity of peritoneal fluid correlates directly with ascitic fluid protein concentration. Patients with an ascitic fluid protein concentration of less than 1 g/dL are at high risk for the development of spontaneous bacterial peritonitis. Two major factors involved in the pathogenesis of spontaneous bacterial peritonitis are seeding of the peritoneal cavity during periods of bacteremia and translocation of bacteria from the gut into peritoneal lymph nodes.

(636–D) (S&F, pp. 1323–1326)

Clues to the diagnosis of secondary bacterial peritonitis include a low ascitic fluid glucose concentration, a high protein concentration, and an elevated lactate dehydrogenase level (LDH). Anaerobic organisms are often present, and peritoneal fluid cultures usually remain positive after 48 hours of antibiotic treatment. In the setting of portal hypertension, the serum ascites/albumin gradient is usually high whether or not a superimposed complication is present.

(637–C) (S&F, p. 1380)

Focal nodular hyperplasia, like hepatocellular adenoma, is associated with oral contraceptive use. It is a tumor-like growth of normal hepatocytes with a central stellate scar. Although hepatic function is not compromised in this condition, it can produce portal hypertension. Neither ultrasonography nor computed tomography can absolutely confirm the diagnosis, although the characteristic central stellate scar with radiating septa may be seen. Liver scans typically are entirely normal because the lesions contain Kupffer cells that take up the radionuclide normally. Small lesions of focal nodular hyperplasia are usually incidental findings and warrant no treatment, although oral contraceptive use should be discontinued to prevent enlargement. Large, symptomatic, or complicated lesions should be resected, which is curative.

(638–C, B, A, D)　　　　**(S&F, p. 1311)**

Cirrhosis is the most common cause of ascites in the United States. In one series, it was present in 85% of patients. Malignancy accounted for 10% of patients in this series. Although tuberculosis is a common cause of ascites in certain parts of Asia (e.g., India), it is an uncommon cause in more developed countries. Pancreatic ascites is relatively unusual.

(639–C)　　　　**(S&F, p. 1143)**

Anti-HBs in the serum of convalescent patients confers almost complete resistance to reinfection with hepatitis B virus of either the same or a different subtype. This is the basis for vaccination with purified HBsAg preparations. In contrast, anti-HBc and anti-HBe do not appear to be protective.

(640–B)　　　　**(S&F, pp. 1367–1368)**

The most likely diagnosis is a hepatocellular carcinoma even with a normal α-fetoprotein level. Up to 20% of hepatocellular carcinomas in high-risk populations are associated with normal levels of this tumor marker. This man is at very high risk because he has presumably had chronic hepatitis B since birth. α-Fetoprotein levels can be normal in up to 50% of low-risk persons with hepatocellular carcinoma.

(641–B)　　　　**(S&F, pp. 1327–1329)**

Salt restriction, dietary education, and diuretics are the mainstay of treatment of cirrhotic ascites. Fluid restriction should be instituted only in the setting of hyponatremia, which is absent in this case.

(642–A)　　　　**(S&F, p. 1330)**

Although placement of a peritoneovenous shunt may permit a decrease in the dosage of diuretics, most patients continue to require diuretics for management of ascites. Bacterial infection is a major complication of peritoneovenous shunting. In a large randomized trial (the Veterans Administration Cooperative Study), shunted patients actually had a higher incidence of infections than medically managed patients and survival was not altered. Although there was an increased interval between hospitalizations, shunting did not reduce the total days spent in hospital.

(643–A, B, C, D)　　　　**(S&F, pp. 1371–1372)**

The risk of hepatocellular carcinoma is dramatically increased in all forms of chronic viral hepatitis and is also particularly high in genetic hemochromatosis. Patients with Wilson's disease are also at some risk, although only if they have cirrhosis.

(644–C)　　　　**(S&F, p. 1310)**

The current model for the mechanism of ascites formation places portal hypertension as the initial prerequisite, followed by nitric oxide synthesis (when portal pressure has reached a critical level), which acts as a vasodilator. The vasodilation leads to a decreased "effective" arterial circulation with concomitant activation of a variety of neurohumoral factors, including norepinephrine, vasopressin, aldosterone, and renin. Thus, there is the paradox of ascites—massive volume overload accompanied by nerve signals and hormone levels suggesting intravascular volume depletion.

(645–A, B, D)　　　　**(S&F, pp. 1170–1773)**

Biliary tract infections account for 40% to 50% of all pyogenic abscesses of the liver. It is difficult to differentiate amebic from nonamebic abscesses by abdominal computed tomography or ultrasonography. Serologic tests, such as the indirect hemagglutination test, are helpful in distinguishing these conditions. Although hepatomegaly may be found in half of patients with pyogenic liver abscesses, right upper quadrant tenderness is unusual. The mainstay of therapy for a pyogenic liver abscess is percutaneous drainage and broad-spectrum intravenous antibiotics, followed electively by correction of the underlying disease.

(646–B)　　　　**(S&F, p. 1206)**

In a patient with alcoholic hepatitis, poor prognosticators are the presence of encephalopathy, a serum bilirubin value greater than 20 mg/dL, and a prolonged prothrombin time. The latter two laboratory values can be applied to a discriminant function ($= 4.6 \times$ [PT − control] + bilirubin [mg/dL]). A discriminant function of more than 32 predicts a 50% one-month mortality. This patient's value was 43.

(647–A)　　　　**(S&F, pp. 1324–1325)**

This is probably a case of bacterial ascites, in which a substantial proportion of cases resolve spontaneously. However, the rate of spontaneous resolution is significantly lower among patients with signs or symptoms compatible with peritonitis. Symptomatic patients should be treated with antibiotics.

(648–C)　　　　**(S&F, pp. 1376–1377)**

Surgical resection of liver metastases secondary to Wilms' tumor has the best survival when compared with other metastatic lesions. This may be due to its relative responsiveness to chemotherapy.

(649–B) **(S&F, pp. 1104–1105, 1108–1109)**

This is a classic presentation of acute Wilson's disease, a disorder of biliary copper excretion that leads to accumulation of toxic concentrations of copper in liver, brain, and other tissues. Patients may present with psychologic, hepatic, or hematologic manifestations, or all three as in this case. Psychologic manifestations may be mild or include frank psychosis. The serum ceruloplasmin is usually low but is not reliable in acute decompensation because it is an acute-phase reactant. A slit-lamp examination may show Kayser-Fleischer rings, but this finding is neither sensitive nor specific for Wilson disease. A 24-hour determination of urinary copper levels would be the most reliable diagnostic tool, with levels as high as 1000 mg/24 hr in cases of fulminant hepatic failure secondary to Wilson disease. In less-advanced cases, a liver biopsy for quantitative copper may be used to confirm the diagnosis.

(650–B) **(S&F, p. 1111)**

Patients who present with fulminant hepatic failure from Wilson disease are usually refractory to treatment with any copper-binding agent. Such patients should undergo emergency orthotopic liver transplantation as a life-saving measure. Data suggest that this should also cure the metabolic defect, which is failure to secrete copper into bile.

(651–A) **(S&F, pp. 1315–1319)**

There is no true gold standard in the diagnosis of spontaneous bacterial peritonitis. If the white blood cell count is more than 250 cells/mm³, there is a greater than 95% chance that bacterial peritonitis is present. The sensitivities of ascitic fluid lactate and pH are less than 50%, whereas that of the Gram stain is less than 10%.

(652–B) **(S&F, p. 1200)**

Acetaldehyde is the immediate metabolic by-product of the oxidation of ethanol. Acetaldehyde is a vasoactive substance and accounts for many of the physiologic effects of ethanol consumption (i.e., flushing, tachycardia). Subjects with low activity of aldehyde dehydrogenase (approximately half of Japanese and Chinese people) are particularly prone to flushing and tachycardia and accordingly usually avoid alcohol.

(653–A, C) **(S&F, pp. 1377–1378)**

The most likely diagnosis in this case is a hepatic adenoma. Long-term oral contraceptive use is a risk factor for the development of this histologically benign tumor. The presence of abdominal pain with anemia suggests that the patient may be bleeding into the tumor, which can cause life-threatening intraperitoneal hemorrhage in some cases. Urgent surgical resection is indicated in this situation. Because about 10% of patients with large adenomas will eventually suffer this complication, resection is usually recommended in these patients even in the absence of bleeding.

(654–D) **(S&F, pp. 1312–1313)**

There are few contraindications to abdominal paracentesis. The most important is the presence of severe uncontrollable coagulopathy. If there are concerns about localizing sites for aspiration of peritoneal fluid in obese patients or those with a history of extensive abdominal surgery, ascitic fluid collections can be localized by ultrasonography.

(655–A) **(S&F, p. 1317)**

Routine culture techniques are less sensitive (50%) than bedside inoculation into blood culture bottles (80%). This is primarily due to the low bacterial concentration and the delay inherent in routine inoculation of ascitic fluid onto agar plates. Use of anaerobic culture bottles will detect intestinal organisms otherwise missed.

(656–C) **(S&F, pp. 1364–1365)**

The primary risk factor for hepatocellular carcinoma is hepatitis B, especially when acquired as an infant. Within high-risk countries, the risk is not evenly distributed throughout the population. People who emigrate from a low-risk country to one with high risk retain the low risk of their country of origin.

(657–D) **(S&F, pp. 1357–1359)**

This patient has fulminant hepatitis B, probably acquired through sexual activity. The surface antigen is already negative, owing to an intense immune response. On admission, he had evidence of stage II hepatic encephalopathy and rapidly deteriorated to stage IV coma. In a large series of patients with fulminant hepatic failure from a variety of causes, cerebral edema was the most common immediate cause of death, followed by major gastrointestinal hemorrhage, hepatocellular failure, and sepsis. Virtually all organ systems may be affected.

(658–B) **(S&F, p. 1205)**

Chronic alcoholism is characterized by a number of laboratory abnormalities, including hyperuricemia, hypomagnesemia, and erythrocyte macrocytosis. Alcoholic liver disease is characterized by leukocytosis, hypoalbuminemia, hyperbilirubinemia, and a disproportionate elevation in the aspartate aminotransferase level when compared with the alanine aminotransferase level.

(659–C) **(S&F, p. 1356)**

Infection with both hepatitis A virus (HAV) and hepatitis B virus (HBV) is a major cause of fulminant hepatic failure (FHF) in western countries. Although the incidence of HAV infection is higher than that of HBV infection, the likelihood of progression to FHF is greater for patients infected with HBV. Acute infection with hepatitis C virus (HCV) is a rare cause of FHF in western countries but may play a significant role in FHF in Japan.

(660–B)   **(S&F, p. 1271)**

The therapy, prednisone or azathioprine, is directed against and hence is effective only against the manifestations of inflammation. Incapacitating symptoms, usually extreme fatigue, along with biochemical or histologic evidence of inflammation, always warrant treatment, whereas severe cytopenia and other measures of hepatic dysfunction such as hyperbilirubinemia or hypoprothrombinemia in the absence of inflammation do not warrant therapy.

(661–A)   **(S&F, pp. 1381–1383, 1508)**

Congenital hepatic fibrosis and adult polycystic disease are both associated with cystic disease of the kidney. Many patients with Caroli's disease also have renal lesions. Although choledochal cysts are congenital, there is no associated renal lesion.

(662–B)   **(S&F, pp. 1311–1312)**

Clinical diagnosis of early ascites is notoriously difficult, and ultrasound is much more sensitive and specific for diagnosis than any of the signs listed. Shifting dullness has a much higher sensitivity and specificity for detecting ascites than the puddle sign (dependent dullness detected with the patient on hands and knees) or the presence of a fluid wave. If no flank dullness is present, there is less than a 10% chance that ascites is present. However, flank dullness is often present without ascites.

(663–C)   **(S&F, p. 1327)**

All of the listed treatments have been used for hepatic hydrothorax. Salt restriction and diuretics represent the mainstay of therapy. By contrast, placement of a chest tube should be reserved for severe respiratory compromise, because it can lead to profound intravascular volume depletion and protein loss. Peritoneovenous shunting has been successfully used, but it is associated with inherent complications. Poorly controlled hepatic hydrothorax is an indication for liver transplantation, which has the best long-term result.

(664–A, B, D)   **(S&F, p. 1100)**

An elevated transferrin saturation and ferritin in an otherwise healthy individual strongly suggests, with a 93% accuracy, that the patient indeed has hereditary hemochromatosis (HHC), whereas normal values can exclude the diagnosis with a 97% accuracy. Hence, only 3 of 100 patients with HHC will be missed using the iron studies as a screening test for HHC. Although the symptoms listed in C are characteristic of HHC, the vast majority of new diagnoses are made in asymptomatic patients on the basis of incidental laboratory abnormalities.

(665–A)   **(S&F, pp. 1381–1382)**

Abdominal ultrasonography is the least expensive, single most valuable test in evaluating a hepatic cyst. It can reliably differentiate between solid and cystic lesions, definitively diagnose certain types of cystic lesions such as congenital and hydatid cysts and, with aspiration, make a microbiologic diagnosis of abscesses. Computed tomography and magnetic resonance imaging may provide additional information in specific circumstances, but at substantially greater cost.

(666–A)   **(S&F, pp. 1358–1359)**

The finding of a pH less than 7.3 in a patient with fulminant hepatic failure secondary to acetaminophen is an ominous finding and necessitates urgent consideration for transplantation. The other abnormalities also have an impact on survival, but to a lesser degree. Because of the excellent post-transplant survival of patients with fulminant hepatic failure, most are listed for transplantation before reaching this stage.

■■■■**Reference**

O'Grady, J. G., Gimson, A. E. S., O'Brien, C. J., et al. Controlled trials of charcoal hemoperfusion and prognostic factors in fulminant hepatic failure. Gastroenterology *94*:1186, 1988

(667–B)   **(S&F, p. 1202)**

The metabolism of acetaldehyde is impaired in alcoholics owing to reduced levels of aldehyde dehydrogenase in the liver. As acetaldehyde concentrations increase in the liver, acetaldehyde becomes attached to cellular proteins, forming acetaldehyde-protein adducts that may contribute to fibrosis by stimulating collagen synthesis.

(668–C)   **(S&F, pp. 1355–1356)**

A wide variety of infections cause fulminant hepatic failure as part of a systemic hemorrhagic fever. These include Lassa and yellow fevers. Hepatitis D superinfection of a patient with hepatitis B may precipitate fulminant hepatic failure. On the other hand, cytomegalovirus infection generally causes only mild hepatic inflammation.

(669–D)   **(S&F, pp. 1322–1323)**

Fever, abdominal pain, and encephalopathy are all common manifestations of spontaneous bacterial peritonitis, with fever present in over two thirds of patients. By contrast, rebound tenderness of the abdomen is present in only 10% of patients.

(670–E)   **(S&F, pp. 1204–1205)**

Most studies have shown that the development of alcoholic liver disease is related to the mean daily intake of alcohol (>40 to 60 g/day for males, >20 g/day for females). Conversely, there are individuals who consume >200 g/day of ethanol and yet do not develop liver disease; thus, other risk factors come into play. Women are more likely to develop liver disease when consuming lower amounts of alcohol as compared with their male counterparts; and unfortunately the disease has a tendency to progress despite abstinence. Nutritional status also appears to be an important factor because liver injury correlates inversely with nutritional status. Many Asian patients are intolerant of alcohol even in low doses, and thus rarely develop alcoholic liver disease. Coexisting infection with hepatitis C virus or hepatitis B virus increases the incidence of liver injury in alcoholics.

(671–D) *(S&F, pp. 1316–1317)*

The value of the serum ascites/albumin gradient is unaffected by infection, diuretic therapy, paracentesis, or albumin infusion. However, hypotension, which reduces splanchnic and portal venous pressures, reduces the gradient, as does hyperglobulinemia, which contributes to oncotic forces. Conversely, triglycerides present in chylous ascites interfere with the albumin assay and falsely increase the gradient.

(672–D) *(S&F, p. 1226)*

All are associated with cholestasis, with the exception of ursodeoxycholic acid. This hydrophilic bile acid promotes bile flow and tends to relieve many of the symptoms associated with profound cholestatic states.

(673–D) *(S&F, pp. 1328–1329)*

Daily weight is the most objective way to follow the response to diuretics. In patients without peripheral edema, weight loss of up to 0.5 kg/day is well tolerated. Abdominal girth, urine volume, and urine sodium are useful adjuncts but may vary considerably from day to day.

(674–C) *(S&F, p. 1270)*

All patients with autoimmune hepatitis have elevated aminotransferase levels, and most have elevated gamma globulin levels as well. Both of these markers correlate with disease severity. Additionally, all patients will have serologic markers of smooth muscle antibody, antinuclear antibody, or anti-LKM1, because demonstration of autoantibodies is required for the diagnosis.

(675–D) *(S&F, pp. 1201–1202)*

Ethanol has a direct affect on the metabolism of fatty acids and lipids, glucose, and proteins. In addition, ethanol directly increases membrane fluidity. Ethanol has little effect on gastric acid secretion.

(676–C) *(S&F, p. 1235)*

Tacrine is a reversible choline esterase inhibitor that improves cognition is patients with Alzheimer's disease. It causes significant (more than three-fold) alanine aminotransferase (ALT) elevations in 25% of patients taking the drug, with women being more susceptible than men. Symptoms are uncommon and usually limited to nausea and vomiting, which resolves on discontinuation of the drug. Patients started on tacrine should be monitored with weekly ALT determinations for three months, and the drug should be stopped if ALT level exceeds three times normal.

(677–A) *(S&F, pp. 1316–1317)*

Portal hypertension results in an abnormally high hydrostatic pressure gradient between the portal bed and the ascitic fluid. To balance, there must be a similarly large difference in oncotic forces between plasma and ascitic fluid, resulting in a large albumin gradient. All of the conditions listed cause ascites through portal hypertension except nephrotic syndrome, which is associated with a normal serum ascites/albumin gradient.

(678–A) *Hepatic adenoma (S&F, p. 1245)*
Peliosis hepatis (S&F, p. 1246)

Peliosis hepatis is characterized by blood-filled cavities in the liver. This lesion is seen in patients with high catabolic states such as tuberculosis or malignancies. In addition, the lesion has been associated with use of anabolic steroids. The disorder may be completely asymptomatic or may be associated with hepatic failure or hemorrhage. Hepatic adenoma, usually associated with the use of oral contraceptives, is also a rare complication of androgen use in weight lifters, female transsexuals, and patients with impotence or aplastic anemia.

(679–B) *(S&F, p. 1230)*

In comparison to other forms of fulminant hepatic failure, acetaminophen-related hepatic failure in alcoholics is characterized by very high levels of alanine aminotransferase (ALT), usually in the range of 2000 to 10,000 IU/L. In contrast, ALT rarely rises above 600 IU/L in patients with alcoholic hepatitis.

■■■■ **Reference**

Lee, W. M. Acute liver failure. Am. J. Med. *96*(Suppl 1A):3s, 1994.

(680–B) *(S&F, p. 1183)*

Clonorchis sinensis is a liver fluke that is common in China and tends to localize in the bile ducts. Infestation with this parasite is characterized by recurrent bouts of cholangitis and is believed to be one of the causes of recurrent cholangiohepatitis in this population. The diagnosis is usually confirmed by the presence of characteristic fluke eggs in the stool, unless complete biliary obstruction is present. Treatment with praziquantel is uniformly effective. There is an increased incidence of cholangiocarcinoma, which may be complicating the current case. *Ascaris* can cause biliary obstruction, but it does not routinely cause recurrent cholangitis.

(681–A, C, D) *(S&F, p. 1211)*

On average, all groups of patients with alcoholic liver disease whether complications are present or not benefit from abstinence. Unfortunately, women, in particular, may show progressive liver disease despite abstinence. The finding of either hepatic inflammation or cirrhosis on biopsy predicted (with equal importance) progression of liver disease. Fatty liver alone had the best prognosis (70%–80%

survival at five years), either hepatitis or cirrhosis alone had an intermediate survival of 50% to 75%, whereas the combination of hepatitis and cirrhosis had the worst five-year survival at 30% to 50%.

(682–C) **(S&F, p. 1292)**

Portal hypertensive gastropathy is, as the name suggests, associated with portal hypertension. Antral vascular ectasias (watermelon stomach) has some similar endoscopic features and is seen in patients without portal hypertension, but the term *portal hypertensive gastropathy* should be reserved for those with evidence of portal hypertension.

(683–A) **(S&F, p. 1223)**

Alcohol lowers the threshold for hepatotoxicity for dose-related hepatotoxins such as acetaminophen and methotrexate and for metabolic idiosyncrasies such as isoniazid; but it has no effect on the risk of hepatotoxicity of chlorpromazine.

(684–D) **(S&F, p. 1357)**

Fulminant hepatic failure is typically complicated by multiple organ system failure. Pulmonary edema is common even with normal cardiac function. Infection is very common because of impaired function of polymorphonuclear leukocytes, defective opsonization, complement deficiency, and low plasma fibronectin levels. Pancreatitis has been found at the time of autopsy in many patients who have died of fulminant hepatic failure, and up to 25% of patients with this disorder have an elevated amylase level. Cerebrovascular accidents are rare in patients with fulminant hepatic failure. Instead, increased intracranial pressure reduces perfusion pressure and may cause herniation of the brainstem.

(685–C) **(S&F, pp. 1324–1325)**

Cefotaxime, a third-generation cephalosporin, has been shown in controlled clinical trials to be superior to a combination of ampicillin and gentamicin for the treatment of spontaneous bacterial peritonitis. Aztreonam has little activity against gram-positive organisms and has been associated with a superinfection rate of nearly 20%. Chloramphenicol is only bacteriostatic against gram-negative rods.

(686–E) **(S&F, p. 1217)**

Obesity, diabetes, hyperlipidemia, estrogens, liver disease secondary to a jejunoileal bypass, and alcoholic liver disease can all produce steatohepatitis, with histologic features that may include fatty necrosis, Mallory bodies, and cirrhosis. There are no reliable biochemical or histologic findings that can reliably distinguish nonalcoholic steatohepatitis (NASH) from alcoholic liver disease, and 40% of NASH patients show fibrosis on liver biopsy.

(687–A, D, E) **(S&F, pp. 1126–1127)**

In acute viral hepatitis, nonspecific constitutional symptoms as well as symptoms referable to the respiratory and gastrointestinal tract may develop. These symptoms include malaise, fatigue, myalgia, anorexia, nausea, and occasionally vomiting. Coryza, headache, photophobia, fever, pharyngitis, and cough may also occur. Hepatomegaly and splenomegaly are seen in 5% to 10% of patients. Hepatic enlargement is generally mild. Stools may be acholic (light gray) because of reduced excretion of bilirubin into the gastrointestinal tract. However, it may take several days before the serum bilirubin value rises to levels producing jaundice. At onset of the icteric phase, the fever declines and the general constitutional symptoms begin to subside.

(688–C) **(S&F, p. 1257)**

This patient presents with acute fatty liver of pregnancy. This disorder occurs in the third trimester of pregnancy and may be fatal if allowed to progress. Although there is no specific therapy, prompt termination of the pregnancy improves both maternal and fetal survival.

(689–E) **(S&F, pp. 1358–1359)**

Despite many attempts to correlate severity of symptoms and laboratory data with prognosis in fulminant hepatic failure (FHF), reliable criteria that can be used to determine whether a patient will survive have not been found. The prognosis of FHF varies depending on the underlying cause, with hepatitis A and acetaminophen toxicity having a more favorable prognosis. For patients without acetaminophen toxicity, adverse prognostic indicators include cryptogenic or drug/toxin liver failure, age younger than 10 or older than 40 years, duration of jaundice of more than one week before encephalopathy, bilirubin level greater than 18 mg/dL, and international normalized ratio (INR) greater than 3.5. For patients in FHF due to acetaminophen toxicity, adverse prognostic indicators include arterial pH less than 7.3, INR greater than 6.5, and creatinine greater than 3.4. Liver histology does not predict outcome and is rarely obtained in this setting. The most reliable predictors of mortality are degree of encephalopathy and prothrombin time.

(690–C) **(S&F, pp. 1310, 1320)**

Chylous ascites occurs when there is disruption of lymphatic drainage into the thoracic duct. This can occur when lymphatic architecture is markedly altered, such as with trauma or lymphoma. Spontaneous lymphatic rupture has been reported in cirrhosis, and there is a 0.5% incidence of chylous ascites among patients with cirrhosis and ascites. Pancreatitis typically produces pigmented ascites, believed to be due to the actions of pancreatic enzymes on erythrocytes.

(691–A, D) **(S&F, pp. 1271–1273)**

Treatment regimens that proved efficacious in the Mayo Clinic trial included prednisone alone or in combination with azathioprine. The prednisone dosage was 60 mg/day, tapering to a maintenance dose of 20 mg/day. When azathioprine was also given at 50 mg/day, the prednisone dosages could be cut in half. In a long-term follow-up study, 66% of patients in remission after successful prednisone therapy suffered a relapse and required re-treatment. After two weeks of medical therapy, if the patient fails to show a normalization of at least one laboratory parameter or if the pretreatment bilirubin level fails to improve, then a high immediate mortality is predicted and the patient should be considered for liver transplantation if there are features of decompensation. Follow-up liver biopsies are usually necessary to determine whether remission has been achieved.

(692–B, D)   ***(S&F, pp. 1138–1139)***

Risk factors for progressing to chronic hepatitis B include age at the time of acquisition, sex, immune status, and possibly ethnic origin. Males are far more likely to progress to chronic disease than females. Age at acquisition appears to be the most important susceptibility factor, with 90% to 95% of neonates born to HBeAg-positive mothers going on to develop chronic infection. Although patients with vertically transmitted hepatitis B may have normal histology, a substantial portion progress to cirrhosis. Any immunosuppressed patient is at risk for developing chronic hepatitis B, including patients receiving cancer chemotherapy, patients with the acquired immunodeficiency syndrome, and patients with chronic renal failure.

(693–A, B, D)   ***(S&F, p. 1372)***

Chronic infection with both hepatitis C virus (HCV) and hepatitis B virus is associated with an increased risk of hepatocellular carcinoma (HCC). HCV is probably the second most common etiologic agent in the development of this disease, being present in 6% to 76% of patients with HCC. In longitudinal studies of post-transfusion hepatitis, HCC was a late development, occurring on average 30 years (range, 15 to 60 years) after HCV infection. In most cases in the United States and Europe, the malignancy was a late complication in patients with known chronic liver disease, but in a Japanese study, up to 30% had the malignancy at the time of presentation. Despite the association of HCV and HCC, the actual risk of an individual with HCV infection developing either cirrhosis or HCC is low. In 1977, 438 young Irish women were accidentally infected with a common source of HCV and, with 18 years follow-up, very few have developed cirrhosis and none has HCC. In Japanese studies, HCV genotype 1b seems to be a more virulent agent, causing higher viral loads and more rapid disease progression.

◼◼◼◼Reference

Cuthbert, J. A. Hepatitis C: Progress and problems. Clin. Microbiol. Rev. 7:505, 1994.

(694–A, C)   ***(S&F, pp. 1141–1142)***

The interferons are a family of glycoproteins with antiviral properties. Interferons stimulate the synthesis and expression of human leukocyte antigens (HLAs) class I on the surface of hepatocytes, which normally have little or no HLA class I display. This permits cytotoxic T cells to recognize and destroy infected cells. Interferon is useful in suppressing hepatitis B viral replication. Thirty to 40 percent of treated patients lose HBV DNA and HBeAg with treatment, but less than 10% lose HBsAg. Effective treatment with interferon transiently worsens liver function and may precipitate liver failure in poorly compensated patients.

(695–B)   ***(S&F, pp. 1135–1136)***

The pattern of self-limited HBsAg-positive infection is one in which HBsAg can be detected only transiently in the blood. It is the most common pattern of primary hepatitis B virus (HBV) infection in adults. HBsAg is usually the first viral marker to appear in the blood after HBV infection. HBeAg is another regular and early marker of HBV infection. A third marker of infection is anti-HBc, which is the antibody directed against the internal antigen of virions. Anti-HBc appears in virtually all patients before the onset of symptoms or hepatic injury, usually three to five weeks after the appearance of HBsAg. Antibody to HBsAg (anti-HBs) usually appears during convalescence after HBsAg has disappeared. In the 10% to 20% of patients who develop arthritis and rash associated with immune complex formation, this antibody tends to appear earlier while replication is still active.

(696–A)   ***(S&F, p. 1373)***

The only potential cure for a patient with hepatocellular carcinoma is surgical resection (including liver transplantation in highly selected cases). Unfortunately, the disease is often multifocal and new tumors often develop after resection. Chemotherapy, chemoembolization, and alcohol injection are palliative.

(697–A)   ***(S&F, p. 1327)***

Complications occur in most cases of umbilical hernias occurring in cirrhotics with ascites. These include skin ulcerations (most common) as well as incarceration and rupture. All are indications for surgery. The absence of ascites before surgery is associated with a five-fold reduction in the rate of hernia recurrence and suggests that ascites should be removed preoperatively. Rupture is a severe complication, with an associated mortality between 10% and 45%.

(698–A, B, C, D)   ***(S&F, pp. 1126–1127)***

Aminotransferase levels increase in the blood as a result of their release from damaged, apoptotic, or necrotic cells. Enzyme elevations always precede jaundice. Alanine aminotransferase levels are usually more abnormal than aspartate aminotransferase levels in both the early and late stages of acute hepatitis and are typically greater in icteric than in anicteric cases. Different hepatitis viruses have different enzyme patterns, including the duration of enzyme abnormalities. Exposure to hepatitis B leads to a more gradual rise in enzyme elevations than does exposure to hepatitis A.

(699–D)   *(S&F, pp. 1205–1206)*

Consumption of ethanol can lead to three histologic findings in the liver: fatty infiltration, steatohepatitis, and cirrhosis. Based on the aspartate aminotransferase (AST)/alanine aminotransferase (ALT) ratio of 3, this patient most likely has asymptomatic alcoholic liver disease. The laboratory finding most suggestive of cirrhosis is thrombocytopenia, which is indicative of hypersplenism. The patient's alcohol consumption is high enough to have advanced liver disease, which may occur in the absence of complications such as ascites, gastroesophageal variceal hemorrhage, or encephalopathy. Chronic hepatitis C usually causes similar elevations in both AST and ALT.

(700–B)   *(S&F, pp. 1201–1203)*

Prohibition did indeed dramatically reduce the rate of death from cirrhosis, which had fallen to half the pre-Prohibition incidence by 1930 and did not equal the 1910 rate until 1973. Men have twice the tolerance of ethanol compared with women and require an average threshold dose of 600 kg before the incidence of liver disease becomes appreciable. Even then, fewer than half of men exceeding the threshold ever develop significant liver disease.

(701–A, B)   *(S&F, pp. 1125–1127)*

Infectious virus may be identified in the feces as early as four days after inoculation of infectious material and continues to increase in magnitude until just before the onset of aminotransferase elevations and jaundice. Hepatitis A may cause cholestatic hepatitis with persistent jaundice and intrahepatic cholestasis. Relapsing hepatitis A has been described in which a second discrete rise in serum aminotransferase levels occurs. Patients remain infectious for approximately ten days after the onset of jaundice. Onset of symptoms is typically abrupt and may occur from 15 to 50 days after exposure.

Reference

Glikson, M. E., Galun, R., Tur-Kaspa, R., and Shouval, D. Relapsing hepatitis A: Review of 14 cases and literature survey. Medicine *71*:14, 1992.

(702–B)   *(S&F, p. 1327)*

Ascites associated with portal hypertension (as in primary biliary cirrhosis) responds best to salt restriction and diuretic therapy. All of the other options produce ascites by peritoneal inflammation.

(703–D)   *(S&F, pp. 1381–1382)*

All of the diseases listed are congenital benign cystic diseases of the liver.

(704–B)   *(S&F, pp. 1367–1368)*

An elevated α-fetoprotein level in the setting of chronic hepatitis B is highly suggestive of hepatocellular carcinoma. This is particularly true for persons born in Asia or the Philippines, where hepatitis B is usually acquired at birth and hepatocellular carcinoma is the most common solid malignancy. An elevated α-fetoprotein level is present in up to 75% of patients with this tumor.

(705–B)   *(S&F, p. 1367)*

Hypoglycemia (type B hypoglycemia, specifically) is one of the most common paraneoplastic syndromes associated with hepatocellular carcinoma (HCC, incidence of about 5%) and should be suspected in all liver disease patients with altered mental status. This type of hypoglycemia is severe and presents early in the course of HCC, often as the cause of the chief complaint. The pathogenesis of hypoglycemia is due to secretion by the tumor of a high molecular weight form of the precursor of insulin-like growth factor.

(706–D)   *(S&F, p. 1209)*

Although the discriminant function for the patient in question 705 is more than 32, suggesting he should benefit from corticosteroid treatment, he has overt gastrointestinal bleeding and anemia. Upper gastrointestinal bleeding from portal hypertension or peptic ulcer disease is usually the cause of bleeding in this group of patients. Corticosteroid therapy should not be started until after his bleeding is stabilized.

(707–B)   *(S&F, p. 1141)*

The most important factors that predict favorable response to interferon-α therapy in hepatitis B are elevated alanine aminotransferase level and low serum hepatitis B viral DNA. Each of these factors suggests a strong host immune response to the infection. Interferon works by boosting the host immune response until it clears the virus. Persons with little or no immune response (such as those who acquired the infection at birth) generally do not benefit from interferon treatment.

Reference

Brook, M. G., Karayiannis, P., Thomas, H. Which patients with chronic hepatitis B virus infection will respond to alpha-interferon therapy? A statistical analysis of predictive factors. Hepatology *10*:761, 1989.

(708–A)   *(S&F, p. 1294)*

The mortality after a variceal hemorrhage is approximately 50% by 6 weeks. Large varices and those with red wale spots seen on endoscopy are more likely to rebleed. However, overall survival is determined primarily by the severity of the underlying liver disease, not by the rebleeding risk. Patients with intercurrent alcoholic hepatitis, portal vein thrombosis, or hepatocellular carcinoma have the worst prognosis.

(709–C)   *(S&F, pp. 1299–1300)*

Long-acting somatostatin analogs such as octreotide (Sandostatin) are as effective as sclerotherapy for treating acute variceal bleeding and are much safer than vasopressin. They work by altering splanchnic hemodynamics and reducing azygous blood flow. Octreotide may be used safely for prolonged intervals.

■■■**Reference**

Saari., A., Klvilaakso, E., Inberg, M., et al. Comparison of somatostatin and vasopressin in bleeding esophageal varices. Am. J. Gastroenterol. *85*:804, 1990.

(710–C)   **(S&F, pp. 1316–1317)**

Although tuberculous ascites is generally associated with a low serum ascites/albumin gradient, the gradient becomes elevated if there is concomitant cirrhosis, reflecting the presence of portal hypertension. Hollow viscus leak and peritoneal malignancy both produce a low serum ascites/albumin gradient.

(711–C)   **(S&F, pp. 1145–1149)**

Hepatitis C is a very common disease in the United States and other industrialized countries. It is estimated that 0.4% to 1.1% of the adult population is chronically infected. Hepatocyte hepatitis C viral RNA remains detectable during the period of biochemical hepatitis. The sensitivity and specificity of the first-generation hepatitis C virus assay was low. Current assays have increased the sensitivity to approximately 99% in chronic infection, but sensitivity in acute infections at the time of clinical presentation remains poor.

■■■**Reference**

Cuthbert, J. A. Hepatitis C: Progress and problems. Clin. Microbiol. Rev. 7:505, 1994.

(712–B)   **(S&F, pp. 1319–1321)**

Laparoscopy is generally most helpful in the diagnosis of causes of ascites associated with peritoneal involvement. Because of the high diagnostic yield of peritoneal fluid cytology and abdominal imaging studies (e.g., ultrasonography, computed tomography) in most conditions, suspected tuberculous ascites is one of the few current indications for diagnostic laparoscopy.

(713–B)   **(S&F, pp. 1321–1322)**

Seeding of ascitic fluid with bacteria is thought to result from bacteremia and/or rupture of mesenteric lymphatics. Bacteremia is prolonged by reticuloendothelial dysfunction, which is common in cirrhosis. Increased gut permeability and seeding of mesenteric lymphatics with bacteria have been demonstrated to favor bacterial peritonitis in experimental models of cirrhosis. Albumin by itself is not protective. However, a low serum albumin correlates with low opsonic activity in peritoneal fluid and therefore with an increased risk of infection.

(714–D)   **(S&F, p. 1206)**

All of the laboratory findings listed are consistent with alcoholic hepatitis, but none is diagnostic. The aspartate aminotransferase value tends to be elevated to a greater degree than the alanine aminotransferase level in alcoholics

with liver disease. This finding is not specific for alcoholic liver disease, because it may be seen in alcoholics with other forms of hepatitis. An elevated gamma glutamyl transpeptidase (GGT) level is highly sensitive for active alcoholic liver disease, but is commonly elevated in many other conditions. Ethanol induces the production of GGT in some individuals, leading to increased serum levels even when no overt liver disease is present.

(715–B)   **(S&F, pp. 1361–1362)**

The development of grade IV encephalopathy secondary to fulminant hepatic failure is an ominous sign. However, the two-day mortality for this group of patients admitted to the hospital is only about 30%. Patients should be evaluated for transplantation before they reach stage IV.

(716–A)   **(S&F, p. 1205)**

Hepatomegaly is the most common physical finding in a patient with acute alcoholic hepatitis. This finding is seen in 80% to 100% of these patients.

(717–C)   **(S&F, pp. 1205–1206, 1209)**

This patient is at high risk of severe alcoholic hepatitis, as indicated by her discriminant function of 38, as calculated by the following formula: total bilirubin + 4.6 × (PT of patient − PT of control). She should receive corticosteroid therapy. She also has a leukocytosis, which may represent an occult infection or hepatic inflammation due to alcoholic hepatitis. Before starting corticosteroid therapy, occult infection must be ruled out. Empirical treatment with antibiotics would be inappropriate. Simple supportive therapy is inadequate in view of her high risk.

(718–A)   **(S&F, pp. 1376–1377)**

Colon cancer metastatic to the liver results in either single or multiple nodular lesions. Other malignancies may also cause mass lesions but more commonly cause diffuse infiltration of the liver parenchyma.

■■■**Reference**

Edmondson, H. A., and Craig J. R. Neoplasms of the Liver. *In* Schiff, L. (ed.), Diseases of the Liver. Philadelphia, J. B. Lippincott, 1992, pp. 1109–1158.

(719–D)   **(S&F, p. 1381)**

In all likelihood, the patient has a hydatid cyst from infection with the tapeworm *Echinococcus granulosus*. Most cysts cause no symptoms, but large ones may rupture either intraperitoneally (producing anaphylaxis) or into the biliary tract (producing cholangitis). The presence of a daughter cyst on the ultrasonogram strongly suggests a hydatid cyst, and great care must be taken to not rupture the lesion and spill the cyst contents into the abdomen. Serologic tests for hydatidosis are positive in only 80% of cases, so when the pretest probability of having hydatid disease is so high, a negative serologic test does not exclude the disease. Results of medical therapy for hydatid disease are disappointing, and the best treatment is careful surgical resection.

(720–D) **(S&F, pp. 1206–1207)**

Histologically, alcoholic cirrhosis can be micronodular, macronodular, or of a mixed pattern. Early alcoholic cirrhosis tends to be micronodular.

(721–A) **(S&F, pp. 1357–1359)**

Multiple metabolic changes occur in fulminant hepatic failure, reflecting the many organ systems involved. Hypoglycemia is a constant danger because of disordered hepatic glycogenolysis and gluconeogenesis combined with the failure of the liver to clear peptide hormones from the blood. Hyperglycemia is not a danger.

(722–B) **(S&F, pp. 1378–1379)**

The patient in this question most likely has a cavernous hemangioma. Although hepatic arteriography is the most accurate method for diagnosis of vascular lesions, a less invasive test for confirming this diagnosis would be the bolus-contrast computed tomography with rapid sequential scans or magnetic resonance imaging, if available. The former study is usually diagnostic if the lesion is more than 3 cm in diameter, whereas magnetic resonance imaging can detect lesions greater than 1 cm in diameter. Liver biopsy should not be done until cavernous hemangioma has been excluded.

(723–B) **(S&F, pp. 1378–1379)**

Thrombocytopenia can be seen in patients with large hemangiomas secondary to sequestration. This is referred to as Kasabach-Merritt syndrome.

(724–C) **(S&F, p. 1247)**

The patient in this case is presenting with fulminant hepatic failure secondary to ingestion of *Amanita phalloides,* which can progress so rapidly that icterus does not have time to develop. This mushroom contains two potent hepatotoxins: phalloidin and α-amanitine. Phalloidin alters membranes of hepatocytes, whereas α-amanitine inhibits hepatocyte ribonucleic acid polymerase and therefore prevents protein synthesis. Although viral hepatitis is the most common cause of acute hepatic failure overall, the patient's history is consistent with toxin-induced liver failure. Acute intermittent porphyria is not associated with liver failure.

(725–D) **(S&F, p. 1271)**

Patients with chronic hepatitis are often depressed and have problems sleeping. Right upper quadrant abdominal pain is frequent and is usually characterized by a dull, aching discomfort that is intermittent and increases late in the day or after strenuous activity. There is often little correlation between the levels of symptoms and the bio-

chemical and histologic evidence of disease. Relief of symptoms by leaning forward in a sitting position suggests retroperitoneal disease such as pancreatitis.

(726–C) **(S&F, p. 1287)**

Cerebral artery aneurysms, congenital heart disease, bile duct and gallbladder anomalies, renal collecting duct defects, and intestinal lymphangiectasia are all seen in association with congenital hepatic fibrosis. Pancreatitis is not.

(727–C) **(S&F, p. 1367)**

Hypercalcemia, erythrocytosis, and hypoglycemia are common paraneoplastic complications of hepatocellular carcinoma, owing to production by the tumor of parathyroid hormone–related protein, erythropoietin, and a precursor of insulin-like growth factor, respectively. Dermatomyositis is sometimes seen but is rare.

(728–D) **(S&F, p. 1075)**

Transferrin, along with albumin and α-fetoprotein, decreases during an acute phase response, whereas the other proteins listed increase.

(729–A) **(S&F, pp. 1206–1207)**

Alcoholic hepatitis is a histopathologic diagnosis characterized by fatty change, necrosis of hepatocytes, and an inflammatory infiltrate. Mallory bodies (condensed cytoskeletal elements) are often present. Councilman bodies are found in viral hepatitis.

(730–B) **(S&F, pp. 1381–1382)**

The patient has a simple cyst of the liver and is minimally symptomatic. No further evaluation or treatment is required. Symptoms that would warrant further study would be the development of jaundice, anemia, or severe abdominal pain or rupture of the cyst.

(731–C) **(S&F, p. 784)**

Many conditions other than cystic fibrosis are associated with elevated levels of sweat electrolytes, including acute respiratory disorders (e.g., croup and viral pneumonia) and chronic respiratory disorders (e.g., α$_1$-antitrypsin deficiency). In many of these situations, the abnormality is transient. Hypothyroidism, not hyperthyroidism, may cause an elevated sweat electrolyte concentration.

(732–A) **(S&F, pp. 1310–1311)**

Spontaneous bacterial peritonitis occurs in pre-existing ascitic fluid (usually in low-protein ascitic fluid due to portal hypertension) but is not the cause of ascites per se. All of the other conditions listed actually cause ascites, albeit through different mechanisms.

(733–C) (S&F, pp. 1302–1303)

The goal is to lower portal pressure below 12 mm Hg because this appears to be the critical level required for bleeding to occur. Although transjugular intrahepatic portosystemic shunt can control active variceal bleeding in 90% of patients, the rate of post-shunt encephalopathy is 20% to 30%. Shunt dysfunction, defined as either stenosis or occlusion, occurs in 48% and 31%, respectively, at one year. Shunt dysfunction is not a benign problem because a third of patients so affected will develop recurrent variceal bleeding within two years.

■■■■**Reference**

Rossle, M., Haag, K., Osch, A., et al. The transjugular intrahepatic portosystemic stent-shunt procedure for variceal bleeding. N. Engl. J. Med. *330*:165, 1994.

(734–D) (S&F, p. 785)

The least reliable method for *in utero* diagnosis of cystic fibrosis is measurement of microvillous enzyme levels in amniotic fluid using monoclonal antibodies, with a false-positive rate of 1% and a false-negative rate of 17%. DNA probes linked to the cystic fibrosis gene can be used in over 80% of affected families, with diagnosis possible as early as 11 to 12 weeks of gestation. Direct mutation analysis is the most reliable and specific test. However, the most common mutation (F508) is present in only about 70% of all affected chromosomes.

(735–C) (S&F, p. 1357)

According to standard criteria, this patient has stage III encephalopathy. Stage I is characterized by either euphoria or depression, mild confusion, slowed mentation, disordered sleep pattern, and slurred speech. Stage II is similar to stage I, but symptoms are more obvious, including drowsiness, inappropriate behavior, and bowel and bladder incontinence. At stage III, the patient develops stupor with somnolence and marked confusion but is still arousable. Frank coma is present at stage IV.

(736–C) (S&F, pp. 1378–1379)

The patient's age, gender, and multiparity along with her symptoms and normal laboratory test all point toward a cavernous hemangioma as the cause of her liver lesion. Hepatocellular adenoma and focal nodular hyperplasia are also possible, although much rarer than a cavernous hemangioma. Hepatocellular carcinoma and metastatic carcinoma are less likely, given the normal liver function test and α-fetoprotein level. The best test in this situation is spiral computed tomography, which would likely show a hypodense central area with an enhancing peripheral zone that is characteristic of a cavernous hemangioma. Magnetic resonance imaging of the liver may also be very specific for hemangioma, especially for small lesions. Arteriography can be pathognomonic for hemangioma with early filling and persistence of irregular lakes.

(737–C) (S&F, p. 1377)

In the proper setting, the diagnosis can be confidently made with a characteristic computed tomographic appearance. Symptomatic lesions can be resected; if rupture occurs, embolization may be required to stop bleeding before resection. Estrogens probably promote growth of the hemangioma.

(738–B) (S&F, p. 1077)

The fat-soluble vitamins include vitamins A, D, E, and K, and all are dependent on adequate fatty acid micellization in the intestine by sufficient bile acids. Vitamin A occurs in nature in three forms. All-*trans* retinol (vitamin A_1) and 3-dehydroretinol (vitamin A_2) are found in mammals, whereas in plants vitamin A occurs as the water-soluble precursor beta-carotene. Vitamin D, produced by the action of ultraviolet light on 7-dehydrocholesterol in the skin of human subjects, is called cholecalciferol (vitamin D_3). The plant form of vitamin D is ergocalciferol or vitamin D_2. Vitamin D is hydroxylated in the liver to 25-hydroxy D and in the kidney to 1,25-dihydroxy D, the active form. Vitamin E (tocopherol) is an antioxidant that protects against lipid peroxidation in membranes. Vitamin K (phylloquinone) is necessary for normal coagulation and is inhibited by warfarin. Cobalamin, or vitamin B_{12}, is not a fat-soluble vitamin, although vitamin B_{12}/intrinsic factor complex is absorbed in the ileum.

(739–B) (S&F, pp. 1141–1142)

In response to interferon-α therapy, the serum aminotransferases will often increase and then decrease to normal, reflecting destruction of infected liver cells by cytotoxic T lymphocytes. The flare of disease activity that occurs in response to interferon therapy often occurs concurrently with the clearance of hepatitis B viral DNA and HBeAg and often leads to long-term remission.

■■■■**Reference**

Perrillo, R. P., Schiff, E. R., Davis, G. L., et al. A randomized controlled trial of interferon alfa-2b alone and after prednisone withdrawal for the treatment of chronic hepatitis B. N. Engl. J. Med. *323*:295, 1990.

(740–C) (S&F, p. 1336)

In surgically created portosystemic shunts, where portal blood is shunted into the vena cava, ingestion of a protein meal causes encephalopathy, thus establishing a role for nitrogenous products in hepatic encephalopathy. Animal studies reveal that an increase in γ-aminobutyric acid–mediated neurotransmission may be involved in the development of hepatic encephalopathy. Supporting this theory are data showing that the use of flumazenil, a benzodiazepine antagonist, may be beneficial in encephalopathy secondary to fulminant hepatic failure. Increased plasma levels of aromatic amino acids (relative to branched-chain amino acids) may lead to the production of false neurotransmitters. Norepinephrine release has no relationship to encephalopathy.

(741–C) **(S&F, pp. 1199–1211)**

Alcoholism is associated with a number of neurologic abnormalities but is not associated with dementia.

(742–C) **(S&F, pp. 1374–1375)**

Of the possibilities listed, the most likely diagnosis is cholangiocarcinoma complicating long-standing sclerosing cholangitis and ulcerative colitis. The factor in the history that suggests a cause other than drug hepatotoxicity is the weight loss. Metastatic colon cancer is a possibility that must be excluded but is less likely to present as biliary obstruction. Cholangiocarcinoma may be difficult to differentiate from an inflammatory stricture of the bile duct.

(743–1-D, 2-C, 3-B, 4-A) **(S&F, p. 1226)**

Drug hepatotoxicity, although rare, tends to be consistent in the mechanism through which liver injury is produced. Acetaminophen, nontoxic at small doses, produces a dose-dependent level of liver injury whereas isoniazid causes an acute hepatitic picture. Oral contraceptives, estrogens, and androgens cause cholestasis (usually without evidence of hepatitis) whereas carbamazepine produces a granulomatous hepatitis.

(744–B, C, D, E) **(S&F, pp. 1123–1165)**

Anemia occurs less frequently in acute viral hepatitis than does leukopenia, even though shortened red blood cell survival appears to be common. Hemolysis has also been seen. Leukopenia is the most common hematologic abnormality. Leukopenia and thrombocytopenia are usually seen during the preicteric phase. α-Fetoprotein level may be elevated in acute hepatitis, commonly during the regenerative phase when the aminotransferase levels are declining. Elevated serum iron levels in acute hepatitis usually reflect release of iron from necrotic hepatocytes.

(745–D) **(S&F, pp. 1145–1146)**

The estimated risk of hepatitis C virus transmission from a single needlestick accident with hepatitis C viral RNA–positive blood is 4% to 10%. This risk is lower than the 7% to 30% for hepatitis B virus transmission and higher than the 0.5% risk for human immunodeficiency virus transmission.

■ Reference

Mitsui, T., Masuko, K., Yamazaki, C., et al. Hepatitis C virus infection in medical personnel after needle stick accident. Hepatology *16*:1109, 1992.

(746–1-B, 2-D, 3-A, 4-C) **(S&F, pp. 1315–1319)**

Primary hepatocellular carcinoma, often associated with portal hypertension, generally produces a high serum ascites/albumin gradient. Lymphatic obstruction, often caused by lymphoma, leads to chylous ascites, in which the triglyceride concentration is markedly elevated. Involvement of the peritoneum by malignancy is associated with abnormal peritoneal fluid cytology. A peritoneal fluid bilirubin concentration greater than 6 mg/dL and greater than the serum bilirubin concentration suggests the presence of a biliary tract leak.

(747–B) **(S&F, p. 1207)**

Fatty infiltration of the liver is the most common histologic finding in patients who drink moderate to large amounts of ethanol. Patients are usually asymptomatic.

(748–1-I, 2-B, 3-F, 4-H, 5-B, 6-B, 7-D, 8-B, 9-B, 10-C, 11-G) **(S&F, p. 1126)**

Viremia is found in all forms of viral hepatitis but is more prolonged in hepatitis B, C, and G. The mortality of acute hepatitis B is between 0.5% and 1.0% for adults, whereas the mortality of acute hepatitis A is less than 0.5% and that of acute hepatitis C is less than 0.1%. Co-infection of patients with hepatitis D virus (which requires hepatitis B virus to replicate) greatly increases the severity of the acute infection but makes chronic infection less likely. All forms of acute viral hepatitis may relapse, but only hepatitis B (with or without D), C, and G viruses produce chronic infection. Data suggest that progression to chronic infection for hepatitis C may exceed 70%. Hepatitis A and E are transmitted by the fecal-oral route, whereas the other viruses are transmitted by parenteral (e.g., intravenous drug abuse) or occult parenteral (e.g., sexual) inoculation. The incubation period of hepatitis B (28 to 160 days) is longer than that for hepatitis A (15 to 50 days) or hepatitis C (14 to 56 days). Vertical transmission may occur for all viruses but is particularly efficient for hepatitis B owing to much higher viral titers in blood and body fluids. Chronic hepatitis G is very common in the United States (up to 2% of volunteer blood donors) but produces little or no known clinical disease. Clinical diagnosis of infection is based on host antibodies to viral antigens in all cases except hepatitis B (for which HBsAg may also be used) and hepatitis G (which currently requires polymerase chain reaction [PCR]). Viral DNA or RNA can be detected by PCR for all viruses, but this test is expensive and subject to false-positive results if not done carefully. PCR thus remains primarily a research tool.

(749–D) **(S&F, p. 1151)**

Chronic hepatitis C is even more common than previously believed. Long-term follow-up studies after posttransfusion hepatitis indicate that at least 70% of patients have persistent or intermittent elevations of alanine aminotransferase. Sensitive assays for the viral genome in liver or blood using polymerase chain reaction (PCR) are positive in 80% to 90% of these individuals. About 20% of chronically infected patients will develop cirrhosis within the next 20 years.

■■■■**Reference**

Alter, M. J., Margolis, H. S., Krawczynski, K., et al. The natural history of community acquired hepatitis C in the United States. N. Engl. J. Med. *327*:1899, 1992.

(750–D)   **(S&F, p. 1270)**

Ten-fold aspartate aminotransferase elevations or five-fold aspartate aminotransferase elevations with two-fold gamma globulin elevations have similarly poor ten-year survival rates if untreated. Unlike other liver diseases, the liver histology in autoimmune hepatitis has powerful prognostic implications because periportal hepatitis alone has a normal five-year survival whereas bridging necrosis implies only a 55% survival at five years (untreated).

(751–A)   **(S&F, pp. 1318–1319)**

Hepatocellular carcinoma often produces ascites by elevation of portal pressure (either due to concomitant cirrhosis or tumor mass effect) rather than by peritoneal involvement. The other malignancies produce ascites by peritoneal implants. Under the latter conditions, peritoneal fluid cytology is virtually always positive.

(752–B, C, E)   **(S&F, pp. 1135–1137, 1148)**

The serologic tests exclude chronic hepatitis B. Given the history of intravenous drug abuse, a unifying diagnosis would be essential mixed cryoglobulinemia associated with hepatitis C. Most "essential" mixed cryoglobulinemia is now recognized to be caused by hepatitis C. In these patients, purpura improves during interferon therapy but symptoms typically return after therapy is discontinued. Porphyria cutanea tarda is associated with liver disease and is characterized by cutaneous lesions but would not explain this patient's renal insufficiency.

■■■■**Reference**

Cuthbert, J. A. Hepatitis C: Progress and problems. Clin. Microbiol. Rev. *7*:505, 1994.

(753–B)   **(S&F, p. 768)**

Annular pancreas involves the second portion of the duodenum in 85% of cases. It is the most common anomaly obstructing the duodenum in infancy, but it may also be asymptomatic and become an incidental finding in surgery or autopsy. Annular pancreas involves the growth of pancreatic tissue into the wall of the duodenum.

(754–B)   **(S&F, pp. 1377–1378)**

Hepatocellular adenomas were extremely rare before the advent of oral contraceptives and still are in men. The relative risk of this benign tumor is increased 25-fold after more than nine years of oral contraceptive use, although the actual risk for individual women taking oral contraceptives is low. Arteriography is often characteristic of a hepatocellular adenoma, but needle biopsy of the lesion is often nondiagnostic because the cells mimic normal hepatocytes. Symptomatic lesions can be resected.

(755–A)   **(S&F, p. 1305)**

Patients with variceal bleeding are probably best managed initially by esophageal variceal ligation. If hemostasis cannot be maintained, and the patient is a candidate for a future liver transplantation, then transjugular intrahepatic portosystemic shunt may decompress the varices and yet not distort the vascular anatomy such that an orthotopic liver transplant is impossible.

(756–A, C, D, E)   **(S&F, p. 1137)**

HBsAg-positive arthritis is symmetric and polyarticular without synovial thickening. The patient often has a rash, and the joint fluid leukocyte count is commonly less than 5000 cells/mm^3 and predominantly mononuclear.

■■■■**Reference**

Cuthbert, J. A. Hepatitis C: Progress and problems. Clin. Microbiol. Rev. *7*:505, 1994.

(757–A)   **(S&F, p. 1366)**

Hepatitis C with cirrhosis is a recognized risk factor for hepatocellular carcinoma. The diagnosis should be suspected in any patient with chronic viral hepatitis who unexpectedly decompensates. Hepatic vein thrombosis is a possible cause of decompensation but is less likely.

■■■■**Reference**

Simonetti R. G., et al. Hepatitis C virus infection as a risk factor for hepatocellular carcinoma in patients with cirrhosis: A case-control study. Ann. Intern. Med. *116*:97, 1992.

(758–B)   **(S&F, p. 1373)**

For resection to be considered, all tumor must be confined to a single lobe. The finding of portal hypertension does not necessarily make a hepatoma nonresectable, although resection is much more difficult when cirrhosis is present.

Pancreas

S&F Section VII

759. Which of the following statements regarding pancreatic disease in patients with cystic fibrosis are TRUE?
  I. The most frequent mutation (F508) is associated with a higher incidence of pancreatic disease than are other mutations.
  II. Pancreatic gland damage is due to obstruction of the main pancreatic duct.
  III. Atrophy and fat replacement of the pancreas is best demonstrated by computed tomography or magnetic resonance imaging.
  IV. Most cystic fibrosis patients develop diabetes at an early age.

  A. I and III
  B. II and IV
  C. I, II, and III
  D. All of the above

760. Pancreatic insufficiency is associated with malabsorption when pancreatic enzyme output is less than what percentage of normal?
  A. 50
  B. 25
  C. 10
  D. 1

761. Treatment options for metastatic pancreatic endocrine tumors include which of the following?
  I. Systemic chemotherapy with streptozocin and doxorubicin
  II. Octreotide
  III. Hepatic artery embolization
  IV. Interferon

  A. I and III
  B. II and IV
  C. I, II, and III
  D. All of the above

762. Each of the following statements about hereditary pancreatitis is true EXCEPT:
  A. It has an autosomal dominant pattern of inheritance.
  B. Pancreatic calcifications are present in up to 50% of patients.
  C. Pancreatic cancer is more common in patients and their kin.
  D. Endoscopic retrograde cholangiopancreatography should be avoided owing to the high risk of pancreatitis.

763. Each of the following is characteristic of multiple endocrine neoplasia–2B syndrome EXCEPT:
  A. Marfanoid habitus
  B. Medullary cancer of the thyroid
  C. Pheochromocytoma
  D. Islet cell tumor of the pancreas
  E. Gastrointestinal tract mucosal neuromas

764. A 47-year-old man with a long history of alcohol abuse is admitted with abdominal pain, intractable nausea, and dehydration. Laboratory tests reveal markedly elevated serum amylase and a normal white blood cell count. Which of the following therapeutic measures is LEAST indicated?
  A. Nasogastric suction
  B. Meperidine
  C. Fluid and electrolyte replacement
  D. Octreotide

765. The patient in question 764 is hospitalized. After two weeks of slow improvement, he develops increasing abdominal pain with a temperature to 102° F and a white blood cell count of 25,000 cell/mm³. Rapid-sequence abdominal computed tomography reveals that over 50% of the pancreas does not enhance after bolus injection of contrast material. The MOST important therapeutic option would be:
  A. Strict NPO and prolonged total parenteral nutrition
  B. Broad-spectrum antibiotics
  C. Endoscopic retrograde cholangiopancreatography to relieve the pancreatic duct obstruction
  D. External drainage of the pancreatic bed

766. Which of the following statements regarding the sweat electrolyte test for cystic fibrosis are TRUE?
  A. Sweat electrolyte concentrations are elevated in about 50% of patients with cystic fibrosis.
  B. It is most accurate during the first week of life.
  C. High- or low-sodium diets may invalidate the results.
  D. A positive test has a chloride concentration greater than the sodium concentration.

767. Extrapancreatic lesions associated with pancreatitis include which of the following:
  I. Subcutaneous fat necrosis
  II. Intramedullary osseous fat necrosis

III. Aseptic epiphyseal necrosis
IV. Demyelination with encephalopathy

A. I and III
B. II and IV
C. I, II, and III
D. All of the above

---

768. The two MOST common functional endocrine tumors of the pancreas are:
A. Gastrinoma and glucagonoma
B. Gastrinoma and insulinoma
C. Gastrinoma and somatostatinoma
D. Gastrinoma and VIPoma

---

769. Clinical conditions that should raise the suspicion of cystic fibrosis include:
I. Meconium ileus
II. Failure to thrive
III. Chronic hepatobiliary disease
IV. Small bowel atresia

A. I and III
B. II and IV
C. I, II, and III
D. All of the above

---

770. At the cellular level, pancreatic secretion can be stimulated by:
A. Activating adenylate cyclase and increasing cyclic adenosine monophosphate
B. Increasing intracellular calcium
C. Both A and B
D. Neither of the above

---

771. Treatment of the uncomplicated distal intestinal obstruction syndrome seen in patients with cystic fibrosis includes which of the following?
I. Oral *N*-acetylcysteine
II. Rectal *N*-acetylcysteine
III. Gastrografin enema
IV. Colonic lavage

A. I and III
B. II and IV
C. I, II, and III
D. All of the above

---

772. With respect to the use of dynamic, contrast medium–enhanced computed tomography for the evaluation of suspected acute pancreatitis, which of the following computed tomographic findings is MOST suggestive of necrotizing pancreatitis as opposed to the less ominous acute interstitial pancreatitis?
A. After intravenous contrast medium enhancement, the enlarged pancreas enhances to the same degree as the spleen.
B. After intravenous contrast medium enhancement, the enlarged pancreas enhances to a lesser extent than the spleen.
C. After intravenous contrast medium enhancement, the enlarged pancreas enhances from 50 Hounsfield units (HU) to 90 HU.
D. After intravenous contrast medium enhancement, the enlarged pancreas enhances from 50 to 90 HU and the dye shows prolonged retention in the pancreas.

---

773. Which of the following statements about pancreatic juice are TRUE?
I. It is isotonic with plasma.
II. It is acidic.
III. The total pancreatic secretion is about 2.5 L/day.
IV. The concentrations of bicarbonate and chloride are constant.

A. I and III
B. II and IV
C. I, II, and III
D. All of the above

---

774. Which of the following statements about pancreas divisum are TRUE?
A. It results from failure of the dorsal and ventral pancreas ducts to fuse.
B. Pancreatic exocrine secretion drains primarily through the duct of Wirsung.
C. It may be seen in up to 10% of the population.
D. It is the most common cause of recurrent pancreatitis in children.

---

775. Each of the following is a risk factor for the development of pancreatic carcinoma EXCEPT:
A. Diabetes mellitus
B. Gallstones
C. Smoking
D. Chronic alcoholic pancreatitis
E. Familial pancreatitis

---

776. Which of the following statements regarding surgical options for pancreatic carcinoma are TRUE?
A. Pancreaticoduodenectomy (Whipple's procedure) is the procedure of choice for small resectable carcinomas of the head of the pancreas.
B. A Whipple procedure, even in experienced hands, has an operative mortality of 15% to 20%.
C. Total pancreatectomy may remove microscopic foci of pancreatic carcinoma separate from the primary lesion.
D. Choledochojejunostomy, cholecystojejunostomy, and gastrojejunostomy are palliative procedures used for large, nonresectable pancreatic carcinomas.

777. Which of the following statements about pancreatic insufficiency are TRUE?
   A. Azotorrhea occurs before steatorrhea and is manifest clinically as muscle wasting.
   B. Clinically overt vitamin B_{12} deficiency is rare.
   C. A reduction in pancreatic amylase secretion commonly results in osmotic diarrhea.
   D. Stool volume is larger with pancreatic insufficiency than in other malabsorptive states.

778. The MOST prominent gastrointestinal symptom in multiple endocrine neoplasia–2A is:
   A. Biliary colic
   B. Nausea and vomiting
   C. Diarrhea
   D. Constipation
   E. Distention

779. Standard criteria for assessing the severity of pancreatitis include each of the following EXCEPT:
   A. Age older than 55
   B. White blood cell count greater than 16,000 cells/mm^3
   C. Aspartate aminotransferase level greater than 250 IU/L
   D. Serum amylase level greater than 500 IU/L
   E. Glucose concentration more than 200 mg/dL
   F. Lactate dehydrogenase value greater than 350 IU/L

780. Each of the following is a prominent clinical feature of the somatostatinoma syndrome EXCEPT:
   A. Diabetes mellitus
   B. Steatorrhea
   C. Mesenteric thrombosis
   D. Cholelithiasis
   E. Weight loss

781. Match each pancreatic function test with its associated feature.
   1. Secretin test
   2. Bentiromide test
   3. Chymotrypsin
   4. Schilling test

   A. Failure of pancreatic enzymes to degrade R protein
   B. *p*-Aminobenzoic acid (PABA) metabolite can be measured in urine or serum.
   C. Measured in feces
   D. Most sensitive and specific test for chronic pancreatitis

782. Intractable pain is a common problem in terminal pancreatic carcinoma. Which of the following statements regarding use of celiac plexus nerve block are TRUE?
   I. Complications such as epigastric pain, paraplegia, and aortic and renal perforation are rare.
   II. Controlled clinical trials have demonstrated improved performance levels with nerve block compared with external beam radiation.

   III. It produces life-long pain relief in more than 70% of patients.
   IV. It is generally performed with a midline "mini-laparotomy."

   A. I and III
   B. II and IV
   C. I, II, and III
   D. All of the above

783. Which of the following statements regarding pancreatic secretion are TRUE?
   I. Acidification of the duodenum is associated with secretin release.
   II. Cholecystokinin potentiates secretin-induced pancreatic bicarbonate secretion.
   III. Cholecystokinin is the major humoral mediator of meal-stimulated enzyme secretion.
   IV. The gastric phase of pancreatic secretion produces the most output.

   A. I and III
   B. II and IV
   C. I, II, and III
   D. All of the above

784. Which of the following endoscopic retrograde cholangiopancreatographic findings are MOST consistent with pancreatic carcinoma?
   I. Single, irregular, focal pancreatic duct stricture
   II. Displacement of Wirsung's duct
   III. Double-duct sign
   IV. Multiple pancreatic duct stenoses with secondary duct dilation

   A. I and III
   B. II and IV
   C. I, II, and III
   D. All of the above

785. Which of the following statements regarding hypocalcemia of acute pancreatitis are TRUE?
   A. Transient hypocalcemia occurs in one third of cases.
   B. Tetany is seen in up to 20% of patients.
   C. The degree of hypocalcemia parallels the severity of pancreatitis.
   D. Hypocalcemia may be a consequence of hypoalbuminemia.

786. Each of the following statements regarding surgical treatment of chronic pancreatitis is true EXCEPT:
   A. The Puestow procedure is best suited for patients with intractable pain and a dilated pancreatic duct.
   B. Total pancreatectomy ensures pain control in patients with a previously failed Puestow or Whipple procedure.

C. Preoperative endoscopic retrograde cholangio-pancreatography is indicated in patients with pancreatic ascites or a pancreatic pleural effusion.

D. Cystoenterostomy is the most common method to surgically drain pseudocysts.

---

787. Complications associated with meconium ileus include:
   I. Peritonitis
   II. Volvulus
   III. Atresia
   IV. Ascites

   A. I and III
   B. II and IV
   C. I, II, and III
   D. All of the above

---

788. Clinical features of pancreatic carcinoma include each of the following EXCEPT:
   A. Cholangitis
   B. Abdominal pain
   C. Weight loss
   D. Jaundice
   E. Pruritus

---

789. Each of the following statements about chemotherapeutic and radiation therapy options for metastatic pancreatic carcinoma are true EXCEPT:
   A. No evidence exists that single-agent chemotherapy either prolongs survival or enhances quality of life.
   B. Combination chemotherapy has been shown to prolong survival and enhance quality of life and should be offered to patients with nonresectable pancreatic cancer.
   C. Radiation therapy offers little palliation except in cases of severe retroperitoneal pain.
   D. Combination chemotherapy and radiation may confer a survival advantage over either modality used alone.

---

790. Clinical presentations of chronic pancreatitis include which of the following?
   I. Malabsorption
   II. Chronic pain
   III. Diabetes
   IV. Jaundice

   A. I and III
   B. II and IV
   C. I, II, and III
   D. All of the above

---

791. Match each complication of pancreatic pseudocysts with its clinical presentation.
   1. Hematemesis   A. Splenic vein thrombosis
   2. Gastric varices   B. Erosion into an artery
   3. Peritonitis   C. Erosion into stomach or
   4. Rapid disappearance   bowel
      of mass   D. Rupture

---

792. Approximately what percentage of patients with Zollinger-Ellison syndrome can be expected to also have multiple endocrine neoplasia–1?
   A. 90%
   B. 50%
   C. 20%
   D. 5%
   E. Less than 1%

---

793. Nutritional management of patients with pancreatic insufficiency resulting from chronic pancreatitis may include each of the following EXCEPT:
   A. Narcotic analgesia
   B. H₂ receptor antagonists
   C. Enzyme supplements
   D. Short-chain fatty acids

---

794. Match each hormone with its stimulus-secretion pathway.
   1. Secretin   A. Activation of adenylate cyclase
   2. Cholesytokinin   and increase of cyclic adeno-
   3. Vasoactive in-   sine monophosphate
      testinal peptide B. Increase in intracellular calcium
   4. Acetylcholine

---

795. Match each pancreatic hormone with its islet cell of origin.
   1. Insulin   A. A cell
   2. Pancreatic polypeptide B. B cell
   3. Glucagon   C. D cell
   4. Somatostatin   D. PP cell

---

796. Which of the following statements regarding rectal prolapse in patients with cystic fibrosis are TRUE?
   A. Patients with an early diagnosis of cystic fibrosis are less likely to develop rectal prolapse.
   B. Onset of rectal prolapse is usually after the age of ten.
   C. Medical management is usually unsuccessful.
   D. About 50% of patients require surgical correction.

---

797. Each of the following statements about pancreatic cystadenocarcinoma is true EXCEPT:
   A. They account for approximately 10% of all pancreatic carcinomas.
   B. A typical patient profile is a middle-aged woman presenting with abdominal pain, weight loss, nausea, and vomiting.
   C. They are generally large, cystic mass lesions arising from the body and tail of the pancreas.
   D. They should be considered for resection even when very large.

798. Which of the following are TRUE statements regarding hepatobiliary disease in patients with cystic fibrosis?
  I. About 20% of patients with cystic fibrosis have evidence of liver disease.
  II. Liver involvement is more common in patients with pancreatic insufficiency.
  III. Neonatal cholestasis is commonly associated with meconium ileus.
  IV. Fatty liver is uncommon in cystic fibrosis.

  A. I and III
  B. II and IV
  C. I, II, and III
  D. All of the above

799. Multiple endocrine neoplasia–1 (MEN-1) is a genetic disorder that includes neoplasms of the pituitary, parathyroid, and pancreatic islet cells. Which of the following clinical manifestations of MEN-1 is MOST common?
  A. Acid hypersecretion
  B. Diarrhea
  C. Hypercalcemia
  D. Hypoglycemia
  E. Galactorrhea

800. Each of the following statements regarding chronic alcoholic pancreatitis is true EXCEPT:
  A. Morphologic changes of chronic pancreatitis are present in one half of alcoholic patients, including those with no prior history of acute pancreatitis.
  B. Chronic alcoholism accounts for 75% of chronic pancreatitis.
  C. Consumption of distilled spirits leads to chronic pancreatitis faster than does consumption of beer or wine.
  D. Alcoholic liver disease is present in up to 50% of patients with chronic pancreatitis.

801. With respect to the initial evaluation of patients with suspected acute pancreatitis, each of the following is one of Ranson's criteria EXCEPT:
  A. Amylase or lipase more than four times normal
  B. Age older than 55 years
  C. White blood cell count greater than 16,000 cells/mm^3
  D. Aspartate aminotransferase level greater than 250 IU/L
  E. Glucose concentration greater than 200 mg/dL

802. Each of the following is a feature of Shwachman's syndrome EXCEPT:
  A. Metaphyseal chondrodysplasia of the hip
  B. Diarrhea and pancreatic insufficiency
  C. Abnormal sweat chloride test
  D. Neutropenia

803. Each of the following statements regarding the radiologic evaluation of acute pancreatitis is true EXCEPT:
  A. Ultrasonography has a sensitivity and specificity over 90% for the diagnosis of cholelithiasis and acute cholecystitis.
  B. Abdominal computed tomography has a sensitivity and specificity over 90% for the diagnosis of acute pancreatitis.
  C. Plain abdominal radiographs are of limited value in the initial evaluation of suspected acute pancreatitis.
  D. The role of angiography is limited to the diagnosis and treatment of hemosuccus pancreaticus.

804. Which of the following statements regarding cystic fibrosis are TRUE?
  I. It is associated with a chloride secretory defect in epithelial cells.
  II. Apical chloride channels are unresponsive to cyclic adenosine monophosphate.
  III. Calcium-mediated chloride secretion is normal.
  IV. Sodium absorption is normal in most tissues.

  A. I and III
  B. II and IV
  C. I, II, and III
  D. All of the above

805. A 45-year-old man was admitted to the intensive care unit ten days ago with severe gallstone pancreatitis. You are asked to see him because of a drop in hemoglobin from 13.6 to 8.2 g/dL. He is tachycardic, and his nasogastric aspirate consists of fresh blood. Upper endoscopy reveals small esophageal and large gastric varices. In addition to his pancreatitis, which of the following conditions is MOST likely to be present?
  A. Chronic viral hepatitis
  B. Alcohol abuse
  C. Cavernous transformation of the portal vein
  D. Splenic vein thrombosis
  E. Hemosuccus pancreaticus

806. In addition to pancreatic carcinoma, CA 19-9 antigen elevation may be present in which of the following disorders?
  I. Gallbladder cancer
  II. Cholangiocarcinoma
  III. Chronic liver disease
  IV. Chronic pancreatitis

  A. I and III
  B. II and IV
  C. I, II, and III
  D. All of the above

807. Zymogen granules are released from the pancreas in direct response to which of the following stimuli?
    I. Cholecystokinin
    II. Food
    III. Cholinergic drugs
    IV. Gastrin

    A. I and III
    B. II and IV
    C. I, II, and III
    D. All of the above

808. The pancreas receives blood from each of the following arteries EXCEPT:
    A. Celiac
    B. Superior mesenteric
    C. Inferior mesenteric
    D. Splenic

809. A patient with acute pancreatitis is found by computed tomography to have a 6-cm pseudocyst adjacent to the stomach. One week later, she is symptomatically improved and able to eat. All laboratory parameters have normalized except for a two-fold elevation in serum amylase level. Which of the following would be the MOST prudent course of action?
    A. Home total parenteral nutrition for six weeks, then follow-up computed tomography and surgery if cyst is unchanged in size
    B. Home total parenteral nutrition for six weeks, then follow-up computed tomography and surgery if cyst is still present, even if smaller
    C. Endoscopic creation of an internal cyst gastrostomy if anatomically feasible
    D. Discharge home with instructions to report any new symptoms, with follow-up computed tomography in three to six months

810. Each of the following statements regarding gallstone pancreatitis is true EXCEPT:
    A. It is twice as common in women as in men.
    B. Gallstones can be detected in stools of over 90% of patients.
    C. The risk of recurrent pancreatitis is about 10% unless gallstones are removed.
    D. The mortality is approximately 12% during the first attack.
    E. Most idiopathic pancreatitis is associated with microlithiasis in bile.

811. In which of the following pancreatic tumors is octreotide therapy of value?
    I. Insulinoma
    II. VIPoma
    III. Glucagonoma
    IV. Nonfunctioning pancreatic endocrine tumor

    A. I and III
    B. II and IV
    C. I, II, and III
    D. All of the above

812. Which of the following pancreatic endocrine tumors is LEAST likely to be malignant?
    A. Gastrinoma
    B. Glucagonoma
    C. Insulinoma
    D. Somatostatinoma
    E. VIPoma

813. Each of the following is characteristic of pancreatic cholera EXCEPT:
    A. Secretory diarrhea, hypochlorhydria, and hypokalemia are usually present.
    B. The neoplastic lesion is usually a large solitary tumor within the body of the pancreas.
    C. Although diarrhea is common, some patients have little or no actual diarrhea.
    D. The diarrhea frequently responds to octreotide therapy.

814. Which of the following histologic types of pancreatic carcinoma is MOST common?
    A. Mucinous cystadenocarcinoma
    B. Mucinous adenocarcinoma
    C. Pancreatic lymphoma
    D. Pancreatic adenoacanthoma
    E. Metastatic pancreatic carcinoma from a distant primary tumor

815. Which type of hyperlipidemia is associated with an increased risk of pancreatitis? (Only one answer is correct.)
    1. Type I
    2. Type II
    3. Type III
    4. Type IV
    5. Type V

    A. 1, 3, and 5
    B. 2, 4, and 5
    C. 1, 2, and 3
    D. 1, 4, and 5

816. Which of the following statements regarding impaired pulmonary function associated with severe acute pancreatitis are TRUE?
    A. Hypoxia frequently occurs in the absence of pulmonary infiltrates.
    B. Hypoxia is largely due to intrapulmonary right-to-left shunting.
    C. The incidence of adult respiratory distress syndrome increases with the severity of pancreatitis.
    D. Diffuse pulmonary infiltrates occur in 50% of patients.

817. Of the following pancreatic endocrine tumors seen in multiple endocrine neoplasia–1, which list BEST reflects the relative frequency?
  A. VIPoma > gastrinoma > insulinoma
  B. Glucagonoma > insulinoma > nonfunctional tumor
  C. Insulinoma > gastrinoma > nonfunctional tumor
  D. Nonfunctional tumor > gastrinoma > insulinoma

818. Each of the following is a prominent clinical feature of glucagonoma EXCEPT:
  A. Rash
  B. Glucose intolerance
  C. Weight loss
  D. Thromboembolic phenomena
  E. Psychiatric disturbances

819. Of the following laboratory tests, all but one have been found to be elevated in more than half of patients presenting with pancreatic carcinoma. Which of these is LEAST likely to be abnormal?
  A. Alkaline phosphatase
  B. Gamma glutamyl transpeptidase
  C. Bilirubin
  D. Carbohydrate antigen (CA 19-9)
  E. Amylase

820. Which of the following statements regarding cystic fibrosis are TRUE?
  A. It is autosomal dominant with variable penetrance.
  B. It occurs in approximately 1 in 300 births.
  C. It is more common in whites than in other racial groups.
  D. Siblings of an index case have a 4% to 5% risk of developing the disease.

821. Pancreatic enzyme replacement in patients with cystic fibrosis is often associated with:
  I. Hyperuricosuria
  II. Perioral irritation
  III. Perianal irritation
  IV. Allergic reactions

  A. I and III
  B. II and IV
  C. I, II, and III
  D. All of the above

822. Acute pancreatitis is associated with each of the following clinical features EXCEPT:
  A. Cardiogenic shock
  B. Pulmonary insufficiency
  C. Low-grade fever
  D. Renal failure
  E. Jaundice

823. Which of the following statements regarding chronic pancreatitis are TRUE?
  A. Alcoholic pancreatitis, in general, has a less favorable prognosis (both morbidity and mortality) than do cases of idiopathic pancreatitis.
  B. Abstinence from alcohol decreases the frequency and severity of pain.
  C. Pain from chronic pancreatitis has a tendency to "burn out" over long periods of time.
  D. Malabsorption occurs when 90% or more of the secretory capacity is lost.

824. Which of the following drugs have been associated with pancreatitis?
  I. Furosemide
  II. Corticosteroids
  III. 6-Mercaptopurine
  IV. Pentamidine

  A. I and III
  B. II and IV
  C. I, II, and III
  D. All of the above

825. A 31-year-old woman presents with a four-hour history of severe abdominal pain. On examination she is in acute distress; her blood pressure is 70/40 mm Hg, and her heart rate is 120 beats per minute. Her abdomen is diffusely tender with no peritoneal signs, and the stool is negative for occult blood. Laboratory examination reveals a hematocrit of 20%, a serum amylase value twice normal, and normal liver function tests. The MOST likely diagnosis is:
  A. Acute pancreatitis
  B. Mesenteric ischemia
  C. Perforated peptic ulcer
  D. Ruptured ectopic pregnancy

826. Which of the following statements regarding mechanisms that protect the pancreas from digesting itself are TRUE?
  I. Pancreatic enzymes are stored as inactive precursors.
  II. Pancreatic enzymes are sequestered in zymogen granules separated from the remainder of the cell.
  III. The enzyme required to activate pancreatic enzymes (enterokinase) is in the duodenum.
  IV. A trypsin inhibitor is present to inhibit the actions of small amounts of trypsin.

  A. I and III
  B. II and IV
  C. I, II, and III
  D. All of the above

827. Which of the following statements regarding chronic pancreatitis are TRUE?
   A. Pancreatic enzyme levels can be normal during an attack of pain.
   B. Diabetic ketoacidosis is a common complication.
   C. Pancreatic calcification on plain radiographs of the abdomen is diagnostic.
   D. Endoscopic retrograde cholangiopancreatography is helpful in the diagnosis of correctable lesions (cysts, strictures).

828. A 47-year-old man with a long history of alcoholism is admitted with abdominal pain and elevated pancreatic enzymes. An abdominal ultrasound evaluation reveals a 4-cm pseudocyst in the head of the pancreas. Appropriate options include which of the following?
   I. Bowel rest
   II. Meperidine for pain control
   III. Hydration and electrolyte correction
   IV. Endoscopic retrograde cholangiopancreatography to assess if the pseudocyst communicates with the pancreatic duct

   A. I and III
   B. II and IV
   C. I, II, and III
   D. All of the above

829. Which of the following statements regarding intestinal manifestations of cystic fibrosis are TRUE?
   A. Small bowel radiography is usually normal.
   B. Lactase deficiency is more common than in the normal population.
   C. Meconium ileus is the presenting manifestation in 10% to 15% of infants.
   D. Meconium ileus predicts future severe pancreatic insufficiency.

Pancreas

■■■—*Answers*

(759–A) (S&F, pp. 786–788)

Ninety-nine percent of homozygotes and 72% of heterozygotes with the F508 cystic fibrosis mutation have pancreatic insufficiency, whereas only 36% of cystic fibrosis patients with other mutations have this problem. Although obstruction of the main pancreatic duct is occasionally found, most pancreatic lesions are caused by obstruction of the smaller ducts by secretions and debris. Although exocrine pancreatic insufficiency is common, clinically relevant diabetes mellitus occurs in less than 5% of patients with cystic fibrosis. Diffuse atrophy of the pancreas with or without fat replacement can usually be visualized by computed tomography or magnetic resonance imaging.

(760–C) (S&F, p. 852)

Significant malabsorption does not occur until pancreatic enzyme output is less than 10% of normal. Fat malabsorption is usually seen before protein or carbohydrate malabsorption.

(761–D) (S&F, pp. 888–890)

The current choice of chemotherapy for metastatic pancreatic endocrine tumors is streptozocin and doxorubicin. Hepatic artery embolization has been successful in small numbers of patients. The antitumor effects of octreotide are minimal, but it has been reported to cause a decrease in tumor size in a limited number of patients. Interferon therapy remains an option for attempting to control symptoms, but it is unclear what percentage of patients respond with reduction of tumor size.

(762–D) (S&F, pp. 800–801)

Hereditary pancreatitis is inherited in an autosomal dominant manner. Males and females are affected with equal frequency and severity. An abdominal radiograph may reveal pancreatic calcification even in early childhood. Calcifications occur during the course of hereditary pancreatitis in approximately 50% of patients. An increased incidence of pancreatic cancer and other intra-abdominal malignancies occurs in patients, and family members without apparent pancreatitis have developed pancreatic adenocarcinoma. Endoscopic retrograde cholangiopancreatography should be employed early for diagnosis and staging and later for preoperative assessment.

(763–D) (S&F, pp. 872–873)

Multiple endocrine neoplasia–2B syndrome is composed of medullary cancer of the thyroid, pheochromocytoma, and multiple mucosal neuromas of the gastrointestinal tract, buccal mucosa, tongue, and conjunctiva, as well as enlarged corneal nerves. Patients have distinct physical characteristics, such as marfanoid habitus, a flat bridge of the nose, and large lips.

(764–D) (S&F, pp. 830–832)

In randomized trials, somatostatin analogs such as octreotide have not been shown to relieve symptoms or to improve the course of pancreatitis.

(765–D) (S&F, pp. 810, 834)

Infected necrosis may be recognized on computed tomography by lack of enhancement of the pancreas after intravenous contrast medium injection in the setting of a patient with systemic signs of infection. It typically occurs within the first 2 weeks of illness, whereas pancreatic abscess usually occurs after at least one month. Mortality is four times higher than with sterile necrosis (38% vs. 9%). Antibiotics alone will not cure the infection. The treatment of choice is débridement with external drainage, either by open surgery or by a percutaneous approach according to the extent and location of the infection.

(766–C, D) (S&F, pp. 784–785)

The diagnosis of cystic fibrosis rests on the finding of abnormal sweat electrolyte levels. Sodium and chloride concentrations in sweat are elevated in 98% to 99% of patients. The test may be falsely elevated during the first week of life. Corticosteroid medications, diuretics, and high- or low-sodium diets may affect the results. Patients with cystic fibrosis have a concentration of chloride greater than that of sodium; the reverse occurs in normal subjects.

(767–D) (S&F, p. 838)

Distant lesions occasionally arise during the course of acute and chronic pancreatitis. Fat necrosis is recognized clinically in less than 1% of cases, whereas autopsy studies reveal a frequency of 10%. Pancreatic encephalopathy may include agitation, hallucinations, confusion, disorientation, and coma. Circulating lipase may produce demyelination of neural tissues, possibly contributing to encephalopathy.

(768–B) (S&F, p. 871)

Pancreatic endocrine tumors are rare. The incidence of insulinoma is approximately one case per million per year, with gastrinomas half as common. Compared with insulinomas, VIPomas are 1/8 as common, glucagonomas are 1/17 as common, and somatostatinomas are extremely rare, with only 50 cases reported in the literature.

(769–D) *(S&F, p. 784)*

Cystic fibrosis is responsible for more than 95% of all infants and children with pancreatic insufficiency, most with meconium ileus, 30% with meconium peritonitis, and 15% with small bowel atresia. Other conditions that should raise suspicion of cystic fibrosis include unexplained chronic pulmonary disease, chronic hepatobiliary disease, hypoproteinemia, azoospermia, and failure to thrive.

(770–C) *(S&F, p. 772)*

Secretin stimulates pancreatic secretion by activating adenylate cyclase and increasing cyclic adenosine monophosphate. Cholinergic agents increase free intracellular calcium in duct cells, which may account for the augmentation of bicarbonate secretion observed with cholinergic and secretin stimulation.

(771–D) *(S&F, p. 792)*

In the past, the uncomplicated distal intestinal obstruction syndrome was thought to be a surgical problem. The syndrome is now usually treated with aggressive medical measures including stool softeners, oral or rectal *N*-acetylcysteine, Gastrografin enemas, and balanced intestinal lavage solutions.

(772–B) *(S&F, p. 810)*

Dynamic, contrast medium–enhanced computed tomography with rapid images of the pancreas immediately after injection of intravenous contrast agent is an extremely effective means of distinguishing necrotizing pancreatitis from the much more benign acute interstitial pancreatitis. A necrotic pancreas fails to enhance, whereas viable pancreatic tissue enhances to the same degree as the spleen. If Hounsfield units (HU) can be measured, then a pancreatic density after contrast medium enhancement of less than 80 HU suggests necrosis and that of less than 50 HU ensures the diagnosis of necrotizing pancreatitis.

(773–A) *(S&F, p. 772)*

Pancreatic juice secreted during stimulation with secretin is clear, colorless, alkaline, and isotonic with plasma. The total daily volume of secretion is about 2.5 L. After stimulation with secretin, bicarbonate concentration increases with a decrease in chloride concentration.

(774–A, C) *(S&F, pp. 768–769)*

Pancreas divisum results from failure of the embryologic dorsal and ventral pancreata to fuse, leading to a situation in which most of the pancreatic exocrine secretion drains through the relatively small duct of Santorini and the accessory papilla. Pancreas divisum has been observed in 5% to 10% of autopsy series and in 2% to 7% of patients undergoing endoscopic retrograde cholangiopancreatography. Idiopathic acute pancreatitis has been associated with pancreas divisum in some clinical series. The relationship between the two remains a matter of controversy.

(775–D) *(S&F, p. 863)*

Diabetes, gallstones, and smoking are each associated with a three- to four-fold increased risk of pancreatic carcinoma. Whereas alcohol consumption is also associated with pancreatic carcinoma, alcoholic pancreatitis (both acute and chronic) is not. Familial pancreatitis is also associated with pancreatic cancer.

(776–A, C, D) *(S&F, pp. 867–868)*

A pancreaticoduodenectomy (Whipple's procedure) is the surgery of choice for resectable carcinomas of the head of the pancreas, and in selected patients (tumor <5 cm, no metastasis by computed tomography, and ASA grade 1 or 2) the operative mortality should be well under 5%. In other cases, total pancreatectomy, which involves *en bloc* resection of the pancreatic bed and adjacent organs, may avoid the need for a difficult pancreaticojejunal anastomosis and allow for removal of microscopic foci of pancreatic carcinoma separate from the primary lesion.

(777–B) *(S&F, pp. 841–842)*

Steatorrhea usually occurs before azotorrhea because pancreatic protease output is better maintained than lipase output. A reduction in pancreatic amylase secretion reduces carbohydrate absorption, but it is unlikely to be clinically important because of starch digestion by salivary gland amylase, increased mucosal absorption caused by reduced proteolytic destruction of brush border hydrolase, and colonic salvage of undigested carbohydrates by their conversion to short-chain fatty acids. At comparable levels of steatorrhea, stool volume is smaller in patients with pancreatic insufficiency than in patients with other malabsorptive disorders. The ability to absorb fluid is much more impaired in patients with malabsorption caused by primary intestinal diseases than in patients with chronic pancreatitis. Although vitamin B_{12} is often poorly absorbed because of reduced degradation of vitamin B_{12}/R protein complexes by pancreatic proteases, clinically overt vitamin B_{12} deficiency is rare. Likewise, clinically evident deficiencies of fat-soluble vitamins A, D, E, and K are rare in patients with pancreatic disease despite the presence of steatorrhea.

(778–C) *(S&F, pp. 872–873)*

Multiple endocrine neoplasia–2A syndrome is composed of medullary carcinoma of the thyroid, parathyroid hyperplasia, and pheochromocytoma. The most prominent gastrointestinal symptom is watery, secretory diarrhea, which is believed to be due to the elaboration of calcitonin. Hypersecretion of prostaglandins, vasoactive intestinal peptide, and, rarely, serotonin may also contribute to diarrhea. The incidence of cholelithiasis is increased with pheochromocytoma; however, biliary colic is not a prominent symptom in this disorder.

(779–D) *(S&F, pp. 810, 828–830)*

In acute pancreatitis, the magnitude of the serum amylase elevation provides little information about the severity of the pancreatitis. The other features listed are Ranson's criteria of severity at admission.

(780–C)   **(S&F, pp. 881–882)**

Somatostatin inhibits the release of numerous gastrointestinal hormones including insulin and glucagon, acid secretion, and pancreatic secretion. Somatostatin also has inhibitory effects on gallbladder contraction and emptying. The clinical features thus include gallbladder disease, weight loss, steatorrhea, and diabetes. Mesenteric thrombosis is not a prominent feature.

(781–1-D, 2-B, 3-C, 4-A)   **(S&F, pp. 778–790)**

The secretin stimulation test is the most accurate test for the diagnosis of chronic pancreatitis, with a sensitivity of 83% and a specificity of 89%. The bentiromide test measures cleavage of ingested N-benzoyl-L-tyrosyl-*p*-aminobenzoic acid (NBT-PABA) into NBT and PABA by chymotrypsin. PABA is measured in the urine after absorption and conjugation by the liver. Because of its convenience, it is the most commonly used noninvasive test of pancreatic function. Chymotrypsin is stable in stool for several days and is easy to measure. Measurement of stool chymotrypsin levels is about 85% sensitive in advanced pancreatic dysfunction but relatively insensitive in mild to moderate disease. Although not evaluated extensively, the dual-label Schilling test may be more sensitive and specific than the NBT-PABA test. Vitamin B_{12} malabsorption may occur in pancreatic disease because of a failure of pancreatic proteases to release vitamin B_{12} from gastric and salivary R proteins.

(782–A)   **(S&F, p. 869)**

Celiac plexus block for intractable retroperitoneal pain in pancreatic carcinoma is generally well tolerated, although rare potential complications include postprocedure abdominal pain and renal or aortic perforation. No controlled studies have been done to show a benefit of celiac plexus nerve block over radiation. Surgery is percutaneous by means of a retrocrural posterior approach. Life-long pain relief is achieved in 70% to 95% of patients.

(783–C)   **(S&F, pp. 776–777)**

Like gastric secretion, exocrine pancreatic secretion is divided into cephalic, gastric, and intestinal phases. Most pancreatic enzyme secretion occurs during the intestinal phase, which is mediated by both hormones and enteropancreatic vagovagal reflexes. Secretin release by the duodenal mucosa depends on the load of titratable acid delivered to the duodenum. Secretin release is triggered by a duodenal pH of below 4.5. Fatty acids longer than eight carbons in length and bile acids also increase secretin release. Although secretin-induced bicarbonate secretion is augmented by cholecystokinin (CCK), CCK alone does not cause bicarbonate secretion. Instead, CCK stimulates pancreatic secretion of digestive enzymes, which is triggered by the presence of fatty acids, peptides, and amino acids in the intestine.

(784–C)   **(S&F, pp. 865–866)**

Endoscopic retrograde cholangiopancreatographic findings in pancreatic carcinoma may be difficult to distinguish from benign pancreatic disease. Single, irregular pancreatic duct strictures, displacement of Wirsung's duct (suggesting a pancreatic head mass), and a double duct sign (suggesting both pancreatic duct and common bile duct strictures) are all suggestive of pancreatic carcinoma. Multiple pancreatic duct stenoses with secondary duct dilation (chain-of-lakes pattern) is more commonly seen in chronic pancreatitis.

(785–A, C, D)   **(S&F, pp. 826, 834)**

Transient hypocalcemia develops in about one third of patients during acute pancreatitis. However, tetany is extremely rare. The degree of hypocalcemia parallels the clinical severity of disease. In many cases, the fall in serum calcium concentration is merely a reflection of decreased binding to serum proteins because of rapidly developing hypoalbuminemia. In more severe cases, pancreatic lipase breaks down lipids to release fatty acids, which form insoluble soaps with calcium.

(786–B)   **(S&F, p. 851)**

The Puestow procedure (longitudinal pancreaticojejunostomy) is usually done in patients with severe pain and an irregular, widely dilated pancreatic duct with alternating segments of narrowing and dilation. Occasionally, a total pancreatectomy is performed for persistence of severe pain after lesser resections; however, even total pancreatectomy does not provide clinically meaningful pain relief in all cases. In cases of pancreatic ascites or pleural effusions, endoscopic retrograde cholangiopancreatography is mandatory to identify the site of the leak. This substantially improves the likelihood of successful surgery and reduces the frequency of recurrence. Creating an anastomosis between the pseudocyst and the stomach (cystogastrostomy), duodenum (cystoduodenostomy), and jejunum (cystojejunostomy) creates prompt drainage of the cyst into the gastrointestinal tract with obliteration of the cyst cavity.

(787–D)   **(S&F, p. 790)**

As many as half of all cases of meconium ileus are complicated by volvulus, atresia, or meconium peritonitis. Clinically, these may present as intra-abdominal calcifications, a meconium pseudocyst, adhesive peritonitis, or meconium ascites.

(788–A)   **(S&F, p. 863)**

The most common complaints of patients with pancreatic carcinoma are pain, weight loss, jaundice, and pruritus, which are present in over 50% of patients. Cholangitis is an uncommon presentation of pancreatic carcinoma, seen in less than 5%.

(789–B)   *(S&F, pp. 868–869)*

Unfortunately, neither single-agent nor combination chemotherapy has been consistently shown to prolong survival or enhance quality of life in patients with advanced pancreatic cancer and should therefore not yet be considered the standard of care. Further studies are needed to confirm an advantage over comfort care alone. Combined chemotherapy with radiation may improve median survival compared with either modality alone, although further studies are required.

(790–D)   *(S&F, pp. 841–842)*

Although half of all chronic pancreatitis cases present with recurrent episodes of acute pancreatitis, pain starts insidiously in 35% and may be continuous or intermittent. About 15% of patients present with diabetes, malabsorption, jaundice, or gastrointestinal bleeding.

(791–1-B, 2-A, 3-D, 4-C)   *(S&F, pp. 854–855)*

Erosion of a pseudocyst into an artery can produce massive hematemesis and shock. Splenic vein thrombosis is common in pancreatitis with or without pseudocyst and may produce gastric varices. Rupture of a pseudocyst into the peritoneal cavity commonly causes chemical peritonitis with intense pain. Rarely, a pseudocyst drains spontaneously into the gastrointestinal tract with spontaneous disappearance of the palpable mass, often with a brief episode of diarrhea.

(792–C)   *(S&F, p. 873)*

Multiple endocrine neoplasia–1 is present in approximately 20% of patients with Zollinger-Ellison syndrome. By contrast, only 4% of patients with insulinoma will also have this syndrome.

(793–D)   *(S&F, pp. 849–850)*

Nutritional therapy for patients with pancreatic exocrine insufficiency often involves control of pain to enhance food intake. The mainstay of therapy is pancreatic enzyme replacement with the aims of reducing symptoms associated with malabsorption and improving nutritional status. It is difficult to eliminate steatorrhea with even large doses of pancreatic enzyme therapy because added lipase tends to be inactivated by gastric acid and pepsin. Gastric inactivation can be reduced with enteric-coated preparations or concomitant H_2 receptor antagonists. Restricting dietary fat to 50 g/day reduces steatorrhea. Feeding medium-chain triglycerides, which do not require pancreatic enzymes for absorption, can increase calorie intake. Short-chain fatty acids (e.g., butyrate, propionate) are unpalatable and offer no nutritional advantage.

(794–1-A, 2-B, 3-A, 4-B)   *(S&F, pp. 775–776)*

The interaction of vasoactive intestinal polypeptide and secretin with acinar cells leads to activation of adenylate cyclase and an increase in cellular cyclic adenosine monophosphate, which mediates their secretory response. A major effect of cholecystokinin and acetylcholine is mobilization and release of intracellular calcium. The mechanism by which an increase in cytosolic calcium mediates secretion is not clear.

(795–1-B, 2-D, 3-A, 4-C)   *(S&F, p. 766)*

Each cell type in the endocrine pancreas appears to secrete a single hormone. B cells are the most numerous (accounting for 50% to 80% of islet cell volume) and secrete insulin. A cells constitute 5% to 20% and secrete glucagon, PP cells account for 10% to 35% and secrete pancreatic polypeptide, and D cells account for 5% to 20% of the islet cell mass and secrete somatostatin.

(796–A)   *(S&F, p. 792)*

Although previously a common complication of cystic fibrosis, rectal prolapse is now reported in only 1% to 2% of patients. Onset is usually in the first years of life and is sometimes the presenting symptom. Patients with an early diagnosis of cystic fibrosis (in infancy) are much less likely to have rectal prolapse as a complication than are those whose diagnosis was delayed until the stools were more voluminous. Medical management is usually successful and only about 10% of patients require surgical correction.

(797–A)   *(S&F, p. 896)*

Pancreatic cystadenocarcinoma accounts for only about 1% of all pancreatic malignancies. The precursor lesion is pancreatic cystadenoma, which accounts for 10% of cystic lesions of the pancreas. A typical patient is a middle-aged woman presenting with abdominal pain, nausea, vomiting, weight loss, and often a palpable abdominal mass. The diagnosis is often elusive and may require laparotomy. Therapy consists of surgical resection. The prognosis is much better than for the more common pancreatic carcinoma, even when a large tumor is present.

(798–C)   *(S&F, pp. 792–794)*

Hepatic involvement in cystic fibrosis (CF) varies from 15% in recent studies to 50% in older studies; however, only about 5% of patients will develop cirrhosis and only 2% progress to clinically important liver disease. Tests of hepatic function in CF may be normal even in overt cirrhosis. The prevalence of liver involvement is much lower in patients who do not have pancreatic insufficiency. Approximately 50% of cholestasis in neonates and young infants is associated with meconium ileus. Fatty liver, often independent of nutritional status, is one of the most common hepatic abnormalities in CF.

(799–C)   *(S&F, p. 873)*

The most common manifestation of multiple endocrine neoplasia–1 (MEN-1) is hyperparathyroidism due to parathyroid hyperplasia, which occurs in more than 85% of cases and is marked by hypercalcemia. Gastrinomas are present in over 50% of MEN-1 patients and may cause acid hypersecretion, peptic disease, and diarrhea. Prolactin-secreting tumors resulting in galactorrhea are present in fewer than half of MEN-1 patients, and insulinomas are found in 21%, most of whom will experience hypoglycemia.

(800–C)   **(S&F, p. 839)**

At autopsy, the morphologic changes of chronic pancreatitis are present in up to 45% of alcoholics who had no symptoms of pancreatic disease during life. In cases of clinically overt chronic pancreatitis, alcoholism was the cause in 75%. The form in which ethanol is ingested does not appear to influence the risk of developing chronic pancreatitis, although the total amount does. In two prospective studies of patients with chronic pancreatitis, 40% to 50% had coexisting alcoholic liver disease.

(801–A)   **(S&F, p. 810)**

Neither amylase nor lipase is part of Ranson's criteria for determining severity of acute pancreatitis on admission. Lactate dehydrogenase level less than 350 IU/L is the fifth criterion.

(802–C)   **(S&F, pp. 797–799)**

Shwachman's syndrome is characterized by exocrine pancreatic insufficiency, hematologic abnormalities, and a normal sweat chloride test. Metaphyseal chondrodysplasia of the femur is common and is a supportive finding for the diagnosis.

(803–C)   **(S&F, pp. 826–828)**

Ultrasonography has a sensitivity of 93% and a specificity of 96% for the diagnosis of cholelithiasis and acute cholecystitis. Abdominal computed tomography has a sensitivity of 92% and a specificity of 90% for identifying changes consistent with the diagnosis of acute pancreatitis. Abdominal computed tomography can predict pancreatic abscess in up to 74% of cases; however, computed tomography cannot determine whether fluid collections, areas of pancreatic phlegmon, or areas of peripancreatic necrosis are infected unless gas is present. Plain films of the abdomen should be obtained in most patients admitted with suspected acute pancreatitis. They may demonstrate the characteristic sentinel loop or colon cut-off sign, but their greatest utility is in identifying other abdominal catastrophes such as a perforated viscus or a thickened intestinal wall (''thumb-printing'') that accompanies bowel infarction. Selective mesenteric angiography is indicated when there is bleeding through the pancreatic duct (hemosuccus pancreaticus). Angiography also offers the option of arterial embolization.

(804–C)   **(S&F, pp. 782–784)**

The abnormal electrolytes present in sweat reflect a secretory defect present in all epithelial cells of endodermal and mesodermal origin. The cellular defect resides in the apical chloride channels, which are present but unresponsive to normal cyclic adenosine monophosphate regulation. Calcium-mediated chloride secretion is normal. However, most evidence supports the presence of defects in β-adrenergic stimulation and protein kinase A– and C–mediated pathways. Sodium absorption is also altered in most tissues. The respiratory epithelium demonstrates a four-fold increase in sodium absorption, whereas the sweat gland has diminished absorption.

(805–D)   **(S&F, p. 838)**

The most likely diagnosis in this clinical situation is splenic vein thrombosis due to peripancreatic inflammation. This condition most often produces isolated gastric varices but may also result in the formation of esophageal varices. Hemosuccus pancreaticus is due to bleeding from the pancreatic duct that gains access to the duodenum through the ampulla of Vater. Cavernous transformation of the portal vein occurs in patients with chronic portal vein thrombosis.

(806–D)   **(S&F, p. 864)**

CA 19-9 is a sialosyl-fucosyl-lactotetraose corresponding to sialylated blood group Lewis a. It is found in normal epithelial cells of the gallbladder, biliary ducts, pancreas, and stomach. The CA 19-9 level is commonly elevated in biliary tract malignancies (55%–65%) and may be elevated in benign conditions such as chronic liver disease and acute or chronic pancreatitis. However, it is genetically absent in 5% to 7% of western individuals.

(807–C)   **(S&F, p. 763)**

After stimulation with cholinergic drugs or cholecystokinin, there is a marked depletion of zymogen granules. Feeding alone produces a less extensive depletion in granules. Gastrin does not directly stimulate zymogen granule release.

(808–C)   **(S&F, pp. 761–762)**

The anterior and posterior superior pancreaticoduodenal arteries arise as branches of the gastroduodenal artery, which is a branch of the celiac artery. The anterior and posterior inferior pancreaticoduodenal arteries arise from the superior mesenteric artery. The splenic artery gives rise to several branches, including the dorsal pancreatic, the pancreatic magna, and the cauda pancreatis.

(809–D)   **(S&F, pp. 836–837)**

Conventional thinking regarding pseudocysts has been that a cyst larger than 5 cm and present for longer than six weeks requires drainage. Although it is true that pseudocysts may rupture or become infected, studies suggest that patients with asymptomatic cysts can be followed expectantly for resolution and drainage reserved for those in whom symptoms occur. Pseudocyst infection is a rare but well-recognized complication that presents with a striking clinical picture of pain, shaking chills, fever (temperature >39° C), and leukocytosis. The treatment of an infected pseudocyst includes broad-spectrum antibiotics and percutaneous or surgical drainage. Pseudocyst rupture into the peritoneal cavity usually produces peritonitis, although pancreatic ascites may also occur. Rarely, the pseudocyst may erode into an adjacent hollow viscus such as the stomach or colon and completely decompress, obviating the need for further treatment; otherwise the treatment of a ruptured pseudocyst is surgical. Hemorrhage occurs from damage to small vessels lining the pseudocyst wall or from erosion of the pseudocyst into nearby major vessels.

(810–C)   **(S&F, p. 818)**

Gallstones are present in 30% to 75% of patients admitted with acute pancreatitis. The peak incidence is in patients 50 to 70 years old, and gallstones occur in women more often than in men (2:1). If the stools of patients with pancreatitis and gallstones are strained for ten days after the onset of an attack of pancreatitis, gallstones are detected in 92%, compared with 12% of patients who have gallstones without pancreatitis, and 0% in patients with alcoholic pancreatitis. The risk of recurrent pancreatitis is about 50% unless all gallstones are removed. The mortality of gallstone pancreatitis is about 12% during the first attack and tends to be lower during subsequent attacks. Up to 75% of patients with idiopathic pancreatitis have crystals in aspirated bile.

(811–C)   **(S&F, pp. 875–876, 878, 880, 884)**

The first three of these pancreatic endocrine tumors typically respond to octreotide by virtue of its inhibitory effect on hormone release. Recent studies using octreotide have shown a 65% reduction in serum insulin levels in patients with insulinoma. Octreotide has also been found to effectively treat the rash, diarrhea, and weight loss of glucagonoma syndrome and is the therapy of choice for VIPoma syndrome. Although most pancreatic endocrine tumors possess somatostatin receptors, the antitumor effects of octreotide are small; and thus it is not generally indicated in the treatment of nonfunctioning pancreatic endocrine tumors.

(812–C)   **(S&F, p. 872)**

Generally, the pancreatic endocrine tumor syndromes have a high rate of malignancy. The malignancy rate is more than 50% in gastrinomas, glucagonomas, somatostatinomas, and VIPomas. Insulinomas, on the other hand, are malignant in less than 10% of cases.

(813–C)   **(S&F, pp. 878–880)**

The pancreatic cholera syndrome is also known as the Verner-Morrison syndrome, the WDHA syndrome (watery diarrhea, hypokalemia, achlorhydria), and the VIPoma syndrome. It is invariably characterized by large-volume secretory diarrhea, hypochlorhydria, and hypokalemia. Thus, a stool output of less than 700 mL/day excludes the diagnosis. A large solitary tumor within the body of the pancreas is usually responsible. Symptoms can be controlled with octreotide.

(814–B)   **(S&F, p. 863)**

Pancreatic cystadenocarcinomas, adenoacanthomas, and pancreatic lymphomas are all rare pancreatic malignancies, each accounting for less than 1% of all pancreatic carcinomas. Lesions metastatic to the pancreas constitute less than 5% of pancreatic malignancies. Pancreatic mucinous adenocarcinoma accounts for 90% of all pancreatic carcinomas.

(815–D)   **(S&F, p. 801)**

The lifetime risk of developing pancreatitis in familial hyperlipidemia is approximately 35% for type I, 15% for type IV, and 30% to 40% for type V.

(816–A, B, C)   **(S&F, pp. 832–833)**

Hypoxia is frequently associated with acute pancreatitis and may occur without visible changes on chest radiographs. The major abnormality responsible is intrapulmonary right-to-left shunting, possibly caused by pulmonary intravascular microthrombi formed as a result of subclinical disseminated intravascular coagulation. The frequency of adult respiratory distress syndrome rises with the increasing clinical severity of the attack and with coexisting hyperlipidemia. Diffuse pulmonary infiltrates and severe hypoxemia develop in only 5% to 10% of patients.

(817–D)   **(S&F, p. 873)**

Pancreatic endocrine tumors occur in more than 80% of patients with multiple endocrine neoplasia–1 (MEN-1). The most common pancreatic endocrine tumor in MEN-1 is the nonfunctional PPoma, which is present in 80% to 100% of MEN-1 patients but is often overlooked owing to the absence of clinical manifestations. Gastrinomas are present in 54% of MEN-1 patients, whereas insulinomas are present in 21%. Glucagonomas and VIPomas are rare, present in 3% and 1%, respectively.

(818–E)   **(S&F, p. 877)**

Cutaneous lesions are one of the most common manifestations of the glucagonoma syndrome, occurring in 64% to 90% of cases. The typical rash is necrolytic migratory erythema and usually precedes diagnosis of the syndrome by six to eight years. Glucose intolerance occurs in 83% to 90% of patients, and weight loss is prominent, occurring in 56% to 96% of patients. Thromboembolic phenomena are also relatively common, occurring in 12% to 35% of cases. Psychiatric symptoms, although mentioned in several reports, are relatively infrequent.

(819–E)   **(S&F, p. 864)**

Biliary obstruction is a common presentation of pancreatic carcinoma. Over 50% of patients have abnormal levels of alkaline phosphatase, gamma glutamyl transpeptidase, bilirubin, and CA 19-9 at presentation. Only 15% present with an abnormal amylase level.

(820–C) **(S&F, p. 782)**

Cystic fibrosis is inherited in an autosomal recessive manner, with a gene frequency of 4% to 5% and clinical expression in 1 of every 2000 to 3000 live births. The risk of a sibling also being affected is 25%. Although reported in various racial groups, cystic fibrosis is more common in whites.

(821–C) **(S&F, p. 789)**

Perioral and perianal irritation are common in infants. Pancreatic extracts have a high purine content, and patients taking large doses can experience hyperuricosuria. There are no reports of allergic reactions to pancreatic extracts; however, hypersensitivity reactions have been described in patients who accidentally inhaled pancreatic extracts.

(822–A) **(S&F, pp. 822–823)**

Hypotension or shock is noted in 30% to 40% of patients and is related to hypovolemia (due to plasma exudation into the retroperitoneal space, fluid accumulation in atonic bowel, vomiting, and hemorrhage) rather than pump failure. Painless acute pancreatitis occurs in less than 2% of cases but has a grave prognosis because the presenting symptom is often shock or coma. The majority of patients with pancreatitis have a temperature between 100° F and 101° F. Higher temperatures suggest a complicating bacterial infection such as cholangitis or a pancreatic abscess. Mild hyperbilirubinemia occurs in up to 40% of patients. It may be related to external compression of the bile duct by the inflamed pancreas or due to alcoholic liver disease; however, a common bile duct stone or ampullary obstruction should be excluded.

(823–A, C, D) **(S&F, pp. 857–858)**

Alcoholic pancreatitis, in general, has a less favorable prognosis in terms of both morbidity and mortality than do cases of idiopathic pancreatitis. Unfortunately, there is no convincing evidence that abstinence from alcohol decreases the severity or frequency of pain in chronic pancreatitis, although individual patients may report relief with cessation of alcohol ingestion. In a longitudinal study involving 245 patients with chronic pancreatitis over a 20-year period, there was a tendency to experience pain relief over time. Fat and protein malabsorption do not occur until more than 90% of the secretory capacity is lost.

(824–D) **(S&F, p. 821)**

A large number of medications have been associated with an increased risk of pancreatitis, including furosemide and hydrochlorothiazide; sulfonamides; oral 5-aminosalicylic acid preparations; antibiotics including metronidazole, tetracycline, and nitrofurantoin; valproic acid; corticosteroids; estrogens; methyldopa (Aldomet); pentamidine; octreotide; and didanosine.

(825–D) **(S&F, p. 828)**

Not all patients with epigastric pain and elevated amylase levels have pancreatitis. The differential diagnosis includes a perforated peptic ulcer, acute cholecystitis, mesenteric vascular occlusion, and a ruptured ectopic pregnancy. The abrupt onset of abdominal pain, shock, and severe anemia is best explained by a ruptured ectopic pregnancy.

(826–D) **(S&F, pp. 772, 774)**

Pancreatic enzymes that could potentially digest the pancreas are stored in an inactive form in membrane-bound zymogen granules. Activation of these enzymes takes place after secretion into the duodenum by the brush border enzyme enterokinase. In addition, the acinar cell secretes a pancreatic secretory trypsin inhibitor that helps prevent premature activation of trypsinogen to trypsin.

(827–A, C, D) **(S&F, pp. 842–846, 853)**

Serum amylase and lipase can be normal during an attack of pain. Diabetes is present in up to 30% of patients; however, diabetic ketoacidosis and diabetic nephropathy are rare. Plain radiographs of the abdomen reveal diffuse or focal pancreatic calcifications in 30% to 60% of patients with chronic pancreatitis. Diffuse calcification is diagnostic of chronic pancreatitis, even if no clinical evidence of pancreatic disease is present. Endoscopic retrograde cholangiopancreatography may be normal in some cases of chronic pancreatitis. In most instances, however, ductal changes and potentially correctable lesions (e.g., stones, strictures, dilation of the duct) are demonstrated.

(828–C) **(S&F, p. 854)**

A 4-cm pseudocyst should be followed for a minimum of six weeks to determine if it is resolving spontaneously before other options are considered. Hydration and pain control are indicated in all patients with acute pancreatitis. Meperidine causes less sphincter of Oddi contraction than morphine and is therefore more useful in this setting. Because it may lead to infection, endoscopic retrograde cholangiopancreatography is only used preoperatively for pseudocysts that fail to resolve spontaneously.

(829–C) **(S&F, p. 790)**

In approximately 80% of patients with cystic fibrosis (CF), small bowel radiography reveals thickened duodenal folds, nodular filling defects, mucosal smudging, dilations, and redundancy. Lactase deficiency is no more common in patients with CF than in control populations of the same ethnic background and age. Meconium ileus is the presenting symptom in 10% to 15% of infants with CF and its expression seems to be regulated genetically. Pancreatic involvement is often milder in infants with meconium ileus than in those lacking this sign. Indeed, infants dying with meconium ileus often have a completely normal pancreas. Meconium ileus may be directly related to the severity of involvement of the intestinal glands.

Topics Involving Multiple Organs

S&F Sections I, II, III, IV, and XI

830. A 44-year-old patient is referred to you. His mother died of endometrial cancer at age 52. His 40-year-old brother recently had a colonoscopy for heme-positive stool and was found to have two adenomas, one of which had carcinoma *in situ*. Which one of the following genetic abnormalities is MOST consistent with this family history?
A. Defect in base-pair mismatch repair enzyme (chromosome 2)
B. Truncated *APC* gene (chromosome 5)
C. Deletion of *p53* (chromosome 17)
D. Deletion of *DCC* (chromosome 18)
E. K-*ras* point mutation

831. On further evaluation the patient in question 830 is found to have cecal colon cancer that is replication error (RER) positive. Which one of the following statements is FALSE?
A. This family does not fit the "Amsterdam criteria" for hereditary nonpolyposis colorectal cancer.
B. This patient needs a subtotal colectomy.
C. The patient's son should have annual colonoscopy starting at age 25 to 30.
D. This patient will have the same prognosis when compared with stage-matched RER-negative cancers.
E. All are true.

832. Regarding use of aspirin to reduce the frequency of colon cancer, which of the following statements are TRUE?
A. Regular, long-term aspirin users have 50% lower cancer rates.
B. NSAIDs other than aspirin also reduce the cancer risk.
C. Cancer risk is not measurably reduced during the first 10 years of use.
D. Higher doses are more effective.
E. Lower cancer mortality is due to an increased number of endoscopies.
F. COX-2 is an important modulator of polyp growth that is inhibited by NSAIDs.

833. A 70-year-old man presents with a one-day history of painless melena. He uses NSAIDs frequently for arthralgias. Five years ago, he had an aortic graft placed because of an enlarging aneurysm. Which of the following statements are TRUE regarding this patient?
I. Angiography would be of little help diagnostically.
II. Surgical exploration is mandatory if no cause of bleeding is found.
III. The finding of a gastric ulcer with a visible vessel would provide an adequate explanation for the clinical presentation.
IV. Upper endoscopy with a pediatric colonoscope would likely identify an aortoenteric fistula if present.

A. I and III
B. II and IV
C. I, II, and III
D. All of the above

834. Which one of the following statements about the gastrointestinal complications of bone marrow transplantation is FALSE?
A. The most common viral pathogen to affect the gastrointestinal system is cytomegalovirus.
B. Hepatitis C is common but rarely progresses to cirrhosis.
C. Post-transplantation lymphoproliferative disorder is associated with Epstein-Barr virus.
D. Veno-occlusive disease occurs in up to 50% of patients.
E. Gastrointestinal graft-versus-host disease requires mucosal biopsy for diagnosis.

835. Which of the following is the MOST useful historical feature in evaluating the cause of constipation?
A. Age at onset
B. Effects of diet
C. Association with pain
D. Stool consistency
E. Activity level

836. Each of the following is associated with erythema nodosum EXCEPT:
A. Infection
B. Leukemia
C. Adenocarcinoma
D. Oral contraceptive use
E. Inflammatory bowel disease

837. A 65-year-old man with a six-month history of watery diarrhea has stool studies revealing a stool sodium concentration of 40 mEq/L, potassium of 90 mEq/L, and osmolality of 290 mOsm/kg. Which of the following is the MOST likely diagnosis?
A. Villous adenoma
B. Chronic salmonellosis
C. Lactulose abuse
D. Excessive antacid use
E. Idiopathic inflammatory bowel disease

838. A 69-year-old man presents with left lower quadrant pain and a low-grade fever over the past two days. Past history is remarkable for a deep venous thrombosis of the left leg five years previously. Physical examination reveals a distended abdomen with normal bowel sounds and moderate left lower quadrant tenderness without rebound or guarding. A plain film of the abdomen is unremarkable. Abdominal computed tomography shows thrombus in the superior mesenteric vein. Which of the following would be the MOST useful therapy?
A. Administer papaverine by means of an angiographic catheter
B. Perform exploratory laparotomy
C. Administer intravenous heparin
D. Perform peritoneal lavage

839. Which of the following are TRUE statements regarding treatment of functional dyspepsia?
A. Prokinetic agents are beneficial in most patients with dyspepsia characterized by reflux-like or dysmotility symptoms.
B. Eradication of *Helicobacter pylori* has been demonstrated to improve symptoms in the majority of dyspeptic patients.
C. Cisapride is superior to domperidone and metoclopramide for the treatment of dysmotility-like dyspepsia.
D. H_2 receptor antagonists have limited value in treating dyspeptic patients but should be tried in most patients anyway.
E. Proton pump inhibitors are superior to H_2 receptor antagonists.

840. A 35-year-old woman with recurrent watery diarrhea has stool studies revealing a stool sodium concentration of 20 mEq/L, stool potassium of 10 mEq/L, and stool osmolality of 290 mOsm/kg. Which of the following is the MOST likely diagnosis?
A. Villous adenoma
B. Vipoma
C. Lactulose abuse
D. Zollinger-Ellison syndrome
E. Idiopathic inflammatory bowel disease

841. Which of the following are TRUE statements regarding upper endoscopy for gastrointestinal hemorrhage?
A. Endoscopy can localize the site of bleeding and offer direct therapy.
B. Endoscopy should be performed within 24 hours of the onset of bleeding.
C. Finding adherent clot or a "visible vessel" in an ulcer crater is associated with a more than 50% chance of re-bleeding.
D. Endoscopy has decreased the mortality in patients with hemorrhage from peptic ulcer disease.
E. Endoscopy is the initial intervention in treating patients with gastrointestinal hemorrhage.

842. Concerning small intestinal Kaposi's sarcoma in patients with acquired immunodeficiency syndrome (AIDS), each of the following is true EXCEPT:
A. It is generally clinically silent with the exception of occasional fecal blood loss.
B. Cutaneous involvement is present in less than 50%.
C. Radiographic manifestations are often nonspecific.
D. Angiography is rarely helpful as a screening measure.
E. Kaposi's sarcoma and lymphoma are the most common small intestinal malignancies in patients with AIDS.

843. A 65-year-old man with a history of lung cancer is completing chemotherapy that is complicated by bone marrow suppression. He has not received any antibiotics. He is now complaining of mild diffuse abdominal pain and diarrhea. Physical examination reveals a low-grade fever and mild diffuse abdominal tenderness, without rebound or guarding. The MOST likely diagnosis is:
A. Diverticulitis
B. Malabsorption
C. Neutropenic enterocolitis
D. Ischemic colitis
E. Giardiasis

844. A 75-year-old man is referred for evaluation of diarrhea. He complains of episodic abdominal pain, which has improved recently, and has three to four loose, oily, foul-smelling stools per day. He has lost ten pounds. A quantitative fecal fat study reveals 60 g/24 hr and a total stool weight of 300 g/24 hr (stool fat concentration = 20 g/100 g stool). The MOST likely diagnosis is:
A. Small intestinal bacterial overgrowth
B. Whipple's disease
C. Pancreatic insufficiency
D. Celiac sprue with localized jejunal lymphoma
E. Zollinger-Ellison syndrome with severe hypersecretion

845. Regarding the patient in question 844, which of the following tests would be the MOST useful initial diagnostic study?
   A. D-Xylose absorption test
   B. Bacterial culture of small intestinal aspirate
   C. ^{14}C-xylose breath test
   D. Right upper quadrant ultrasonography

846. Which one of the following endoscopic findings is associated with the highest risk of ulcer re-bleeding?
   A. Flat red spot in an ulcer base
   B. Adherent clot in ulcer base
   C. Giant (more than 3 cm) ulcer
   D. Exudative ulcer base
   E. Oozing rim of clean-based ulcer

847. A 30-year-old man is brought to the emergency department by the police after swallowing a large amount of cocaine in a condom. On physical examination he has normal vital signs and a normal pupil examination and is alert and oriented. The MOST appropriate course of action is:
   A. Endoscopic removal
   B. Emergent surgical removal
   C. Induction of emesis
   D. Observation
   E. Acid suppression

848. A 65-year-old man presents with the recent onset of darkening of the skin of his neck and axillae and multiple skin tags on his body. On physical examination he has velvety, hyperpigmented skin on his neck and axillae and diffuse skin tags. His abdominal examination is normal. The MOST likely underlying gastrointestinal malignancy is:
   A. Carcinoid
   B. Lymphoma
   C. Gastric adenocarcinoma
   D. Gastrinoma
   E. Esophageal squamous carcinoma

849. A 55-year-old man with recently diagnosed small cell carcinoma of the lung presents with a one-year history of constipation, bloating, and intermittent nausea and vomiting. He is on no medications and has no other past medical history. A barium enema and small bowel follow-through showed no obstruction or intraluminal lesions. Physical examination shows a distended abdomen without masses, normal bowel sounds, and normal rectal examination. The MOST likely diagnosis is:
   A. Gastrointestinal tract metastasis
   B. Biliary colic
   C. Pseudo-obstruction
   D. Partial small bowel obstruction
   E. Mesenteric ischemia

850. A 56-year-old woman with a history of scleroderma is referred for evaluation of diarrhea and anemia. Her physical examination shows features of scleroderma. Examination of the stool is negative for blood, leukocytes, ova, parasites, and bacterial pathogens. A flexible sigmoidoscopy and barium enema examination are unrevealing. Which of the following diagnoses BEST explains the clinical features?
   A. Collagenous colitis with iron-deficiency anemia
   B. Jejunal diverticula with bacterial overgrowth and resulting folate deficiency
   C. Jejunal diverticula with bacterial overgrowth and resulting vitamin B_{12} deficiency
   D. *Clostridium difficile* enterocolitis

851. Anorexia nervosa usually begins in women at what stage of life?
   A. Prepuberty
   B. Menarche
   C. Four to five years after menarche
   D. Young adulthood (20 years or older)

852. Which of the following are TRUE statements regarding respiratory symptoms secondary to esophageal disease?
   A. Respiratory symptoms are thought to be mediated by vagal reflexes.
   B. The absence of heartburn symptoms in an asthmatic patient argues strongly against gastroesophageal reflux (GER) as the cause of the bronchospasm.
   C. Asthma that is worsened by bronchodilators is typical of GER-induced bronchospasm.
   D. A normal direct laryngoscopic examination effectively excludes GER as a cause of upper respiratory symptoms.

853. A 36-year-old woman comes to the emergency department with a one-day history of maroon-colored stools and mild dizziness. She is otherwise asymptomatic. Her only past medical history is Ehlers-Danlos syndrome. On physical examination, she is orthostatic and has minimal periumbilical tenderness. A nasogastric aspirate yields nonbloody "bilious" fluid that is heme negative. Which of the following are TRUE statements regarding this patient?
   A. Admission to the intensive care unit is warranted.
   B. The history of Ehlers-Danlos syndrome is not relevant.
   C. The test for occult blood on the nasogastric aspirate is not relevant.
   D. An upper gastrointestinal source is possible.

854. Which of the following factors is NOT associated with a higher mortality in patients with acute upper gastrointestinal bleeding:
   A. Fresh blood on nasogastric lavage

B. Hematocrit less than 30% on admission
C. Hematochezia
D. Coexisting illness
E. Age

---

855. Specify whether the following statements are TRUE or FALSE.
A. In sporadic colon cancers, accumulation of genetic abnormalities over time is an important aspect of carcinogenesis.
B. A replication error–positive (RER+) phenotype accounts for 15% to 20% of sporadic colon cancers.
C. A replication error–positive (RER+) phenotype accounts for virtually 100% of hereditary nonpolyposis colon cancers.
D. A replication error–positive (RER+) phenotype results from mutations in DNA mismatch repair genes, especially *hMSH2* and *hMLH1*.

---

856. A 40-year-old woman presents to her primary care physician with a complaint of constipation of several years' duration. The history is not helpful, and the physical examination is normal. The stool is negative for occult blood, and a blood cell count is normal. Which of the following is the LEAST likely explanation for her problem?
A. Irritable bowel syndrome
B. Chronic idiopathic constipation
C. Victim of previous sexual abuse
D. Colorectal carcinoma
E. Munchausen's syndrome

---

857. Referring to the case in question 856, which of the following is LEAST indicated?
A. Recommend a high-residue diet
B. Ask her to prepare a diary of her bowel habits
C. Reassure her of the low probability of a life-threatening illness
D. Perform flexible sigmoidoscopy
E. Establish a good patient–doctor relationship by scheduling follow-up visits

---

858. Concerning patients with factitious diarrhea, which one of the following statements is FALSE?
A. They are usually women.
B. They often surreptitiously abuse laxatives.
C. They typically have obvious psychological abnormalities.
D. They may have stool osmolarity of less than 100 mOsm/kg.
E. They are often affiliated with the health-care profession.

---

859. A 26-year-old nurse who is 34 weeks pregnant calls complaining of a one-week history of nausea, vomiting, headache, and ankle swelling. She reports her blood pressure to be 180/113 mm Hg. She has had no prior problems with the pregnancy. Which of the following is the MOST likely cause of her vomiting?
A. Hyperemesis gravidarum
B. Acute fatty liver of pregnancy
C. Nausea and vomiting of pregnancy
D. Superior mesenteric artery syndrome
E. Gastroesophageal reflux

---

860. A 31-year-old man is brought to your office by his mother who complains that her son vomits, without antecedent nausea, during or shortly after meals. This problem has been present intermittently for 12 years. She reports that his older sister also has had this problem. Which of the following diagnoses is MOST likely?
A. Intestinal malrotation
B. Idiopathic gastroparesis
C. Psychogenic vomiting
D. Superior mesenteric artery syndrome
E. Jamaican vomiting sickness

---

861. A 70-year-old man presents complaining of the onset of upper abdominal pain after doing yard work that morning. He has associated nausea and diaphoresis. The pain does not radiate. He has a past history of hypertension and diabetes. Examination is remarkable for diaphoresis and a nontender abdomen. Which of the following is the LEAST likely diagnosis?
A. Cholecystitis
B. Myocardial ischemia
C. Penetrating ulcer
D. Diverticulitis
E. Pancreatitis

---

862. Patients with upper gastrointestinal bleeding who are found to have a gastric ulcer with a visible vessel by endoscopy have a re-bleeding rate of approximately:
A. 1%
B. 10%
C. 25%
D. 50%
E. 80%

---

863. Injuries due to ingestion of button batteries depend on each of the following EXCEPT:
A. Battery size
B. Congenital anomalies of the gastrointestinal tract
C. Delayed passage through or impaction in the esophagus
D. Failure of the battery to pass within 72 hours

---

864. Match the hyperbilirubinemia with the associated characteristic.

| 1. Type I Crigler-Najjar syndrome | A. Very slow sulfobromophthalein clearance |

2. Type II Crigler-Najjar syndrome
3. Dubin-Johnson syndrome
4. Rotor's syndrome

B. Autosomal recessive, plasma bilirubin concentration greater than 20 mg/dL
C. Autosomal dominant with plasma bilirubin value less than 20 mg/dL
D. Autosomal recessive with coarse pigment in centrilobular hepatocytes

865. Match each form of intestinal ischemia with the associated risk factor.
1. Superior mesenteric artery emboli
2. Nonocclusive mesenteric ischemia
3. Superior mesenteric artery thrombosis
4. Mesenteric venous thrombosis

A. Stable angina
B. Polycythemia vera
C. Cardiogenic shock
D. Ventricular aneurysm

866. Which of the following are important factors in determining the extent of injury after caustic ingestion?
   I. Type of agent
   II. Concentration
   III. Amount ingested
   IV. Fasting versus fed state

   A. I and III
   B. II and IV
   C. I, II, and III
   D. All of the above

867. Indicate whether each of the following statements about constipation is TRUE or FALSE:
   A. In the United States, nonwhite patients report constipation more frequently than whites.
   B. In the United States, stool frequency is inversely related to dietary fiber.
   C. Constipation increases with age.
   D. In healthy, sedentary subjects, a program of regular exercise will decrease whole-gut transit time.
   E. In the United States, women report constipation more frequently than men.

868. Intermittent solid food dysphagia is MOST characteristic of which of the following lesions?
   A. Pulsion diverticulum
   B. Distal esophageal stricture
   C. Schatzki's ring
   D. Zenker's diverticulum

869. All of the following are true statements about Dieulafoy's lesion (ex ulceratio simplex) EXCEPT:
   A. It is due to a small mucosal defect overlying an aberrantly large, persistent-caliber submucosal artery.
   B. Its most common site is in the proximal stomach, on average 6 cm distal from the cardioesophageal junction where arteries are largest.

C. It is rarely accompanied by abdominal pain.
D. Like Cameron ulcers, Dieulafoy's lesion is much more common in women than men.

870. All of the following statements about intestinal lymphangiectasia are true EXCEPT:
   A. Although probably present for years, the disease most commonly becomes manifest in the elderly.
   B. Most patients affected by intestinal lymphangiectasia absorb more than 80% of ingested fat.
   C. Hypogammaglobulinemia and profound lymphocytopenia are characteristic.
   D. The diagnosis can be made by endoscopic biopsy.

871. Which of the following statements about the globus sensation are TRUE?
   I. It is a experienced by up to half of the general population.
   II. It is frequently associated with odynophagia.
   III. When carefully examined, upper esophageal sphincter function is normal.
   IV. The symptoms are worse with meals.

   A. I and III
   B. II and IV
   C. I, II, and III
   D. All of the above

872. Each of the following statements regarding dysphagia is true EXCEPT:
   A. Dysphagia noted within one second of swallowing a bolus suggests an oropharyngeal problem.
   B. Dysphagia due to achalasia is usually associated with weight loss.
   C. Daily dysphagia can be seen with esophageal rings or webs.
   D. Malignant esophageal strictures typically present as dysphagia in the absence of pyrosis.

873. Initial evaluation of diarrhea in a patient with acquired immunodeficiency syndrome (AIDS) should include each of the following EXCEPT:
   A. Careful history and physical examination
   B. Three stool samples for ova and parasites
   C. Stool for culture
   D. Flexible sigmoidoscopy
   E. Acid-fast stain of stool

874. The MOST frequent infiltrating disease involving the liver in acquired immunodeficiency syndrome is:
   A. Cytomegalovirus
   B. Histoplasmosis
   C. *Mycobacterium avium-intracellulare*
   D. Kaposi's sarcoma
   E. Lymphoma

875. Each of the following is a common gastrointestinal problem during pregnancy EXCEPT:
A. Nausea and vomiting
B. Gastroesophageal reflux
C. Cholelithiasis
D. Pancreatitis
E. Constipation

876. Which of the following is characterized by nausea, abdominal pain, jaundice, and fulminant hepatic failure during the third trimester of pregnancy?
A. Acute cholecystitis
B. Cholestasis of pregnancy
C. Acute fatty liver of pregnancy
D. Hyperemesis gravidarum

877. Empirical treatment of odynophagia in patients with the acquired immunodeficiency syndrome would BEST be done with:
A. Acyclovir
B. Fluconazole
C. Omeprazole
D. Sucralfate
E. Foscarnet

878. A frequent gastrointestinal complication of epidermolysis bullosa is:
A. Small bowel obstruction
B. Pancreatitis
C. Rectal ulceration
D. Esophageal stricture
E. Peptic ulcer disease

879. Each of the following drugs has been shown to be effective in the treatment of diabetic gastroparesis EXCEPT:
A. Metoclopramide
B. Bethanechol
C. Cisapride
D. Erythromycin
E. Domperidone

880. Match malabsorption of the following vitamins or minerals with the associated clinical syndrome
1. Vitamin A   A. Follicular keratosis
2. Thiamine   B. Acrodermatitis
3. Zinc   C. Cheilosis
4. Iron   D. Secondary hyperparathyroidism
5. Vitamin D   E. Peripheral neuropathy

881. Each of the following statements regarding short-chain fatty acids (SCFAs) is true EXCEPT:
A. The predominant SCFAs in humans are acetate, propionate, and butyrate.
B. SCFAs increase colonic efflux of sodium and water.

C. The colon can salvage as much as 500 kcal of unabsorbed carbohydrate daily by converting them to SCFAs.
D. SCFAs are produced by bacterial fermentation of undigested carbohydrates.

882. Breath hydrogen testing can be used to detect colonic fermentation of each of these sugars EXCEPT:
A. Sorbitol
B. Glucose
C. Fructose
D. Lactulose
E. Lactose

883. A middle-age man presents to the emergency department with altered mental status. He is alert but disoriented. On physical examination, he is tachycardic with postural hypotension. He has lateral gaze paralysis. The family reports that he has had recent difficulty walking and has been drinking large amounts of alcohol. This patient would most likely benefit from:
A. Lactulose therapy
B. Intravenous infusion of thiamine and glucose
C. Intravenous infusion of cobalamin (vitamin B_{12})
D. Intramuscular injection of folate

884. Match each drug with an associated effect:
1. Flumazenil   A. Amnesia
2. Fentanyl   B. Adjunctive sedation for alcoholic
3. Midazolam   patients
4. Droperidol   C. Short-acting sedative
                              D. Benzodiazepine antagonist

885. Estrogens cause jaundice by:
I. Inhibiting the hepatocyte plasma membrane Na^+/K^+ pump
II. Decreasing membrane fluidity
III. Perturbing the function of organic anion transporters

A. I only
B. II only
C. I and II
D. II and III
E. All of the above

886. Each of the following is characteristic of rumination EXCEPT:
A. Esophageal, gastric, and small bowel motility are normal.
B. Patients regurgitate food, chew the bolus again, and reswallow.
C. It may occur in infancy.
D. Psychological disturbances are often present.
E. Hiatal hernia repair is indicated if medical therapy fails.

887. Each of the following drugs may produce constipation EXCEPT:
    A. Codeine
    B. Dicyclomine
    C. Phenothiazines
    D. Magnesium-containing antacids
    E. Aluminum-containing antacids

888. Which of the following urinary tract problems are associated with constipation?
    I. Urgency and nocturia
    II. Hydronephrosis
    III. Urinary tract infection
    IV. Glomerulonephritis

    A. I and III
    B. II and IV
    C. I, II, and III
    D. All of the above

889. A liver disease associated with hypothyroidism is:
    A. Primary sclerosing cholangitis
    B. Primary biliary cirrhosis
    C. Fatty liver
    D. Wilson's disease
    E. Hemachromatosis

890. With respect to polyarteritis nodosa, all of the following are true EXCEPT:
    A. It is a necrotizing vasculitis of small- and medium-sized arteries.
    B. Hepatitis B–related polyarteritis nodosa is a late complication of chronic hepatitis B and primarily involves the hepatic artery.
    C. Abdominal pain is the most common gastrointestinal symptom, with hemorrhage, perforation, and bowel infarction occurring in approximately 10% of cases.
    D. Mesenteric arteriography characteristically shows aneurysmal dilations of medium-sized visceral arteries.

891. Which of the following drugs increase the risk of gastric or duodenal ulceration?
    I. Corticosteroids
    II. Bismuth subsalicylate
    III. Nonacetylated salicylates
    IV. Digoxin

    A. I and III
    B. II and IV
    C. I, II, and III
    D. None of the above

892. Each of the following is a common finding in peritonitis associated with ambulatory peritoneal dialysis EXCEPT:
    A. Fever

    B. Abdominal pain
    C. Cloudy peritoneal fluid
    D. Gram-positive cocci in peritoneal fluid culture

893. The MOST common abnormality of the liver in diabetes mellitus is:
    A. Iron deposition
    B. Steatosis
    C. Cholestasis
    D. Fibrosis
    E. Cirrhosis

894. Which of the following are TRUE statements concerning cholangiopathy of the acquired immunodeficiency syndrome?
    A. Many cases are associated with cytomegalovirus, *Cryptosporidium,* or Microsporidia.
    B. Ductular changes consist of papillary stenosis, sclerosing cholangitis–like lesions, or long strictures.
    C. Sphincterotomy will usually result in both symptomatic and enzymatic improvement.

895. Each of the following is a possible complication of upper endoscopy EXCEPT:
    A. Perforation
    B. Bleeding
    C. Pancreatitis
    D. Bacteremia

896. Each of the following is a true statement about Gilbert's syndrome EXCEPT:
    A. It is present in 5% to 7% of white adults in the United States.
    B. It is characterized by increased serum conjugated bilirubin.
    C. Bilirubin concentration may rise two-fold to three-fold after fasting.
    D. It is a benign syndrome that requires no further workup.
    E. Unlike most other liver diseases, postprandial concentrations of bile acids are normal.

897. Which of the following antiemetic medications is LEAST likely to cause adverse central nervous system effects?
    A. Scopolamine
    B. Tetrahydrocannabinol
    C. Domperidone
    D. Metoclopramide
    E. Prochlorperazine

898. Which of the following gut segments is LEAST well supplied by collateral circulation?
    A. Duodenum
    B. Jejunum

C. Splenic flexure
D. Rectum

899. Which of the following are TRUE statements concerning neurologic diseases and the gastrointestinal tract?
A. Acute head trauma causes an increased risk of upper gastrointestinal tract bleeding.
B. Corticosteroid administration increases the risk of gastrointestinal bleeding in trauma patients.
C. Spinal cord injury disrupts both sensory and motor function of the rectum, often causing chronic constipation.

900. Which of the following are common causes of diarrhea in intensive care unit patients?
A. Hyperosmotic tube feeding
B. Pseudomembranous colitis
C. Medications
D. Intestinal ischemia
E. Defective anal continence

901. Each of the following is characteristic of visceral pain EXCEPT:
A. It is dull in character.
B. It is well localized.
C. It is midline.
D. It is cramping, burning, or gnawing.
E. Patients often try to have a bowel movement in an effort to relieve it.

902. Juxtapapillary or periampullary diverticula are associated with an increased frequency of which of the following?
I. Cholelithiasis
II. Recurrent choledocholithiasis after cholecystectomy
III. Biliary and pancreatic anomalies
IV. Duodenal carcinoma

A. I and III
B. II and IV
C. I, II, and III
D. All of the above

903. Which of the following physiologic events do NOT normally occur in response to filling of the rectum with stool from the sigmoid colon?
A. Contraction of the external anal sphincter
B. Relaxation of the rectum
C. Contraction of the puborectalis muscle
D. Contraction of the internal anal sphincter
E. Conscious sensation of rectal filling

904. Each of the following statements concerning the effects of human immunodeficiency virus infection on hepatitis B is true EXCEPT:
A. Previously lost HBsAg may reappear.

B. Anti-HBs may be lost more rapidly.
C. Expression of HBeAg is increased.
D. Clinical liver disease is more severe.
E. Serum levels of DNA polymerase are increased.

905. Each of the following is a cutaneous manifestation associated with BOTH Crohn's disease and ulcerative colitis EXCEPT:
A. Pyoderma gangrenosum
B. Erythema nodosum
C. Erythema multiforme
D. Oral aphthous ulceration
E. Pyostomatitis vegetans

906. Which of the following statements regarding the response to fasting is TRUE?
A. The postabsorptive period begins after ingested food has been absorbed.
B. In early starvation, glucose is produced by gluconeogenesis from fatty acids.
C. During short-term starvation, the predominant fuel consumed by the brain is glucose.
D. During long-term starvation, adipose tissue provides 50% of energy requirements.

907. Dyspepsia is best defined as:
A. Persistent or recurrent abdominal discomfort centered in the epigastrium.
B. Persistent or recurrent pain, belching, nausea, or bloating centered in the abdomen.
C. Burning substernal discomfort after meals.
D. There is no single definition for dyspepsia.

908. All of the following may be useful in the treatment of gastric bezoars EXCEPT:
A. Papain
B. Pancreatic enzymes
C. Acetylcysteine
D. Cellulase

909. Which of the following statements regarding diet and dyspepsia are TRUE?
A. Coffee, tea, and other caffeinated beverages may cause chronic unexplained dyspepsia.
B. Food allergies have not been causally linked to dyspepsia.
C. Fat content of foods may affect the severity of dyspepsia.
D. Spicy diet has been causally linked to chronic dyspepsia.

910. Protein-losing enteropathies can be expected to lower multiple serum proteins, especially those with long half-lives. Particularly useful proteins used to test for this condition include each the following EXCEPT:
A. IgA

B. Albumin
C. IgG
D. IgM
E. Transferrin

---

911. Which voluntary muscle is the MOST important in maintaining fecal continence?
A. Internal anal sphincter
B. Puborectalis muscle
C. Levator ani muscle
D. External anal sphincter

---

912. Which of the following are TRUE statements about human immunodeficiency virus (HIV)-induced anal ulcer?
A. At least half of anal ulcers in HIV-positive patients have no identifiable cause.
B. They are rarely painful and often asymptomatic.
C. Treatment with ganciclovir often results in healing.
D. They may be caused by syphilis, tuberculosis, herpes simplex, or neoplasms.

---

913. Each of the following is a gastrointestinal manifestation of systemic sclerosis (scleroderma) EXCEPT:
A. Esophageal dysmotility
B. Delayed gastric emptying
C. Pancreatitis
D. Fatty liver
E. Intestinal fibrosis

---

914. Each of the following is a gastrointestinal manifestation of amyloidosis EXCEPT:
A. Dysphagia
B. Gastric outlet obstruction
C. Biliary colic
D. Pseudo-obstruction
E. Diarrhea

---

915. The following conditions are all gastrointestinal manifestations of hyperthyroidism EXCEPT:
A. Cholestasis characterized by conjugated hyperbilirubinemia and an elevated alkaline phosphatase level is the most common liver manifestation.
B. Diarrhea is due to accelerated small bowel transit.
C. Dysphagia is due to proximal esophageal myopathy.
D. Weight loss and abdominal pain mimic an intra-abdominal malignancy.

---

916. Long-term total parenteral nutrition may result in a variety of specific nutritional deficiencies. Match the following micronutrient deficiency with the clinical features it may cause.

1. Essential fatty acids   A. Myalgias, cardiomyopathy
   B. Eczematous dermatitis

2. Thiamine   C. Night blindness
3. Vitamin A   D. Wernicke's encephalopathy, refractory lactic acidosis
4. Selenium

---

917. The MOST common cause of diarrhea in critically ill patients receiving tube feedings is:
A. Antibiotics
B. Hypertonic formulations
C. Excessive rate of infusion
D. Sorbitol in elixirs

---

918. Match the diagnosis with the most appropriate diet. Use each answer only once.

1. Diverticulitis   A. Clear-liquid diet
2. Difficulty chewing   B. Full liquid diet
3. Abdominal surgery preparation   C. Mechanical soft diet
4. Dysphagia for solids   D. Low-fiber diet

---

919. Which of the following is MOST likely to stimulate gut pain receptors?
A. Cutting
B. Stretching
C. Burning
D. Crushing
E. Tearing

---

920. Which of the following tests is MOST likely to demonstrate an aortoenteric fistula?
A. Abdominal computed tomography
B. Angiography
C. Abdominal ultrasonography with Doppler imaging
D. Endoscopy

---

921. The MOST common cause of odynophagia and dysphagia in patients with the acquired immunodeficiency syndrome is:
A. *Candida*
B. Cytomegalovirus
C. Herpes simplex
D. Lymphoma
E. Reflux esophagitis

---

922. In which of the following situations during colonoscopy is the risk of perforation greatest?
A. Hydrostatic balloon dilatation of a colonic anastomotic stricture
B. Removal of a 1.5-cm pedunculated polyp in the ascending colon
C. Diagnostic colonoscopy in a patient with severe diverticulosis
D. Hot biopsy forceps use on a diminutive cecal polyp

---

923. Which of the following foods have been shown to lower pressure of the lower esophageal sphincter?
   I. Chocolate

II. Onions
III. Carminatives
IV. Sugars

A. I and III
B. II and IV
C. I, II, and III
D. All of the above

924. Which one of the following statements about collagenous colitis is FALSE?
A. It is characterized by a thickened subepithelial collagen band.
B. It affects primarily elderly women.
C. Plasma cells are prominent within the lamina propria.
D. It causes a secretory diarrhea.
E. It is linked with collagen vascular diseases.

925. Early deaths after caustic ingestion most commonly result from which of the following complications?
A. Mediastinitis and peritonitis
B. Gastrointestinal hemorrhage
C. Severe alkalosis
D. Adult respiratory distress syndrome

926. Match the following vascular causes of gastrointestinal hemorrhage with the associated characteristic:
1. Vascular ectasias
2. Osler-Weber-Rendu disease
3. Watermelon stomach
4. Colonic hemangioma

A. Associated with portal hypertension
B. Frank gastrointestinal bleeding unusual
C. Common cause of bleeding in elderly
D. Associated with cutaneous lesions

927. Common causes of diarrhea of unknown origin include all of the following EXCEPT:
A. Surreptitious abuse of laxatives
B. Defective anal continence masquerading as diarrhea
C. Collagenous colitis
D. Neuroendocrine tumor
E. Irritable bowel syndrome

928. Each of the following statements concerning the acute abdomen during pregnancy is true EXCEPT:
A. Appendicitis is the most common indication for operation.
B. Accurate diagnosis is more difficult during pregnancy.
C. Surgical intervention for appendicitis entails a high risk of fetal loss and should be delayed until after delivery if possible.
D. Acute abdominal pain in pregnant patients occurs with the same frequency and from the same

causes as acute abdominal pain in nonpregnant, age-matched women.
E. The enlarged uterus displaces abdominal organs and can alter clinical manifestations.

929. Infectious causes of pancreatitis in patients with the acquired immunodeficiency syndrome include each of the following EXCEPT:
A. Cytomegalovirus
B. *Campylobacter*
C. *Mycobacterium avium-intracellulare*
D. *Cryptococcus*
E. Herpes simplex virus

930. Each of the following is a common cause of childhood fecal incontinence EXCEPT:
A. Hirschsprung's disease
B. Mental retardation
C. Childhood encopresis
D. Neural tube defects

931. Each of the following is a true statement regarding the role of the chemoreceptor trigger zone (CTZ) in vomiting EXCEPT:
A. Dopamine receptors in the CTZ play a role in mediating vomiting.
B. The CTZ is located in an area where the blood-brain barrier is virtually nonexistent.
C. The vomiting center is under the control of the CTZ.
D. The CTZ is important in mediating nausea and vomiting associated with uremia.

932. Match each laxative agent with an associated side effect:
1. Psyllium
2. Mineral oil
3. Anthraquinones
4. Lactulose

A. Vitamin A deficiency
B. Flatulence
C. Melanosis coli
D. Small bowel obstruction

933. Which of the following are TRUE statements concerning an acute abdomen?
A. Diagnostic error is twice as common in men as in women.
B. Diagnostic error is highest in females aged 1 through 20 years.
C. Elderly patients are less likely to have a condition requiring surgery.
D. Incorrect diagnosis is common in patients older than age 50.

934. Which of the following is the MOST common cause of peritonitis?
A. Appendicitis
B. Perforated peptic ulcer
C. Gangrenous bowel or gallbladder
D. Postoperative complication

935. Metabolic and endocrine disorders that can induce constipation include each of the following EXCEPT:
A. Diabetes mellitus
B. Sarcoidosis with hypercalcemia
C. Hyperthyroidism
D. Hyperparathyroidism
E. Hypothyroidism

936. Which of the following statements concerning esophageal foreign bodies are TRUE?
A. The most common cause of impaction in adults is a food bolus above a stricture or ring.
B. Papain should be tried before endoscopy to digest an impacted meat bolus.
C. Pointed objects should be removed endoscopically by grasping the pointed end and pulling it snug against the endoscope tip before removal.
D. Glucagon may help relax the esophagus before endoscopic removal.

937. While awaiting endoscopic removal of a sharp object in the stomach, the patient should be maintained in which position?
A. Supine
B. Upright
C. On the abdomen
D. Left lateral decubitus
E. Right lateral decubitus

938. Each of the following is a true statement about anismus EXCEPT:
A. It is a common mechanism of functional outlet obstruction.
B. It is caused by spasm of the internal anal sphincter.
C. It most commonly occurs in young boys and adult women.
D. It is common in patients who have been sexually abused.
E. The only successful treatment is biofeedback.

939. Match the disease process with the micronutrient deficiency with which it is associated:
1. Diabetes mellitus
2. Acrodermatitis enteropathica
3. Anemia
4. Cardiomyopathy

A. Selenium
B. Zinc
C. Chromium
D. Copper

940. Which of the following descriptions of abdominal pain is MOST characteristic of acute appendicitis:
A. Sudden onset, periumbilical, diffuse, severe pain
B. Gradual onset, right lower quadrant, diffuse, moderate pain
C. Gradual onset, periumbilical initially, then right lower quadrant, moderate pain

D. Sudden onset, right lower quadrant, localized severe pain
E. Sudden onset, epigastric initially, then diffuse severe pain

941. Which of the following statements concerning non-Hodgkin's lymphoma in patients with the acquired immunodeficiency syndrome are TRUE?
A. They are primarily T-cell neoplasms.
B. The gastrointestinal and hepatobiliary tracts are uncommon sites of primary involvement.
C. The prognosis is determined mainly by the extent of underlying immunocompromise.

942. Match each cutaneous syndrome with its associated gastrointestinal pathology.
1. Peutz-Jeghers syndrome
2. Acanthosis nigricans
3. Necrolytic migratory erythema
4. Gardner's syndrome
5. Blue rubber bleb nevus syndrome

A. Cavernous hemangiomas
B. Adenomatous polyps
C. Adenocarcinoma
D. Hamartomas
E. Glucagonoma

943. Each of the following is a characteristic presenting feature of acute mesenteric ischemia EXCEPT:
A. Abdominal pain
B. Abdominal tenderness
C. Heme-positive stool
D. Leukocytosis

944. Which one of the following statements regarding adaptation during starvation is TRUE?
A. Cholesterol present in adipose tissue represents the major fuel reserve in the body.
B. Resting metabolic rate decreases by 25% at 7 days and 50% at 30 days.
C. Energy expenditure declines progressively after 30 days of continued starvation.
D. Adipose tissue consumes less than 5% of resting metabolic rate.

945. All of the following may be seen with the refeeding syndrome EXCEPT:
A. Volume overload
B. Hypoglycemia
C. Hypophosphatemia
D. Diarrhea

946. Which of the following statements regarding bleeding from colonic diverticula are TRUE?
I. Bleeding is usually painless and often massive.
II. Bleeding will stop spontaneously in about 80% of cases.
III. Bleeding usually arises from a single diverticulum.

IV. If bleeding does not stop or recurs, a right hemi-colectomy should be performed.

A. I and III
B. II and IV
C. I, II, and III
D. All of the above

947. A previously healthy college student presents with a 24-hour history of an illness characterized by profuse watery diarrhea and occasional abdominal cramping. She is nauseated but has not vomited and feels somewhat better over the last four hours. On physical examination, she is afebrile and not orthostatic and her abdominal examination is benign. The best management strategy at this time is:
A. Ciprofloxacin, 500 mg orally b.i.d. for 7 days
B. Tetracycline, 500 mg orally q.i.d. for 7 days
C. Ampicillin, 500 mg orally q.i.d. for 7 days
D. Metronidazole, 250 mg orally t.i.d. for 7 days
E. None of the above

948. Which of the following statements pertaining to defecation and fecal incontinence are TRUE?
A. Rectal distention by gas or stool results in a reflex relaxation of the internal anal sphincter.
B. Rectal distention by gas or stool results in a reflex contraction of the puborectalis muscle.
C. Diabetic patients often have diarrhea, but the incidence of overt incontinence is not different from age-matched subjects.
D. Most cases of idiopathic fecal incontinence are due to peripheral neuropathy.

949. Each of the following is a common physical sign of a perforated ulcer EXCEPT:
A. Fever
B. Abdominal wall rigidity
C. Absent bowel sounds
D. Subcutaneous emphysema
E. Abdominal pain

950. Which one of the following statements regarding the management of gastroparesis diabeticorum is FALSE?
A. Phenothiazines, although not directly stimulating gastric emptying, nonetheless have a beneficial effect on relief of nausea.
B. Metaclopramide's effect of accelerating gastric emptying often diminishes after four to six weeks, although the patient may remain asymptomatic.
C. The most common side effects of cisapride are headaches, abdominal cramping, and diarrhea.
D. Erythromycin, a motilin agonist, accelerates gastric emptying in gastroparesis diabeticorum, at least for the short term.

951. A 24-year-old woman who is six weeks pregnant is admitted to the hospital with persistent nausea and vomiting. She is found to be volume depleted, hypokalemic, and hyponatremic. Which of the following statements regarding this patient are TRUE?
A. The likely diagnosis is hyperemesis gravidarum.
B. The vomiting is likely to persist throughout her pregnancy.
C. The vomiting is likely to occur with subsequent pregnancies.
D. The fetus is likely unaffected.
E. Antiemetics are contraindicated.

952. Jaundice associated with the presence of eosinophilia should heighten the suspicion of each of the following EXCEPT:
A. Sarcoidosis
B. Parasitic disease
C. Amyloidosis
D. Drug toxicity

953. Chronic diarrhea in diabetic patients may be due to several conditions that either are a direct complication of diabetes or are associated with diabetes. These conditions include each of the following EXCEPT:
A. Small intestinal dysmotility
B. Pancreatic diseases (pancreatitis, pancreatic carcinoma)
C. Celiac sprue
D. Crohn's disease
E. Bacterial overgrowth

954. Which of the following is NOT a factor that signals satiety?
A. Gastric distention
B. Fatty acids
C. Cholecystokinin
D. Deoxycholic acid

955. Each of the following statements regarding globus sensation is true EXCEPT:
A. Globus is usually associated with dysphagia.
B. Globus may be variably described as "tightness," "choking," a "lump," or "strangling" sensation.
C. Manometric studies are typically normal in patients with globus.
D. Histrionic features are absent in the majority of patients with globus.

956. Which one of the following statements regarding enteral and parenteral feeding is TRUE?
A. Parenteral nutrient requirements are better known than enteral requirements.
B. Enteral nutrition is associated with a higher rate of cholelithiasis.

C. Adequate parenteral nutrition maintains the structural and functional integrity of the intestine.

D. Enteral feeding helps prevent translocation of bacteria across the gut wall.

---

957. Patients with upper gastrointestinal bleeding who are found to have a clean ulcer base by endoscopy have a re-bleeding rate of approximately:

A. 1%
B. 10%
C. 20%
D. 40%
E. 80%

---

958. Which of the following are TRUE statements about complications of upper gastrointestinal endoscopy?

A. Complications from gastrointestinal endoscopy are common.

B. Patients with prosthetic heart valves should receive prophylactic antibiotics before diagnostic endoscopy.

C. Respiratory depression is a common side effect of midazolam.

D. Transmission of infection can occur as a result of endoscopy.

---

959. Examples of disorders associated with increased production of bilirubin include each of the following EXCEPT:

A. Polycythemia vera
B. Ineffective erythropoiesis
C. Resorption of hematomas
D. Dubin-Johnson syndrome

---

960. In which part of the stomach are diverticula MOST likely to occur?

A. Antrum
B. Body
C. Fundus
D. Cardia

---

961. Which of the following statements concerning acquired immunodeficiency syndrome (AIDS) and diarrhea are TRUE?

A. Effective treatment exists to eliminate *Cryptosporidium*-induced diarrhea.

B. Infection by enteric bacterial pathogens are more frequent and more virulent in AIDS patients.

C. Infiltration of the colon on rectal biopsy by *Mycobacterium avium-intracellulare* establishes the cause of the diarrhea.

---

962. Which one of the following statements regarding weight-loss diets is FALSE?

A. Prolonged fasting results in marked hypokalemia, hypophosphatemia, and profound postural hypotension.

B. Very low-calorie diets (<800 kcal/day) are safe if patients are supervised.

C. Most patients can successfully follow a balanced low-calorie diet (1000 to 1200 kcal/day).

D. Use of artificial sweeteners has no significant effect on body weight.

E. Nonabsorbable fat substitutes (e.g., sucrose polyester) can cause vitamin malabsorption.

---

963. Most of the complications of intestinal bypass surgery for weight reduction result from:

A. Decreased oral intake
B. Malabsorption
C. Dysmotility
D. Dumping syndrome

---

964. The average asymptomatic person has 200 mL of intestinal gas. How many milliliters of intestinal gas are found in patients who complain of abdominal distention that they attribute to gas?

A. Less than 200 mL
B. 200 to 300 mL
C. 300 to 400 mL
D. 400 to 500 mL
E. More than 500 mL

---

965. The MOST common gastrointestinal symptom in acquired immunodeficiency syndrome is:

A. Odynophagia
B. Diarrhea
C. Early satiety
D. Abdominal pain
E. Vomiting

---

966. With respect to the value of abdominal computed tomography (CT) in patients with jaundice, which of the following statements are TRUE?

A. CT is less sensitive than endoscopic retrograde cholangiopancreatography and percutaneous transhepatic cholangiography at detecting bile duct obstruction.

B. Bowel gas may obscure the common bile duct.

C. Most gallbladder stones are visualized.

D. Obesity limits image quality.

---

967. All of the following statements about dietary treatment of lymphatic obstruction with medium-chain triglycerides (MCTs) are true EXCEPT:

A. Compared with long-chain triglycerides, MCTs are hydrolyzed to fatty acid more rapidly.

B. MCTs are water soluble.

C. After intestinal absorption, MCTs are incorporated into chylomicrons and transported by mesenteric lymphatics.

D. MCTs can be used to increase calorie intake.

E. Compared with long-chain triglycerides, MCTs are more ketogenic and should not be given to patients with diabetes.

968. Which of the following is NOT associated with gastrointestinal bleeding?
A. Amyloidosis
B. NSAID usage
C. Corticosteroids
D. Scleroderma
E. Juvenile polyps

969. After the esophagus, the MOST frequent site of perforation from an ingested foreign body is:
A. Stomach
B. Proximal duodenum
C. Ileocecal region
D. Sigmoid colon
E. Rectum

970. A black mass found in the stomach during esophagogastroduodenoscopy is MOST likely:
A. A phytobezoar
B. An exophytic gastric cancer
C. A Gummi Bear bezoar
D. A trichobezoar
E. A polybezoar

971. Which of the following statements regarding NSAID use are TRUE?
A. Chronic NSAID use may present as an iron-deficiency anemia.
B. Intramuscular or intravenous administration of an NSAID greatly reduces the risk of ulceration.
C. Enteric coatings substantially reduce the risks of aspirin use.
D. Eighty percent or more of NSAID-induced gastric ulcers have an associated antral gastritis.

972. Match the diet or supplement with the condition that most commonly precludes its use. Use each answer only once.
1. Full-liquid diet   A. Severe malnutrition
2. Clear-liquid diet   B. Insulin-dependent diabetes
3. High-fiber diet   C. Crohn's disease of terminal
4. Medium-chain tri-   ileum
   glycerides   D. Lactose intolerance

973. A 39-year-old woman presents with a six-month history of defecation producing greasy, foul-smelling stools. She has lost 15 pounds. On physical examination, her vital signs are normal but she is thin and has shiny, taut skin and a blackened painless first digit. Appropriate treatment for her gastrointestinal disorder would be:
A. Prednisone
B. Cyclosporine
C. Tetracycline
D. Azathioprine
E. Omeprazole

974. Each of the following statements regarding glutamine is true EXCEPT:
A. Glutamine is an essential amino acid.
B. Glutamine shortens the shelf-life of parenteral nutrition formulas.
C. Glutamine enhances intestinal adaptation to massive resection.
D. During catabolic states, glutamine uptake by the intestine increases.

975. Which of the following organs has the lowest energy requirement per gram of tissue?
A. Small bowel
B. Liver
C. Brain
D. Kidney

976. Which of the following disorders develop as a result of abnormal esophageal motility?
  I. Zenker's diverticulum
 II. Epiphrenic diverticulum
III. Midesophageal diverticulum
 IV. Schatzki's ring

A. I and III
B. II and IV
C. I, II, and III
D. All of the above

977. Which of the following is the most useful historical feature in evaluating the cause of fecal retention and soiling in children?
A. Deliberate withholding of stool by the child to control parents
B. Effects of diet
C. Association of defecation with pain
D. Stool consistency
E. Activity level

978. Which of the following is NOT a *Diagnostic and Statistical Manual of Mental Disorders–IV* criterion for diagnosing anorexia nervosa?
A. Primary or secondary amenorrhea
B. Intense fear of gaining weight, even though underweight
C. Disturbance in the way one's body is perceived
D. Self-induced vomiting, use of laxatives or diuretics, strict dieting or fasting, or vigorous exercise to prevent weight gain

979. Each of the following is an indication for surgical management of an enteric fistula EXCEPT:
A. Presence of an end fistula
B. Bowel obstruction distal to fistula
C. Presence of a high-output fistula
D. Persistent drainage despite treatment of infection

980. Which of the following are TRUE statements regarding energy balance and expenditure in obesity?
  A. Hyperphagia is not the primary cause of obesity.
  B. Obese persons expend more energy when active than lean persons.
  C. The basal metabolic rate of obese subjects is greater than for lean subjects.
  D. Obese persons have relatively efficient energy metabolism.

981. Which of the following diseases is NOT associated with gastroparesis?
  A. Anorexia nervosa
  B. Pernicious anemia
  C. Scleroderma
  D. Diabetes
  E. Polymyositis

982. A particularly worrisome foreign body that small children are prone to ingest is:
  A. Safety pins
  B. Toothpicks
  C. Matches
  D. Small batteries
  E. Nails

983. Match the following causes of diarrhea with the associated clinical finding.
  1. Zollinger-Ellison syndrome   A. Flushing
  2. Amyloidosis   B. Reflux esophagitis
  3. Systemic mastocytosis   C. Autonomic neuropathy
  4. Whipple's disease   D. Fever
  5. Collagenous colitis   E. Female sex and age older than 70

984. A 72-year-old woman with a history of chronic atrial fibrillation presents with the sudden onset of periumbilical pain worsening over a four-hour period. On physical examination, the abdomen is distended and minimal periumbilical tenderness is present. Plain films of the abdomen show no evidence of perforation. Because of the concern of acute mesenteric ischemia, an angiogram is performed. It shows no evidence of vascular occlusion. Which of the following tests would be MOST likely to confirm the diagnosis of nonocclusive mesenteric ischemia?
  A. Look for "thumbprinting" on the scout film of the angiogram
  B. Order a Doppler ultrasound evaluation to measure flow in the mesenteric vessels
  C. Perform abdominal computed tomography to look for thickened bowel wall
  D. Look for mesenteric vasospasm on the angiogram

985. Which one or more of the following are TRUE statements about colonic ischemia?
  A. It is usually associated with a period of low cardiac output.

  B. It is often associated with frank blood in stool.
  C. An angiogram will usually pinpoint a specific cause.
  D. Clinical findings can mimic inflammatory bowel disease.

986. Match the vitamin with the clinical disease caused by its deficiency.
  1. Thiamine   A. Megaloblastic anemia
  2. Niacin   B. Pellagra
  3. Folic acid   C. Scurvy
  4. Vitamin C   D. Beriberi

987. Factors that predispose to gastric bezoar formation include all of the following EXCEPT:
  A. Previous gastric surgery
  B. Diabetes mellitus
  C. Opiates
  D. High-fiber diet
  E. Crohn's disease
  F. Vagotomy and pyloroplasty

988. Which of the following statements regarding energy needs are TRUE?
  A. Resting metabolic rate (RMR), basal energy expenditure (BEE), resting energy expenditure (REE), and basal metabolic rate (BMR) are interchangeable terms.
  B. Total energy expenditure (TEE) is the sum of resting energy expenditure, the thermic effect of food digestion, and the thermic effect of physical activity.
  C. Forty percent of TEE is due to physical activity.
  D. Using height, weight, age, and sex, the Harris-Benedict equation can be used to determine TEE.

989. A 45-year-old woman presents to the emergency department with violent retching of sudden-onset, small-volume emesis in association with epigastric pain. Multiple attempts at passing a nasogastric tube are unsuccessful. An upright chest film shows an air bubble above the diaphragm. Which of the following is the MOST likely diagnosis?
  A. A perforated duodenal ulcer
  B. An esophageal stricture
  C. Adenocarcinoma arising in the gastric cardia
  D. Gastric volvulus

990. A 76-year-old woman presents with fever and crampy left lower quadrant pain. Computed tomography (CT) of the abdomen reveals a 6-cm left lower quadrant mass. Of the following CT characteristics, which is MOST specific for diagnosing an abdominal abscess?
  A. Low-density appearance
  B. Gas seen within the mass

C. Enhancement of center with intravenous contrast agent

D. Obliteration of tissue planes

---

991. A needle aspirate of the mass demonstrates purulent material, and the patient is treated with intravenous ampicillin, gentamicin, and metronidazole. A catheter is advanced into the abscess and is connected to suction with drainage of 150 mL of pus over 24 hours. At what point can the catheter be removed?

A. When fever has resolved

B. When drainage is no longer significant

C. When the abscess cavity has collapsed

D. All of the above are required

---

992. Gas production by colonic bacteria can be used to diagnose carbohydrate malabsorption. The gas produced by these bacteria that is useful in diagnostic testing is:

A. Hydrogen

B. Methane

C. Nitric oxide

D. Carbon dioxide

E. Nitrogen

---

993. When a person who has fasted is re-fed protein, early nitrogen accumulation occurs in:

A. Kidney

B. Liver

C. Skeletal muscle

D. Smooth muscle

---

994. All of the following are associated with hypothyroidism EXCEPT:

A. Reflux esophagitis

B. Gastric hypomotility

C. Increased incidence of gallstones

D. Constipation

E. Increased gastric acid secretion

---

995. Match each prokinetic agent with its mechanism of action:

1. Erythromycin	A. Central and peripheral dopamine antagonist
2. Cisapride	
3. Ondansetron	B. Central and peripheral serotonin antagonist
4. Metoclopramide	
	C. Motilin agonist
	D. Release of acetylcholine from the myenteric plexus

---

996. Involvement of the esophagus with progressive systemic sclerosis (PSS, scleroderma) accounts for significant morbidity in these patients. All of the following statements regarding esophageal involvement with PSS are true EXCEPT:

A. CREST syndrome (PSS with limited cutaneous involvement) rarely involves the esophagus.

B. Dysphagia may be due to absent peristalsis or peptic stricture of the esophagus.

C. Gastroesophageal reflux disease, due to lax lower esophageal sphincter tone and impaired gastric emptying, is often associated with Barrett's metaplasia of the esophagus.

D. Despite Barrett's metaplasia, the incidence of adenocarcinoma of the esophagus in PSS patients is not increased.

---

997. Treatable diseases that cause protein-losing enteropathy and endoscopically visible damage to the intestinal mucosa include each of the following EXCEPT:

A. Sprue, both celiac and tropical types

B. Eosinophilic gastroenteritis

C. Graft-versus-host disease

D. Bacterial overgrowth

E. Whipple's disease

---

998. What proportion of patients with Barrett's esophagus cannot sense the presence of acid in their esophagus?

A. 10%

B. 33%

C. 66%

D. 90%

---

999. Which of the following prognostic indicators predicts UNLIKELY spontaneous closure of a gastrointestinal fistula?

A. Low output (<500 mL/day)

B. Acute duration

C. Long fistula tract

D. Partial obstruction distal to the fistula

E. Anastomotic breakdown as the cause of the fistula

1000. The major mechanism by which hyperthyroidism causes diarrhea is:

A. Increased intestinal secretion

B. Small bowel inflammation

C. Hypermotility of the small bowel

D. Gastrin stimulation

E. Bile salt malabsorption

1001. Chronic functional abdominal pain (CFAP) is a distinct medical condition best diagnosed by the presence of positive symptom criteria. All of the following are part of the Rome diagnostic criteria for CFAP EXCEPT:

A. Frequently recurrent or continuous abdominal pain for at least 6 months

B. Incomplete or no relationship of the pain with physiologic events (e.g. with eating, defecation, or menses)

C. Some loss of daily functioning

D. Some objective evidence of systemic disorder (e.g., weight loss, anemia, elevated sedimentation rate)

E. No evidence for organic disease and insufficient evidence for other functional gastrointestinal disorders to explain the abdominal pain

---

1002. With which of the following conditions are patients LEAST likely to present with complaints of odynophagia?
A. Caustic ingestion
B. Herpetic esophagitis
C. Severe peptic esophagitis
D. Esophageal carcinoma

1003. Dermatitis herpetiformis is associated with which disease?
A. Crohn's disease
B. Lymphoma
C. Celiac sprue
D. Pernicious anemia
E. Achalasia

1004. Which one or more of the following statements about melanosis coli are TRUE?
A. It is caused by anthracene laxative abuse.
B. It is caused by diphenolic laxative abuse.
C. The pigment identified in the colon is melanin.
D. It mainly affects the cecum and rectosigmoid region.
E. It requires at least three to five years of laxative abuse to develop.

1005. Which of the following statements about nutritional assessment are TRUE?
A. Measuring arm circumference and triceps skinfold thickness is an easy and sensitive way to determine a change in arm muscle circumference.
B. At least 20% of the population is malnourished by anthropometric criteria.
C. Albumin correlates well with disease and complications and is not an index of nutrition *per se.*
D. Immune competence as measured by delayed cutaneous hypersensitivity is reduced in malnutrition, making anergy a good predictor of malnutrition.

1006. Match the following clinical types of functional constipation with its most characteristic set of symptoms.

1. Simple constipation (as in irritable bowel syndrome)
2. Slow transit
3. Outlet delay (dyssynergia, anismus)
4. Fecal impaction
5. Pseudo-obstruction

A. Straining, stool frequency may be normal, increased, or decreased
B. Recurrent or constant distension, vomiting
C. Soiling
D. Abdominal pain and difficult defecation, exacerbated by stress and reversible by diet
E. Invariably infrequent bowel actions, never loose stools

1007. Which of the following is LEAST likely to control active bleeding from esophageal varices?
A. Intravenous vasopressin and nitroglycerin
B. Transjugular intrahepatic portosystemic shunt
C. Endoscopic sclerotherapy
D. Intravenous octreotide
E. Endoscopic variceal ligation

1008. Of the following organisms, which one is LEAST likely to be found in an abdominal abscess in a patient presenting *de novo* to the hospital?
A. Bacteroides
B. *Escherichia coli*
C. Enterococcus
D. Staphylococcus

1009. Which of the following statements about defecation are TRUE?
  I. The "call to stool" can be duplicated by distention of a balloon in the rectum.
 II. Defecation is initiated by inhibition of the puborectalis muscle and the external anal sphincter.
III. Once defecation is initiated, it can be completed by propulsive contractions in the colon and rectum alone.
IV. The defecation mechanism requires an intact spinal cord above the level of T12.

A. I and III
B. II and IV
C. I, II, and III
D. All of the above

1010. A 66-year-old woman presents complaining of frequent soiling to the point she must wear diapers. Her past medical history is significant for diabetes mellitus controlled with oral hypoglycemics for the past 15 years. Which of the following statements are TRUE?
  I. Her incontinence is probably due to reduced anal sphincter pressure and impaired sensation.
 II. Incontinence occurs in approximately 20% of patients with long-standing diabetes mellitus.
III. Her incontinence may improve with biofeedback training.
IV. Her incontinence is most likely caused by her diabetic diarrhea.

A. I and III
B. II and IV
C. I, II, and III
D. All of the above

1011. The most abundant gas in normal flatus is nitrogen. People with excess flatus produce most of the extra gas:
A. In the small bowel from bacteria colonizing the region

B. In the duodenum by the reaction $H^+ + HCO_3^- \rightarrow CO_2 + H_2O$

C. By air swallowing

D. In the colon from the fermentation of carbohydrates producing H_2, CO_2, and CH_4

E. In the duodenum due to N_2 recruited because of the high luminal CO_2

1012. The gastrointestinal disease MOST frequently associated with tylosis is:

A. Esophageal cancer

B. Peptic ulcer disease

C. Adenomatous polyps

D. Gastric cancer

E. Achalasia

1013. Which of the following malignancies may complicate caustic ingestion?

  I. Nasopharyngeal carcinoma

  II. Gastric carcinoma

  III. Duodenal carcinoma

  IV. Esophageal carcinoma

A. I and III

B. II and IV

C. I, II, and III

D. IV only

E. All of the above

1014. Which of the following radiologic studies is of LEAST practical value in the diagnosis of abdominal abscess?

A. Chest radiograph with abdominal films

B. Abdominal ultrasonography

C. Computed tomography of the abdomen

D. Magnetic resonance imaging of the abdomen

1015. Administering fat-free parenteral nutrition can cause biochemical evidence of essential fatty acid deficiency within:

A. Two days

B. Two weeks

C. Two months

D. Six months

1016. Which of the following neurologic conditions is LEAST likely to be associated with constipation?

A. Parkinson's disease

B. Multiple sclerosis

C. Subacute combined degeneration

D. High spinal cord lesions

E. Low spinal cord lesions

1017. With regard to peritoneal malignancies, which of the following are TRUE?

A. Mesothelioma is the most common tumor.

B. The peritoneal fluid is characteristically bloody.

C. Therapeutic paracentesis is preferable to diuretics for management of ascites.

D. Pseudomyxoma peritonei has a better prognosis than other metastatic tumors.

1018. Which of the following statements concerning diabetic gastroparesis are TRUE?

A. Delayed gastric emptying, as evidenced by an abnormal saline load test, is an early complication in type I diabetics.

B. The severity of symptoms correlates well with the objective findings of motility disturbance.

C. Clinical symptoms include nausea, bloating, postprandial vomiting, and early satiety.

D. Clinical symptoms are more common with long-standing disease and increased age.

1019. Which one of the following lesions does NOT warrant endoscopic therapy in patients with upper gastrointestinal bleeding?

A. Actively bleeding gastric ulcer

B. Esophageal varices

C. Duodenal ulcer with a visible vessel

D. Duodenal ulcer with a flat pigmented spot

E. Lesion of Dieulafoy

1020. All of the following are true statements about peritoneal mesothelioma EXCEPT:

A. Most cases are benign.

B. Diagnosis usually requires laparoscopy or laparotomy.

C. Spouses of asbestos workers are at risk.

D. Optimal treatment for malignancy is chemotherapy and radiation.

1021. Hyperparathyroidism is associated with an increased risk of:

A. Gastritis

B. Pernicious anemia

C. Colon polyps

D. Peptic ulcer disease

E. Malabsorption

1022. Obesity is properly defined as:

A. Body mass index (wt/ht^2) greater than 27.8 kg/m^2

B. Body mass index (wt/ht^2) greater than 27.8 lbs/ft^2

C. 1.4 times UBW (usual body weight)

D. 1.4 times IBW (ideal body weight)

1023. Which of the following statements concerning caustic ingestion are TRUE?

  I. The lower esophageal sphincter is the most common site of esophageal stricture formation.

  II. Oropharyngeal lesions are more frequent after solid lye ingestion.

III. A careful visual examination of the oropharynx generally predicts the extent of esophageal injury.
IV. Hoarseness and stridor after caustic ingestion should be evaluated with direct laryngoscopy.

A. I and III
B. II and IV
C. I, II, and III
D. All of the above

1024. Which of the following statements about microscopic or collagenous colitis are TRUE:
A. The most frequent presenting symptom is watery diarrhea in middle age.
B. Intraepithelial lymphocytes and an infiltration of plasma cell in the lamina propria are the histologic hallmarks.
C. A thickened band of collagen may be present beneath the surface epithelium, but thickened collagen *per se* is not sufficient to produce diarrhea.
D. Both radiographic and colonoscopic appearances are usually completely normal.

1025. The incidence of hiatal hernia among the elderly of North America approximates:
A. 10%
B. 25%
C. 60%
D. 90%

1026. Medical options for treating cholestatic liver disease include:
I. Naloxone
II. Rifampin
III. Ursodiol
IV. Omeprazole

A. I and III
B. II and IV
C. I, II, and III
D. All of the above

1027. Which of the following abdominal abscess locations is LEAST favorable for catheter drainage?
A. Between the duodenum and vena cava
B. Within the pelvis
C. Between the liver and diaphragm
D. Periappendicular

1028. Which of the following pharmacologic therapies has been found to reduce mortality in patients with acute bleeding from esophageal varices?
A. Metoclopramide
B. Somatostatin
C. Vasopressin
D. Propranolol
E. None of the above

1029. Which of the following can be determined by rectal manometry?
I. The threshold for sensation of rectal distention
II. The competence of the rectoanal inhibitory reflex
III. The rectoanal contractile response
IV. Rectal compliance

A. I and III
B. II and IV
C. I, II, and III
D. All of the above

1030. Lavage of the peritoneum with 1 L of normal saline can be diagnostically useful in the setting of suspected peritonitis when clinical, biochemical, and radiographic information is nondiagnostic. Each of the following findings in the lavage fluid supports the diagnosis of peritonitis EXCEPT:
A. White blood cell count greater than 500 cells/mm^3
B. Albumin less than 0.5 g/dL
C. Bilirubin greater than serum bilirubin
D. Bacteria on Gram stain

1031. Which of the following is LEAST likely to metastasize to the gastrointestinal tract?
A. Breast cancer
B. Lung cancer
C. Thyroid cancer
D. Ovarian cancer
E. Malignant melanoma

1032. Which of the following laboratory values is LEAST likely to explain constipation?
A. Thyroid stimulating hormone level of 9.7 IU/L (normal, 1.0 to 4.0)
B. Serum calcium concentration of 11.5 mg/dl (normal, 8.4 to 10.4)
C. Serum potassium concentration of 2.9 mmol/L (normal, 3.6 to 5.0)
D. Serum gastrin level of 225 pmol/L (normal, less than 100)
E. Fasting glucose concentration of 224 mg/dl (normal, 70 to 110)

1033. In persons of normal weight, death from starvation usually occurs when what percentage of body weight has been lost?
A. 20
B. 30
C. 40
D. 50

1034. Each of the following conditions would be expected to present with the sudden onset of severe pain EXCEPT:
A. Rupture of ectopic pregnancy

B. Boerhaave's syndrome
C. Cholecystitis
D. Dissecting aortic aneurysm
E. Perforated ulcer

1035. A 20-year-old man presents with dark stools for the past week. He gives a history of frequent nosebleeds throughout childhood. On physical examination, he is pale, and multiple telangiectases are noted on his lips, tongue and digits. Rectal examination reveals melena. The MOST likely diagnosis is:
A. Henoch-Schönlein purpura
B. Osler-Weber-Rendu disease
C. CREST syndrome
D. Hemophilia
E. Hemolytic-uremic syndrome

1036. The syndrome characterized by adenomatous polyps, epidermal cysts, osteomas, fibromas, and desmoid tumors is:
A. Peutz-Jeghers syndrome
B. Gardner's syndrome
C. Cronkhite-Canada syndrome
D. Cowden's syndrome
E. Muir-Torre syndrome

1037. A 62-year-old man presents with complaints of halitosis, recurring upper respiratory illness, and worsening dysphagia. A barium swallow demonstrates a large Zenker's diverticulum. Which of the following would be valid reasons to recommend that the patient have surgery?
I. Relief of dysphagia
II. Decrease the risk of recurrent aspiration and infection
III. Freshen the patient's breath
IV. Prevent the development of carcinoma within the diverticulum

A. I and III
B. II and IV
C. I, II, and III
D. All of the above

1038. In diagnosing the presence of protein-losing enteropathy, the single test providing the BEST combination of simplicity and reliability is:
A. 24-Hour α_1-antitrypsin clearance
B. 24-Hour ^{131}I-albumin clearance
C. Upper endoscopy with biopsy of the stomach and small intestine
D. Spot α_1-antitrypsin in the stool
E. ^{51}Cr-albumin elimination test

1039. Peripheral parenteral nutrition is most commonly limited by:
A. Inadequate nutrient delivery

B. Volume restriction
C. Thrombophlebitis
D. Hyperglycemia

1040. In patients with fecal incontinence, anal manometry can directly measure which of the following?
A. Rectal sensation and compliance
B. Motor nerve supply and skeletal muscle responses
C. Basal and squeeze pressures in the anal canal
D. Rectal compliance

1041. Which one of the following tissues can BEST oxidize lipid as a fuel?
A. Erythrocytes
B. Renal medulla
C. Peripheral nerve
D. Skeletal muscle
E. Brain

1042. Conditions that can cause protein-losing enteropathy by decreasing lymphatic drainage from the intestine include each the following EXCEPT:
A. Hepatic cirrhosis
B. Tricuspid insufficiency
C. Constrictive pericarditis
D. Carcinoid syndrome
E. Atrial septal defect

1043. Which of the following have been shown to be of value in treating patients with fecal incontinence?
A. Metamucil
B. Lomotil
C. Loperamide
D. Tincture of opium

1044. Each of the following statements about peritoneal tuberculosis is true EXCEPT:
A. The lymphocyte count in the peritoneal fluid is usually elevated.
B. Laparoscopy is virtually always diagnostic.
C. Fever is uncommon.
D. Ascites may resolve with diuretics if cirrhosis is present.

1045. Oral aphthous ulcers are associated with all of the following conditions EXCEPT:
A. Inflammatory bowel disease
B. Thrush
C. Behçet's syndrome
D. Pernicious anemia
E. Prolonged fever

Section VII

Topics Involving Multiple Organs

Answers

(830–A)   **(S&F, pp. 1912–1916)**

The genetic basis of colon cancer is becoming better understood. This patient's family history is most consistent with Lynch II syndrome, in which colorectal cancer is seen in association with a number of other malignancies, often including endometrial and ovarian cancers. The genetic defect in Lynch II syndrome is failure to correct base-pair mismatches during DNA replication, causing point mutations affecting one of several editing enzymes. Although the brother's adenomas could have been due to an attenuated *APC* gene, the endometrial cancer in his mother makes it much more likely that the genetic syndrome is Lynch II. The young ages of both the mother and the brother strongly suggest that this kindred may be part of a Lynch family even though only two members have cancer.

References

Bronner, C. E., Baker, S. M., Morrison, P. T., et al. Mutation in the DNA mismatch repair gene homologue hMLH1 is associated with hereditary nonpolyposis colon cancer. Nature 368:258, 1994.

Giardiello, F. M., Krush, A. J., Petersen, G. M., et al. Phenotypic variability of familial adenomatous polyposis in 11 unrelated families with identical APC gene mutation. Gastroenterology 106:1542, 1994.

Leach, F. S., Nicolaides, N. C., Papadopoulos, N., et al. Mutations of a mutS homolog in hereditary nonpolyposis colorectal cancer. Cell 75:1215, 1993.

Lynch, H. T., Smyrk, T. C., Watson, P., et al. Genetics, natural history, tumor spectrum, and pathology of hereditary nonpolyposis colorectal cancer: An updated review, Gastroenterology 104:1535, 1993.

Nicolaides, N. C., Papadopoulos, N., Liu, B., et al. Mutations of two PMS homologues in hereditary nonpolyposis colon cancer. Nature 371:75, 1994.

Spirio, L., Olschwang, S., Groden, J., et al. Alleles of the APC gene: An attenuated form of familial polyposis. Cell 75:951, 1993.

(831–D)   **(S&F, pp. 54–60)**

Patients who are replication error positive (RER +) have a much better prognosis than those who are RER negative. RER + cancers tend to accumulate genetic abnormalities by a series of point mutations, whereas RER − cancers tend to accumulate their genetic abnormalities by deleting large segments of DNA.

Reference

Thibodeau, S. N., Bren, G., and Schaid, D. Microsatellite instability in cancer of the proximal colon. Science 260:816, 1993.

(832–A, B, C, F)   **(S&F, pp. 353–354)**

Aspirin and certain other NSAIDs have been shown to reduce the rate of colon cancer in controlled clinical trials by up to 50%. This effect does not become evident until after 10 to 20 years of regular use, presumably reflecting slow progression of the adenoma–carcinoma sequence. Maximum effects are seen with four to six aspirin tablets per week. The presumed mechanism is inhibition of cyclooxygenase-2 (COX-2), an inducible form of this enzyme that regulates growth in colonic epithelial tissues and is increased in most colorectal cancers. The beneficial effects of aspirin on cancer mortality are largely offset by increased mortality from cerebrovascular accidents.

Reference

Garewal, H. S. Aspirin in the prevention of colorectal cancer. Ann. Intern. Med. 121:303, 1994.

(833–C)   **(S&F, pp. 200–201)**

Upper endoscopy should be the first step in the management of this patient but would not likely visualize an aortoenteric fistula if present, even if the distal duodenum is visualized. It would, however, identify other reasons for the bleeding. Angiography is usually not helpful unless there is active bleeding at the time of the injection. Abdominal computed tomography is the single best imaging study to identify an aortoenteric fistula, but only one third of these lesions is identified preoperatively.

(834–B)   **(S&F, pp. 381–384)**

Bone marrow transplantation may produce all of the gastrointestinal problems associated with liver transplantation and several others as well. As in liver transplantation, cytomegalovirus is the most common viral pathogen, and hepatitis C may progress to cirrhosis within 5 to 10 years. Unlike liver transplantation, hepatic veno-occlusive disease (VOD) is very common, occurring in up to 50% of patients, with severe disease in 25%. VOD commonly presents as ascites within three weeks of marrow transplantation. Acute graft-versus-host disease (GVHD) may occur anywhere in the gastrointestinal tract between the gastroesophageal junction and the anus. Because differentiation from infectious enteritis is difficult clinically, mucosal biopsy is usually needed even if the patient has known GVHD on skin biopsy.

(835–A)   **(S&F, p. 184)**

When evaluating constipation, the most important historical information is the time of onset. Most patients who have congenital causes have had difficulties with their bowel habits from birth. Constipation of recent onset is frequently due to a new pathologic process, either organic or psychological. Colonic malignancy is the most worrisome possibility but is unlikely if the constipation has been present for two years or more. Association with pain, consistency of the stools, and dietary and exercise habits may provide clues to the etiology but are less useful.

(836–C) **(S&F, p. 443)**

Erythema nodosum is a common inflammatory process of the subcutaneous fat with a marked predilection for women. Lesions appear as approximately 1-cm shiny, tender, deep red nodules on the anterior shins. The most common causes are infections (streptococcal, fungal, and tuberculous), medications (especially oral contraceptives), and leukemia. Seven percent of patients with Crohn's disease and 4% of patients with ulcerative colitis develop erythema nodosum. There is no known association with adenocarcinoma.

(837–A) **(S&F, pp. 128–130)**

This patient's stool osmotic gap is 30 mOsm/kg [290 – 2(40 + 90)]. High electrolyte concentrations in the setting of a stool osmolarity gap of less than 50 is a classic finding of secretory diarrhea. The only disease listed that causes a secretory diarrhea is villous adenoma.

(838–C) **(S&F, pp. 2015–2017)**

Intravenous heparin significantly reduces progression and recurrence of thrombosis as well as mortality. Exploratory laparotomy should be limited to patients who present with peritoneal findings or those who develop progressive deterioration on heparin therapy. Angiographic administration of papaverine may be helpful in patients believed to have marginally viable bowel at the time of laparotomy.

(839–A, D) **(S&F, pp. 114–115)**

Gastric emptying, particularly of solids, appears to be delayed in 30% to 80% of dyspeptic patients. Cisapride improves symptoms in 65% to 90% of patients, compared with only 13% to 42% for placebo. Whereas cisapride works well for all patients, H_2 receptor antagonists work best for patients with reflux-like or ulcer-like symptoms. Available data are insufficient to implicate *Helicobacter pylori* in dyspepsia. Eradication of *H. pylori* does not improve symptoms significantly better than placebo and may make some patients feel worse. These trials are complicated by a very high placebo response rate (30%–60%). Trials of cisapride have shown symptom improvement in 60% to 90% of patients compared with 5% to 60% on placebo. However, there are few studies comparing cisapride with other prokinetic agents, and those few that exist suggest similar effectiveness. Domperidone is the most extensively studied agent for treating dysmotility-like dyspepsia but is not available in the United States. Use of H_2 receptor antagonists for dyspepsia is widespread, with response rates (35%–80%) better than placebo in only about one half of reported trials. Patients with ulcer-like dyspepsia may benefit most from use of H_2 receptor antagonists. Limited data suggest that the clinical response to omeprazole is only 15% to 20% when care is used to exclude patients with reflux-like symptoms. Because of their excellent safety profile, most experts would advocate limited trials of H_2 receptor antagonists for ulcer-like or reflux-like dyspepsia, while reserving prokinetic agents for patients with dysmotility-like dyspepsia.

(840–C) **(S&F, p. 135)**

This patient's stool osmotic gap is 230 mOsm/kg [290 – 2(20 + 10)]. A gap of more than 125 mOsm in the setting of a stool sodium of less than 60 mEq/L suggests the presence of a nonabsorbable, osmotically active substance such as lactulose, magnesium, sorbitol, or polyethylene glycol. The other choices can cause diarrhea but generally with little or no osmotic gap.

(841–A, B, C) **(S&F, pp. 200–201)**

Endoscopy is the most accurate means of localizing a gastrointestinal bleeding site and can provide a direct treatment by coaptive coagulation or injection therapy. Because endoscopy can potentially improve patient outcome, it should be performed early in the course of hemorrhage. Stigmata associated with a high risk of rebleeding (>50% in 48 hours) include an adherent fresh clot in an ulcer base, a pigmented protuberance (signifying a visible vessel), or a visible vessel itself. Endoscopy has been shown to decrease patient transfusion requirements and hospital stay, but not patient mortality. Initial therapy in a patient who is bleeding should always be volume assessment and resuscitation. Once the patient's condition has been stabilized, diagnostic tests to identify the source of bleeding can be started.

(842–B) **(S&F, pp. 387–405, 1860)**

Immunosuppression such as in acquired immunodeficiency syndrome (AIDS) is associated with increased risk of small intestinal malignancy. Kaposi's sarcoma and lymphoma are the most common forms in AIDS patients. Kaposi's sarcoma is often clinically silent and rarely causes any gastrointestinal symptoms, with the exception of occasional fecal blood loss. The radiographic findings of small intestinal involvement are nonspecific, being consistent with a variety of submucosal infiltrative diseases. Skin lesions of Kaposi's sarcoma are almost universally present in patients with gastrointestinal tract involvement.

(843–C) **(S&F, pp. 87–88)**

A common cause of abdominal pain, fever, and diarrhea in neutropenic patients is neutropenic enterocolitis (typhlitis). The pathogenesis is unknown. Any part of the bowel may be involved with edema, inflammation, necrosis, and ulceration. Treatment is supportive. However, surgery may be required for acute complications such as perforation. The main determinant of survival is normalization of the granulocyte count.

(844–C) **(S&F, p. 136)**

Whereas all of the diseases listed can cause steatorrhea, the severe fat malabsorption seen in this patient is most typical of pancreatic insufficiency. Zollinger-Ellison syndrome does not generally cause this degree of malabsorption, although some fat malabsorption can occur because of acid inactivation of pancreatic enzymes. Likewise, small intestine mucosal diseases cause fluid malabsorption as well as steatorrhea, so stool is more watery and voluminous and the fat concentration is accordingly lower. A fecal fat output greater than 14 g/24 hr and a fecal fat concentration greater than 8 g/100 g stool suggests pancreatic insufficiency.

(845–A)   **(S&F, pp. 1504–1511)**

Because the suspicion of pancreatic insufficiency is high, the best initial approach is to exclude small intestinal disease. The best screening test for this is the D-xylose absorption test, the result of which is typically normal in patients with pancreatic insufficiency. Choices B and C address the possibility of bacterial overgrowth, an unlikely diagnosis in this patient. Esophagogastroduodenoscopy with small bowel biopsy (not listed as an option) could be considered but is expensive. Endoscopic retrograde cholangiopancreatography (ERCP) (not listed as an option) would be reasonable, but its expense dictates exclusion of small bowel disease first. ERCP has a high sensitivity for detection of ductal irregularities consistent with chronic pancreatitis, which is the most likely cause of this patient's pancreatic insufficiency.

(846–B)   **(S&F, pp. 206–207)**

A "visible vessel" or adherent clot correlates with an approximately 50% risk of rebleeding within 48 hours. In contrast, a flat red spot or oozing from an otherwise clean-based ulcer is associated with less than 4% chance of rebleeding. Ulcer size does not correlate with risk of rebleeding unless other stigmata such as clot or visible vessel are present.

(847–D)   **(S&F, p. 334)**

Persons smuggling drugs may ingest packaged quantities of cocaine or narcotics, often in latex condoms, expecting them to pass. Numerous reports have dealt with their management. Administration of cathartics is controversial. Endoscopic removal is unwise because of the potential for rupture on manipulation. Initial observation is warranted. If the offending boluses remain in the intestine for more than 48 hours, surgery is often advised. Development of symptoms may warrant prompt surgical removal.

(848–C)   **(S&F, p. 447)**

Acanthosis nigricans is a velvety hyperplasia and hyperpigmentation of the skin of the neck and axillae, often associated with multiple skin tags. The condition is sometimes hereditary and often associated with obesity or other endocrinopathies. When acanthosis nigricans develops abruptly in middle or old age, an underlying malignancy should be suspected. Usually the skin changes coincide with symptoms or signs of the tumor but may precede it in 25% of cases. Abdominal adenocarcinomas account for 85% of the associated malignancies, with gastric carcinoma representing over 60%.

(849–C)   **(S&F, p. 418)**

A striking paraneoplastic syndrome that affects the gastrointestinal tract is disordered motility with intestinal pseudo-obstruction. This rare condition is most frequently associated with small cell carcinoma of the lung, but it also has been described with pulmonary carcinoid and undifferentiated tumor of unknown primary. The onset of symptoms may predate the discovery of the tumor by several years.

(850–C)   **(S&F, p. 315)**

Patients with progressive systemic sclerosis or scleroderma have small bowel dysmotility with delayed transit and associated jejunal diverticula. As a result, bacterial overgrowth ensues, resulting in vitamin B_{12} deficiency and anemia. Folate is produced and released by the bacteria within the gut. Treatment includes monthly vitamin B_{12} injections and intermittent courses of broad-spectrum oral antibiotics.

(851–C)   **(S&F, p. 288)**

Anorexia nervosa usually begins in the teen years, primarily in women, and most often four to five years after menarche. Bulimia begins at a later age than anorexia nervosa, usually before 25 years. However, presentation to medical attention may not take place until the woman is in her third or fourth decade of life.

(852–A, C)   **(S&F, pp. 103–104)**

Although gastroesophageal reflux (GER) has been thought to cause upper respiratory symptoms by recurrent bouts of microaspiration, this mechanism has been inconsistently demonstrated in human subjects. Better evidence exists in support of a vagally mediated reflex as the cause of GER-induced bronchospasm. The typical symptoms of pyrosis and regurgitation are frequently absent in suspected cases of GER-induced asthma; indeed, half of all adult asthmatics demonstrate an abnormally high frequency and duration of acid reflux when studied by ambulatory pH monitoring. Bronchodilators lower the lower esophageal pressure and thereby worsen GER. Thus, late-age and late-onset wheezing that develops in a patient with no prior history of allergies and that is made worse by bronchodilators is suggestive of GER-induced asthma. Some patients with respiratory symptoms due to GER will have abnormalities noted at laryngoscopy, including vocal cord edema, erythema or hyperemia, vocal cord ulcers, and/or granulomatous changes.

(853–A, C, D)   **(S&F, p. 200)**

The unstable vital signs and the presence of maroon stools warrant close monitoring. Patients with Ehlers-Danlos syndrome may bleed from vascular malformations, and thus the history provides a clue as to the possible source of bleeding. A nonbloody aspirate does not exclude bleeding from a postpyloric lesion. False-negative results can be seen in up to 16% of patients with a confirmed upper gastrointestinal source of bleeding. Furthermore, nasogastric aspirates that are reported to be "bilious" only contain bile about half of the time. Testing of nonbloody aspirates for occult blood is unreliable, because trauma caused by tube passage often releases small amounts of blood.

(854–B)   ***(S&F, pp. 198–199)***

The admitting hematocrit can be normal even in patients with massive bleeding because red blood cells and plasma are lost in the same amounts from the intravascular space. The hematocrit does not fall until extracellular fluid enters the intravascular compartment to restore volume. Patients who require more than 5 units of blood have been found to have a higher mortality. Hematochezia is seen with upper gastrointestinal bleeding only if bleeding is brisk.

Reference

Silverstein, F. E., Gilbert, D. A., Tedesco, F. J., et al. The national ASGE survey on upper gastrointestinal bleeding: II. Clinical prognostic factors. Gastrointest. Endosc. 27:80, 1981.

(855–All are true)   ***(S&F, p. 60)***

Vogelstein's 1988 paper documented the importance of the accumulation of genetic abnormalities as opposed to the sequence of abnormalities in the genesis of colorectal cancer. The replication error–positive (RER +) phenotype appears to be associated with deficiencies in the *hMLH1* gene complex, which serves a genetic proofreading function. Inability to repair base-pair mismatches during DNA replication is therefore thought to be a major mechanism by which these genetic abnormalities may accumulate. Though DNA-mismatch repair gene mutations are universal in hereditary nonpolyposis colorectal cancer; they have also been found in sporadic cancers of the esophagus, stomach, pancreas, and colon.

References

Bronner, C. E., Baker, S. M., Morrison, P. T., et al. Mutation in the DNA mismatch repair gene homologue hMLH1 is associated with hereditary nonpolyposis colon cancer. Nature 368:258, 1994.
Vogelstein, B., Feron, E. R., Hamilton, S. R., et al. Genetic alterations during colorectal-tumor development. N. Engl. J. Med. 319:525, 1988.

(856–D)   ***(S&F, pp. 1543–1544)***

Patients with irritable bowel syndrome and chronic idiopathic constipation commonly present with no specific historical or physical findings. One half of women with functional gastrointestinal disorders are victims of sexual abuse. Somatic reactions to sexual abuse include abdominal pain and constipation. Patients with Munchausen's syndrome may deny that they defecate and often undergo surgery for the false diagnosis of constipation. Constipation of recent onset is frequently due to significant pathology. When constipation has been present for two years or more, colonic malignancy is unlikely to be the cause.

(857–D)   ***(S&F, pp. 180, 1536–1548)***

Constipated patients seen by a primary care physician should be reassured if the history and physical examination are not suggestive of any specific diagnosis, a complete blood cell count is normal, and stools are negative for occult blood. The most common diagnosis in this setting is irritable bowel syndrome. A trial of high-fiber diet should precede any further investigation. A diary may be helpful because a difference in stool frequency may be found between recalled and recorded data. Occasionally, obsessive-compulsive disorder may be recognized by how data are recorded. Also, keeping a diary may help this patient identify associations with events in her life. If hidden psychological trauma is the cause, only through a solid patient–doctor relationship will this be ventilated. Endoscopic evaluation is needed only if her condition is refractory to these approaches.

Reference

Camilleri, M., Thompson, W. G., Fleshman, J. W., Pemberton, J. H. Clinical management of intractable constipation. Ann. Intern. Med. 121:520, 1994.

(858–C)   ***(S&F, pp. 144–146)***

Patients with factitious diarrhea are usually women and often have no obvious psychological problems; thus the diagnosis can at times be very difficult. Tests for surreptitious laxative abuse (including alkalinization of stool to detect phenolphthalein and stool electrolytes to calculate an osmotic gap) may be helpful. A stool osmolarity of less than 100 mOsm/kg suggests that water has been added to simulate diarrhea.

(859–B)   ***(S&F, pp. 121–123)***

Of the conditions listed, only acute fatty liver of pregnancy is associated with hypertension and peripheral edema. Liver function tests should be checked in this patient and liver biopsy considered if the aminotransferase levels are elevated. The characteristic histologic finding is microvesicular fat. The only effective treatment is immediate delivery of the fetus.

(860–C)   ***Timing of emesis (S&F, p. 119)***
                    Psychogenic vomiting (S&F, pp. 123–124)

Psychogenic vomiting is characterized by long-standing vomiting that occurs during or shortly after meals. There is often a family history of vomiting, and the vomiting is of little concern to the patient. Vomiting during meals may also occur in patients with pyloric channel ulcers, owing to pylorospasm.

(861–D)   ***(S&F, pp. 82–88)***

Common causes of upper abdominal pain include diseases of the liver, gallbladder, pancreas, stomach, and proximal intestine. However, acute diseases of the chest may closely mimic primary diseases of the abdomen. Myocardial ischemia (as this patient was later found to have), pneumonia, and pulmonary embolus should be considered. Diverticulitis usually presents with lower abdominal pain.

(862–D) *(S&F, pp. 206–207)*

The presence of a visible vessel (sentinel clot) in the ulcer crater indicates a high risk of rebleeding (43%–55%), even if the lesion is not actively bleeding at the time of endoscopy. Accordingly, such lesions should be treated with endoscopic hemostatic therapy and monitored closely for at least 24 hours, ideally in an intensive care setting. Approximately one third will require urgent surgery for rebleeding if treated with acid-reducing drugs alone. The presence of an adherent clot or flat red spot in the ulcer crater indicates an intermediate risk of rebleeding (10%–22%). Such patients should remain hospitalized for at least 24 hours after bleeding subsides.

(863–D) *(S&F, pp. 340–341)*

Batteries larger than 15 mm are more likely to result in injury. Any structural abnormalities may prevent or delay passage and increase the risk of local tissue damage. The majority of button batteries pass through the gastrointestinal tract within 18 to 72 hours, but perforation of the esophagus can occur in as little as six hours. The only reported fatalities have occurred with esophageal impaction.

(864–1-A, 2-C, 3-D, 4-B) *(S&F, p. 223)*

Other than Gilbert's syndrome, hereditary disorders of hepatic bilirubin metabolism are uncommon. They are characterized by impaired excretion of bilirubin in the setting of reduced or absent hepatic UDP-glucuronyltransferase activity. Only type I Crigler-Najjar syndrome is associated with a poor prognosis, with death in infancy common from kernicterus. The inheritance pattern is autosomal recessive for all but type II Crigler-Najjar syndrome, in which it is autosomal dominant.

(865–1-D, 2-C, 3-A, 4-B) *(S&F, pp. 2013–2015)*

Emboli that lodge in the superior mesenteric artery generally originate from mural thrombi in the left atrium or ventricle. Thus, patients at risk for superior mesenteric artery emboli would include those with chronic atrial fibrillation or known left ventricular aneurysm. A variety of conditions are associated with nonocclusive mesenteric ischemia. Major precipitating factors include acute pulmonary edema, cardiac arrhythmia, and shock. Superior mesenteric artery thrombosis occurs in regions affected by atherosclerosis. Patients at risk generally have atherosclerotic disease involving the coronary, cerebrovascular, or peripheral arterial circulation. The list of conditions associated with mesenteric venous thrombosis is long (cf. Table 118–1). Prominent causes include hypercoagulable states, such as oral contraceptive use; myeloproliferative disorders (e.g., polycythemia vera); and deficiencies of antithrombin III, protein S, and protein C.

(866–D) *(S&F, pp. 335–336)*

The severity of caustic injury to the gastrointestinal tract is dependent on several variables: type of agent (strongly alkaline and acidic agents are more injurious); concentration; quantity; physical state (fed versus fasting); and the duration of exposure.

(867–A-T, B-F, C-T, D-F, E-T) *(S&F, pp. 176–177)*

Self-reported constipation in the United States is higher in blacks and women and increases with age. In contrast to conventional wisdom, within a population there is no correlation between stool frequency and dietary fiber, nor does vigorous exercise increase stool frequency in healthy people.

(868–C) *(S&F, p. 99)*

The complaint of intermittent solid food dysphagia is typical for patients with Schatzki's ring, which is also referred to as a mucosal or B-ring. They may also present with sudden complete esophageal obstruction without antecedent symptoms.

(869–D) *(S&F, p. 2029)*

Dieulafoy's lesion, a nonulcerating erosion of a persistent caliber (unusually large) artery through the gastric mucosa, is typically found about 6 cm distal to the gastroesophageal junction, where the arteries are largest in caliber. Bleeding is not usually heralded by gastrointestinal symptoms, and emergency surgery may be necessary to localize a bleeding site, because endoscopy may miss the lesion if it is not actively bleeding at the time. A variety of endoscopic techniques are available to achieve hemostasis, but the long-term efficacy of these interventions remains to be established. Dieulafoy's lesion is more common in men than women by a 2:1 ratio.

(870–A) *(S&F, pp. 371–372)*

Intestinal lymphangiectasia is probably a congenital disorder resulting from a malunion of intestinal lymphatics and is characterized by dilatation of intestinal lacteals and the formation of lymphenteric fistulas. These structural changes cause leakage of lymph containing chylomicrons, protein, and lymphocytes into the intestinal lumen, leading to steatorrhea, protein-losing enteropathy, and enteric lymphocyte losses. Clinical manifestations include asymmetric or symmetric peripheral edema and nonbloody diarrhea, with about half of patients eventually developing chylous effusions. Fat malabsorption is usually mild, and most patients absorb more than 80% of ingested fat. Weight loss and fat-soluble vitamin deficiencies are uncommon unless severe steatorrhea or anorexia is present. Most patients have minimal gastrointestinal symptoms, but some complain of abdominal pain, distention, nausea, vomiting, and diarrhea. The diagnosis of intestinal lymphangiectasia can be confirmed by a peroral jejunal biopsy demonstrating dilated submucosal lacteals.

(871–A) **(S&F, pp. 97–98)**

Globus sensation (formerly globus hystericus) is a feeling of a lump or tightness in the throat unrelated to swallowing. Up to 46% of the general population have experienced the sensation at one time or another. Globus sensation typically occurs between meals, and swallowing solids or large liquid boluses may offer temporary relief. Dysphagia and odynophagia are not present. Modern manometric studies have consistently shown the upper esophageal sphincter to be functioning normally.

(872–C) **(S&F, pp. 98–99)**

Oropharyngeal or "transfer" dysphagia is typically noted within one second of a swallow and occurs equally with liquids and solids. Achalasia is usually associated with weight loss, in contrast to esophageal rings, webs, and peptic strictures. Daily complaints of dysphagia are not typically noted with rings or webs. Instead, the symptoms typically occur intermittently. Dysphagia with weight loss and pyrosis is more suggestive of a benign peptic stricture than a malignant one.

(873–D) **(S&F, pp. 393–394)**

A careful history and physical examination is always indicated when evaluating any patient with diarrhea. Initial workup of diarrhea in patients with the acquired immunodeficiency syndrome should include three stool specimens for ova and parasites, stool for culture, and acid-fast stain for *Cryptosporidium*. If these tests provide no diagnosis, sigmoidoscopy with biopsies of any abnormal area (or random biopsy of rectal mucosa if no abnormalities are apparent) should be performed.

(874–C) **(S&F, p. 401)**

Mycobacterium avium-intracellulare infection is the most common specific hepatic disease in persons with the acquired immunodeficiency syndrome, with an incidence of up to 46%. The pathologic hallmark is the presence of poorly formed granulomas containing acid-fast bacilli with foamy histiocytes.

(875–D) **(S&F, pp. 416–417)**

Nausea with or without vomiting is a common, usually self-limited symptom of early pregnancy. Hyperemesis gravidarum is reserved for first-trimester patients with persistent, severe nausea and vomiting leading to a reduction of 55 or more in body weight and disturbed fluid and electrolyte balance. Gastroesophageal reflux occurs in 30% to 80% of women during pregnancy and typically worsens as pregnancy progresses. Numerous studies have shown abnormal esophageal motility and diminished lower esophageal sphincter pressures. Constipation is also common and may reflect smooth muscle inhibition by progesterone. Gallbladder motility is decreased by estrogen and progesterone during pregnancy, possibly accounting for the increased incidence of cholelithiasis in pregnant women. In contrast, pancreatitis is infrequent.

(876–C) **(S&F, p. 225)**

Several cholestatic disorders are associated with pregnancy. These include hyperemesis gravidarum, which is generally a self-limited disorder of the first trimester occurring in approximately 10% of cases. Liver failure is not a feature of this illness. Intrahepatic cholestasis of pregnancy typically occurs in the third trimester, presents as pruritus, and is only infrequently associated with jaundice. A far more serious syndrome is acute fatty liver of pregnancy. This metabolic disorder characteristically occurs in the third trimester and is characterized by infiltration of hepatocytes with microvesicular fat. When jaundice is present it is usually accompanied by nausea, abdominal pain, and encephalopathy. The disorder may be fatal unless the pregnancy is brought to an end. Preeclampsia, a microvascular disorder of the third trimester heralded by hypertension and proteinuria, affects the liver in approximately 10% of cases. A particularly severe form, the HELLP syndrome, is associated with hemolysis and thrombocytopenia.

(877–B) **(S&F, pp. 397–398)**

An empirical initial approach in the management of odynophagia in most patients with the acquired immunodeficiency syndrome is reasonable and should be directed at eradicating candidal infection. Therefore, either ketoconazole, fluconazole, or topical antifungal agents should be used. Ketoconazole may be less effective than fluconazole because of the high prevalence of achlorhydria in human immunodeficiency virus infection, which impairs its absorption. If symptoms persist after empirical therapy, endoscopy with brushings and biopsy should be performed.

(878–D) **(S&F, p. 442)**

Epidermolysis bullosa is a heterogeneous group of disorders of skin fragility characterized by the formation of blisters with minimal trauma. They have been divided into dystrophic, junctional, and simplex forms. Oral erosions, caries, and gingival involvement are almost universal. Besides oral erosions, esophageal strictures are the most common gastrointestinal complication in the dystrophic form. They commonly occur in the upper third of the esophagus but also may be found in the lower third. Strictures are most likely induced by repeated trauma from food and gastric contents.

(879–B) **(S&F, pp. 414–415)**

Prokinetic agents increase gastric motor activity and are useful in the treatment of gastroparesis. Metoclopramide and domperidone are dopamine antagonists and stimulate acetylcholine release in the myenteric plexus. These agents increase gastric tone and accelerate emptying. Cisapride increases acetylcholine release from postganglionic neurons of the gut and stimulates gastric emptying. Erythromycin has been shown to be a motilin receptor agonist. In contrast, cholinergic drugs (such as bethanechol) have no effect on either phase 3 of the migratory motor complex or on gastric transit times after meals.

(880–1-A, 2-E, 3-B, 4-C, 5-D) (*S&F, p. 240*)

Depletion of vitamin A causes night blindness and follicular keratosis. Thiamine deficiency causes beriberi and Wernicke's syndrome, with the latter particularly common in alcoholics. Wernicke's syndrome is characterized by dementia, disturbed ocular motility, ataxia, and peripheral polyneuropathy. Zinc depletion results in acrodermatitis enteropathica, a disorder often confused with psoriasis. Alopecia and pustular and vesicular lesions over extensor areas are prominent. Iron deficiency is a classic cause of cheilosis. Vitamin D malabsorption leads to hypocalcemia and secondary hyperparathyroidism.

(881–B) (*S&F, pp. 260–261*)

The predominant short-chain fatty acids (SCFAs) in humans are acetate, propionate, and butyrate. They are produced primarily by bacterial fermentation of undigested carbohydrates (mostly starch and fiber) in the colon. About 90% of the 25 g of unabsorbed carbohydrates that enter the colon each day are metabolized to SCFAs and absorbed as energy substrates. The colon can salvage as much as 500 kcal of unabsorbed carbohydrate daily. This process is particularly important for recapturing lost calories in patients with malabsorption. SCFAs normally provide 60% to 70% of the energy needs of the colonic mucosa. Absorption of SCFAs is coupled with sodium-proton exchange and increases colonocyte sodium and water influx. Diarrhea associated with refeeding malnourished patients, antibiotic use, and abdominal surgery may be related to cellular energy deficits and impaired sodium absorption caused by SCFA deficiency.

(882–B) (*S&F, pp. 155–156*)

Sorbitol is a sugar alcohol found in many low-calorie sweeteners that is passed into the colon and fermented by colonic bacteria. Fructose and lactose are important dietary carbohydrates that are frequently malabsorbed and fermented by colonic bacteria. Lactulose is useful clinically both in treating patients with hepatic encephalopathy and in measuring oral-cecal transit time because it is fermented by colonic bacteria as well. Glucose is the correct answer because whereas it is useful in breath hydrogen testing to detect bacterial overgrowth in the jejunum, glucose is so efficiently absorbed that it never reaches the colon. The only important exception is in the case of a patient with a gastrocolic fistula.

(883–B) (*S&F, p. 268*)

This patient has classic findings of Wernicke's encephalopathy. The encephalopathy results from a thiamine deficiency and is common in patients with poor nutrition who abuse alcohol.

(884–1-D, 2-C, 3-A, 4-B) (*S&F, p. 302*)

Flumazenil can reverse all behavioral effects of diazepam or midazolam and shortens the recovery period after conscious sedation. It does not reverse respiratory depression and must be used with caution in patients who are benzodiazepine dependent or who have a history of seizures. Fentanyl, an opioid analgesic, has an analgesic effect lasting 30 to 60 minutes. However, respiratory depression may persist longer than the analgesic effect, as with most narcotic sedatives. Midazolam, a short-acting benzodiazepine central nervous system depressant, has both sedative and amnestic effects. Sedation after intravenous use is achieved in three to five minutes, and up to 80% of patients receiving intravenous midazolam have no recall of the endoscopic procedure. Droperidol, a neuroleptic agent, has both sedative and antiemetic effects. Patients with active substance abuse or who are at risk for paradoxical agitation with benzodiazepine administration appear to benefit significantly from addition of droperidol to the usual conscious sedation narcotic and benzodiazepine.

(885–E) (*S&F, p. 225*)

A number of drugs produce a histologically bland intrahepatic cholestasis. Estrogens inhibit the hepatocyte plasma membrane Na^+/K^+ pump, an important modulator of solute transport from blood to bile, and perturb the function of organic anion transporters by decreasing membrane fluidity. Cholestasis secondary to oral contraceptives usually develops within two months of the initiation of therapy. Jaundice is usually accompanied by pruritus, whereas fever, rash, and arthralgias are absent. Anabolic steroids can produce a syndrome clinically indistinguishable from that of estrogen-induced cholestasis. The clinical features of cholestasis due to total parenteral nutrition are similar.

(886–E) (*S&F, p. 124*)

Rumination is the process of regurgitating food (one mouthful at a time) from the stomach to the mouth, chewing the food, and then reswallowing it. When present in infants, it is often associated with failure to thrive, marasmus, and even death. Rumination is often accompanied by reflux, but surgery should be avoided. It may respond to various behavior modification therapies.

(887–D) (*S&F, p. 183*)

Many drugs induce constipation. Among the most common are opiates, anticholinergics, hematinics (especially iron), diuretics, and antacids (calcium and aluminum compounds). Magnesium-based antacids commonly produce diarrhea.

(888–C) (*S&F, pp. 184, 174–195*)

Urinary tract problems are common among constipated patients and may disappear after successful treatment of constipation. Urinary tract infections are more frequent among constipated patients. Constipation is also associated with frequency, urgency, hesitancy, stress incontinence, nocturia, and enuresis. Bladder calculi, increased bladder capacity, atonic bladder, vesicoureteral reflux, and dilatation of the upper renal tract may also occur. Glomerulonephritis is not associated with constipation.

(889–B) **(S&F, p. 413)**

Hypothyroidism is encountered in about 25% of patients with primary biliary cirrhosis. Hashimoto's disease is the most common cause in these cases. Pernicious anemia may also occur in patients with primary biliary cirrhosis who also have hypothyroidism.

(890–B) **(S&F, p. 425)**

Polyarteritis nodosa, a disease of small- and medium-sized arteries, exhibits a mean age of presentation of 45 years. Abdominal pain is present in 44% of afflicted individuals. Small bowel involvement is common (especially the jejunum), and ischemic injury to the small bowel causes hemorrhage (6%), perforation (5%), and infarction (1.4%). Other commonly involved gastrointestinal organs include the gallbladder and pancreas. Hepatitis B–related polyarteritis nodosa is an early complication of hepatitis B and is indistinguishable from classic polyarteritis nodosa.

(891–D) **(S&F, pp. 343–349, 630)**

Most studies indicate that corticosteroids alone do not significantly increase ulcer risk. However, corticosteroids potentiate the ulcer risk of NSAIDs when given in combination. The toxicity of aspirin (acetylsalicylic acid) to the gastroduodenal mucosa is in large part attributed to its acetyl group, which inactivates the cyclooxygenase enzyme and leads to a suppression of mucosal prostaglandins. Salicylate compounds that lack the acetyl group (such as the nonacetylated salicylates) do not affect mucosal cyclooxygenase. In short-term blinded clinical studies (up to three months) of nonacetylated salicylate usage, no gastroduodenal ulcers have been noted. Likewise, bismuth subsalicylate (Pepto-Bismol) lacks an acetyl group. At pH less than 3.5, gastric acid reacts with the complex, forming bismuth oxychloride and liberating salicylate. Many drugs may cause dyspeptic symptoms, including digoxin and theophylline. There is no evidence, however, that these drugs increase ulcer risk.

(892–A) **(S&F, pp. 2039–2040)**

In the setting of ambulatory peritoneal dialysis, over two thirds of peritonitis is caused by gram-positive cocci, mostly skin flora. Although 75% of patients have abdominal pain and tenderness, only a third are febrile. Virtually all will have a cloudy peritoneal effluent.

(893–B) **(S&F, p. 416)**

The most prominent abnormality of the liver in diabetes is steatosis. It is present in 21% to 78% of patients. When present, it reflects long-term poor glucose control. Thirteen percent of 1392 patients with fatty liver studied in Japan had diabetes. The degree of fatty metamorphosis parallels the obesity of diabetics. With increasing amounts of fat, steatohepatitis with Mallory hyaline and fibrosis may be seen. An association between steatonecrosis and type 5 hyperlipoproteinemia in insulin-dependent diabetes has been described; however, the pathogenesis is not clear.

(894–A, B) **(S&F, p. 403)**

The etiology of cholangiopathy associated with the acquired immunodeficiency syndrome (AIDS) is unknown, although many cases are associated with cytomegalovirus, *Cryptosporidium,* or both. Microsporidia has also been identified in isolated cases. Ductular changes include papillary stenosis, a sclerosing cholangitis–like lesion, or long extrahepatic strictures. Sphincterotomy for papillary stenosis in AIDS cholangiopathy usually results in symptomatic improvement in patients. However, liver function tests will usually continue to rise, probably reflecting progression of intrahepatic disease.

(895–C) **(S&F, pp. 305–306)**

Perforation of the esophagus or stomach is rare (0.03%—0.1% of procedures) and usually occurs during blind passage of the endoscope. Predisposing factors include cervical osteoarthritic spurs, surgical anastomoses, strictures, inflammation due to caustic ingestion or neoplasm, or balloon dilatation during therapeutic endoscopy. Bleeding is exceedingly rare (0.03% of procedures) but can occur due to Mallory-Weiss tear or after sclerotherapy, polypectomy, or stricture dilatation. Bacteremia can also occur, particularly with high-risk upper endoscopic procedures of esophageal dilatation and sclerotherapy.

(896–B) **(S&F, pp. 221–223)**

Of the hereditary unconjugated hyperbilirubinemias, Gilbert's syndrome is the most common. It affects 5% to 7% of white adults in the United States and is characterized by decreased hepatic clearance of unconjugated bilirubin. The bilirubin concentration can be further increased with fasting or dehydration and is decreased after the administration of phenobarbital. The diagnosis is usually established by repeated finding of normal liver function tests, including normal serum bile acid levels, in an otherwise healthy individual. It is a benign condition requiring no further workup.

(897–C) **(S&F, pp. 125–126)**

Domperidone does not readily cross the blood–brain barrier and causes fewer central nervous system effects than the other drugs listed.

(898–C) **(S&F, p. 2009)**

The splenic flexure and sigmoid colon, in particular, have limited collateral circulation. Ischemic events in these two "watershed areas" are more common than in the duodenum and rectum, which are supplied by abundant collateral circulation.

(899–A, C) **(S&F, pp. 427–429)**

Acute head trauma is associated with a high incidence of upper gastrointestinal tract pathology. In one study, acute gastroduodenal lesions were found in 75% of patients and overt bleeding in 45%. Most lesions develop within one week of injury. Prophylaxis with either antacids, sucralfate, or H$_2$ receptor antagonists should be considered. In this study, no correlation between corticosteroid use and upper gastrointestinal tract bleeding was observed. Chronic constipation affects many patients with spinal cord injury. Damage to the upper motor neurons in the spinal cord eliminates both the sensation of rectal fullness and the voluntary control of defecation. The postprandial gastro-colic reflex is often absent and splanchnic outflow may be decreased, further impairing the coordination of intestinal and colonic motility.

(900–A, B, C, D, E)   ***(S&F, p. 147)***

Diarrhea in patients in intensive care units is common, and although careful etiologic studies have not determined the exact frequency of the various potential causes of diarrhea, all of the problems listed are common factors.

(901–B)   ***(S&F, pp. 81–82)***

Visceral pain occurs when noxious stimuli affect an abdominal viscus. It is dull, poorly localized, and felt near the midline because abdominal organs receive sensory afferents from both sides of the spinal cord. The quality is often described as cramping, burning, or gnawing. In contrast, parietal pain is generally intense and more precisely localized to the site of the lesion. Parietal pain is usually aggravated by movement.

(902–C)   ***(S&F, p. 314)***

Juxtapapillary diverticula are believed to arise from disordered motility with an increased incidence of sphincter of Oddi dysfunction. Sphincteric dysfunction may contribute to increased biliary contamination and hence pigment stones. Pancreatic and biliary anomalies have also been noted more frequently, but duodenal carcinoma is not more common.

(903–D)   ***(S&F, p. 161)***

When stool fills the rectum, a normal subject consciously senses the filling as a vague "call to stool." The striated skeletal muscles of the external anal sphincter and the puborectalis contract while the smooth muscles of the rectum and internal anal sphincter relax, allowing the sensitive mucosa of the proximal anal canal to determine if the rectal contents are solid, liquid, or gas.

(904–D)   ***(S&F, pp. 401–402)***

Human immunodeficiency virus (HIV) and hepatitis B virus (HBV) interact in many ways. Several reports describe reappearance of HBsAg in HIV-infected patients previously believed to be immune, either from reinfection or reactivation. In addition, there is accelerated loss of naturally acquired anti-HBs. There is an increased prevalence of HBeAg, with elevated levels of viral DNA polymerase and increased titers of anti-HBc. Thus, a large proportion of patients with both HIV and HBV have a

chronic carrier state with highly infectious serum and body fluids. The severity of clinical liver disease is usually reduced, perhaps reflecting immunosuppression caused by the HIV.

(905–D)   ***(S&F, pp. 443–444)***

Both ulcerative colitis and Crohn's disease have many cutaneous manifestations. Skin lesions are more common and often more specific in Crohn's disease. The most common lesions seen in Crohn's disease are granulomatous lesions of the perianal or perifistular skin. Oral lesions are mainly seen in Crohn's disease and include aphthous ulceration, angular cheilitis, and granulomatous cheilitis. Oral aphthous ulceration is not seen in ulcerative colitis. Pyostomatitis vegetans, a rare oral manifestation that is more common in ulcerative colitis, consists of superficial pustules coating a friable erythematous and eroded mucosa. Pyoderma gangrenosum, erythema multiforme, and thrombophlebitis are nonspecific findings seen in both diseases.

(906–A)   ***(S&F, pp. 239–241)***

The metabolic response to fasting can be divided into five phases: the postabsorptive period, early starvation, short-term starvation, long-term starvation, and terminal starvation. The postabsorptive period begins after ingested food has been absorbed, ends at the onset of the early starvation phase, and is characterized by a decline in portal vein glucose and insulin concentrations and stimulation of hepatic glycogen breakdown to produce glucose (glycogenolysis). During the early starvation period, the liver produces glucose from hepatic glycogen breakdown (glycogenolysis) and plasma precursors (gluconeogenesis). Lipolysis mobilizes fatty acids (oxidized for fuel) and glycerol (oxidized or used for gluconeogenesis). During short-term starvation, the predominant fuel consumed by the brain changes from glucose to ketone bodies and the predominant fuel consumed by muscle changes from fatty acids to ketone bodies. During long-term starvation, the body relies almost entirely on adipose tissue for fuel. Terminal starvation occurs after 60 or more days of fasting.

(907–A)   ***(S&F, pp. 105–106)***

Although dyspepsia may be associated with other symptoms, the only consistent symptom is persistent or recurrent abdominal discomfort centered in the upper abdomen. Associated clinical manifestations can include belching, nausea, early satiety, and bloating, but these are not required for the diagnosis. Patients may be subdivided into having reflux-like, ulcer-like, and dysmotility-like dyspepsia according to the characteristics of the discomfort.

(908–B)   ***(S&F, p. 334)***

Pancreatic enzymes have no reported ability to break down gastric bezoars. Papain and acetylcysteine have been reported to be effective in breaking down some gastric bezoars. A diet high in fiber may help prevent bezoar formation.

(909–B, C)   **(S&F, pp. 106–107)**

No conclusive evidence exists that caffeinated beverages, spicy foods, or food allergies are associated with chronic dyspepsia, although many patients will report consistent worsening of their symptoms with certain foods. Fat content of foods may affect the severity of dyspepsia by altering gastrointestinal motility. Long-chain fatty acids and other fats delay gastric emptying, possibly exacerbating symptoms of early satiety, nausea, and bloating in the subset of patients with dysmotility-associated dyspepsia. Although coffee, alcoholic beverages, and acidic foods may exacerbate heartburn, they have not been linked to dyspepsia despite the fact that spicy foods and distilled alcoholic beverages may cause gastric mucosal irritation visible on endoscopy. Many patients presenting with dyspeptic symptoms turn out to have lactose intolerance. However, the degree of dyspepsia correlates poorly with lactose consumption, suggesting it is not responsible in most cases.

(910–E)   **(S&F, pp. 369–370)**

Transferrin has a relatively short half-life and its level in serum depends on the iron status of the individual. Levels of albumin and immunoglobulins (except IgE) are especially useful.

(911–B)   **(S&F, pp. 161–162)**

The puborectalis muscle is believed to be the most important voluntary muscle in maintaining continence of stool. When contracted, it draws the rectum forward, producing an angulation between the axis of the rectum and the axis of the anal canal of approximately 90 degrees. This angle seems to be crucial for maintaining continence of solid stool, allowing increases in abdominal pressure that otherwise might threaten fecal continence. The external anal sphincter tires after a few minutes and can delay defecation only briefly.

(912–A, D)   **(S&F, p. 399)**

Human immunodeficiency virus (HIV)–positive patients may have anal ulcerations from a variety of causes, including sexually transmitted diseases such as syphilis, herpes simplex, and cytomegalovirus. The ulcers are often extremely painful, especially on defecation. Biopsies for culture and histology are helpful in ruling out specific causes. The treatment of cytomegalovirus-induced ulcers with ganciclovir is disappointing. Studies suggest that the injection of corticosteroids into the lesion may relieve the pain of HIV-induced ulcers.

(913–D)   **(S&F, pp. 422–424)**

Numerous gastrointestinal abnormalities may accompany systemic sclerosis. Esophageal involvement includes impaired peristalsis and lower esophageal sphincter hypotension, which frequently leads to esophagitis and strictures. Small bowel hypomotility and impaired gastric emptying may occur, owing to collagen deposition in the mucosa, and can lead to bacterial overgrowth, pseudo-obstruction, and intussusception. Idiopathic calcific pancreatitis has also been reported.

(914–C)   **(S&F, p. 430)**

Systemic amyloidosis may cause gastrointestinal symptoms from the mouth to the anus. Esophageal, gastric, and intestinal dysmotility from infiltration can result in dysphagia (similar to achalasia), gastric outlet obstruction, intestinal pseudo-obstruction, diarrhea, constipation, megacolon, or fecal incontinence. Biliary colic is not commonly seen in amyloidosis.

(915–A)   **(S&F, pp. 411–412)**

Hyperthyroidism does indeed often cause mild liver test abnormalities, but the characteristic findings are of a mild elevation in aminotransferases and an unconjugated hyperbilirubinemia. An elevated alkaline phosphatase level in hyperthyroidism is usually of bone, not liver, origin.

(916–1-B, 2-D, 3-C, 4-A)   **(S&F, p. 268)**

In addition to the deficiencies listed, specific micronutrient deficiencies have been identified as causing neutropenia and anemia (copper), glucose intolerance (chromium), nasolabial and perineal acrodermatitis (zinc), and tachycardia, tachypnea, central scotomas, and irritability (molybdenum).

(917–A)   **(S&F, p. 263)**

Diarrhea occurs in 30% to 50% of critically ill patients receiving tube feedings. Antibiotic use correlates most closely with the prevalence of diarrhea. Diarrhea may occur in as many as 40% of acutely ill patients receiving antibiotics and tube feeding but is found in only 3% of patients who are not receiving antibiotics. *Clostridium difficile* toxin is detectable in the stool of about 50% of patients receiving antibiotics. Other factors that may contribute are low serum albumin levels and nonabsorbable carbohydrates such as sorbitol (found in elixirs of common medications such as acetaminophen, theophylline, and cimetidine). Rarely, infectious diarrhea from contaminated enteral formulas will occur.

(918–1-D, 2-C, 3-A, 4-B)   **(S&F, p. 255)**

Clear-liquid diet consists of clear fluids or nondairy foods that are liquid at room temperature, such as broth, juices, coffee, tea, gelatin, and ices, and is used to prevent dehydration and minimize dietary residue before gastrointestinal and surgical procedures or to assess gastrointestinal tract tolerance before instituting a more rigorous diet. A full-liquid diet consists of foods that liquefy at room temperature (particularly milk and milk products like custards, milk shakes, and ice cream) and is used in the transition from clear liquids to solid foods and in patients who cannot chew. Mechanical soft diet contains minced or ground meat or poultry and flaked fish, whereas the regular soft diet contains moist and tender meat, poultry, or fish. Both diets include soft pureed fruits and vegetables, are low in fiber, and are nutritionally adequate. The mechanical soft diet is effective for patients who cannot chew their food or have mild dysphagia. The regular soft diet can be used during the transition period between a liquid and regular hospital diet. The low-fiber diet restricts fiber and other foods, such as prune juice, that increase stool volume. This diet includes cooked vegetables, cooked fruits, and tender meats. Low-fiber diets decrease the weight and bulk of the stool and delay intestinal transit. This diet is indicated to avoid obstruction when the intestinal lumen is pathologically narrowed because of inflammatory changes or tumor. Low-fiber diets are also used to decrease flow into the colon during acute diverticulitis, ulcerative colitis, or infectious enterocolitis.

(919–B) **(S&F, pp. 80–81)**
Abdominal viscera are insensitive to many stimuli that would ordinarily evoke external pain, such as cutting, tearing, or crushing. Visceral pain is primarily caused by stretch or tension. Inflammation and ischemia are other processes that can produce intra-abdominal pain.

(920–A) **(S&F, pp. 2031–2032)**
Aortoenteric fistula occurs after 1% to 2% of abdominal aortic grafts, usually within 24 months of surgery. Bleeding is typically intermittent and not easily demonstrated by angiography. Abdominal computed tomography typically shows loss of demarcation of the aortic wall at the proximal anastomosis of the graft, indicative of localized infection. Endoscopy is essential to exclude other causes of upper gastrointestinal bleeding but rarely detects the fistula, which is typically in the third portion of the duodenum.

(921–A) **(S&F, pp. 396–397)**
The majority of patients with the acquired immunodeficiency syndrome with odynophagia and dysphagia have *Candida* esophagitis alone or in association with infection with other pathogens, specifically cytomegalovirus (CMV) or herpes simplex virus (HSV). Less frequently, CMV and HSV may cause esophagitis without *Candida*. Some patients develop large nonspecific ulcerations of the esophagus in the absence of an identifiable pathogen. These may reflect direct damage from the human immunodeficiency virus.

(922–A) **(S&F, p. 306)**
The incidence of bowel perforation during colonoscopy is low for diagnostic colonoscopy (0.2%–0.4%) and for polypectomy or other electrosurgical injury such as hot biopsy forceps (0.3%–1%). The highest incidence of perforation occurs in hydrostatic balloon dilatation of colonic anastomotic strictures (4.6%). Mechanical perforation at sites of weakness in the colonic wall (e.g., diverticulosis or inflammation with fixation of bowel wall) may predispose to perforation; however, the rate is still quite low (0.2%–0.4%).

(923–D) **(S&F, p. 101)**
All of the foods listed have been shown to aggravate pyrosis by lowering the lower esophageal sphincter pressure. Additional foods and drugs such as fats, alcohol, tobacco, and calcium channel blockers can worsen pyrosis by the same mechanism.

(924–E) **(S&F, pp. 143–144)**
Collagenous colitis affects primarily elderly women (15:1 female-to-male ratio) and is not associated with collagen vascular diseases. Plasma cells and neutrophils invade the lamina propria. It causes a mild secretory diarrhea. Diagnosis can be made by the finding of a thickened collagen band in the subepithelium, which differentiates this disease from the clinically similar disease microscopic colitis. These disorders have also been called lymphocytic colitis in the past, but this name is now falling from favor.

(925–A) **(S&F, pp. 335–336)**
The most common cause of early death after caustic ingestion is perforation that leads to mediastinitis and peritonitis.

(926–1-C, 2-D, 3-A, 4-B) **(S&F, pp. 2024, 2028–2030)**
At least 25% of patients older than the age of 60 have vascular ectasias in the right colon. It is probably the most frequent cause of recurrent lower intestinal bleeding in this age group. Osler-Weber-Rendu disease (hereditary hemorrhagic telangiectasia) is characterized by telangiectases on the lips, oral and nasopharyngeal mucosa, or hands. Almost half of cases of "watermelon stomach" (gastric antral vascular ectasias) are associated with portal hypertension. It is unknown if portal hypertension is causative, however. With the exception of cavernous hemangiomas of the rectum, which may cause massive bleeding, colonic hemangiomas typically produce occult blood loss.

(927–D) **(S&F, pp. 147–148)**
Although many patients with diarrhea of unknown origin are suspected to have neuroendocrine tumors, this is a very uncommon diagnosis. All of the other entities listed are much more likely.

(928–C) **(S&F, p. 87)**
Appendectomy for uncomplicated appendicitis results in a 3% fetal loss rate that increases to 20% with perforated appendicitis; therefore, early diagnosis and surgical intervention are indicated.

(929–B) **(S&F, p. 399)**
Potential infectious causes of pancreatitis in acquired immunodeficiency syndrome are multiple. The most common is cytomegalovirus (CMV), followed by *Mycobacterium tuberculosis, M. avium-intracellulare, Cryptococcus,*

and herpes simplex virus. Infectious pancreatitis may not always be clinically obvious and should be suspected in any patients with abdominal pain and elevated amylase level. *Campylobacter* has not been associated with pancreatitis.

(930–A) **(S&F, p. 170)**

Childhood incontinence occurs in 1% to 2% of otherwise healthy seven-year olds. Congenital anomalies associated with incontinence include neural tube defects (e.g., myelomeningocele or spina bifida) and anal atresia. Mentally retarded children tend to be slow at achieving bowel control, and some never achieve this goal. In most cases, incontinence in childhood is a part of the syndrome of encopresis ("functional incontinence"). In these children, bowel movements are irregular, bulky, and painful. This results in fecal retention, rectal distention, and reflex anal relaxation, which promotes soiling. Hirschsprung's disease results from an aganglionic segment within the rectum and sigmoid colon that prevents normal relaxation of the internal anal sphincter after rectal distention. It typically presents in infancy with symptoms of obstruction. Overflow incontinence is not a feature of this disease.

(931–C) **(S&F, pp. 118–119)**

The chemoreceptor trigger zone (CTZ) is not able to cause vomiting without the mediation of an intact vomiting center. The CTZ is essentially an emetic chemoreceptor.

(932–1-D, 2-A, 3-C, 4-B) **(S&F, p. 187)**

Bulk-forming agents (e.g., psyllium) are high in fiber. If taken without water, these products may expand in the intestinal tract and cause obstruction. They also cause flatulence, but less so than lactulose. Lactulose is a hyperosmotic laxative. It exerts an osmotic effect and is metabolized by bacteria in the colon to volatile fatty acids that lower the pH and increase colonic peristalsis. It may cause flatulence, cramps, and electrolyte disturbances. The major lubricant laxative is mineral oil. Adverse reactions include foreign body reactions and lipoid pneumonia in the event of aspiration. Chronic use may cause deficiencies of fat-soluble vitamins A, D, and K. Chronic abuse of stimulant laxatives such as anthraquinone derivatives may produce a brownish discolored colonic mucosa known as melanosis coli.

(933–B, D) **(S&F, pp. 82–85)**

When evaluating an acute abdomen, diagnostic error is more common in women, with the highest rate occurring in females ages 1 through 20 years. The elderly are more likely to have a condition requiring surgery and are also more likely to have an incorrect initial diagnosis owing to the larger number of likely causes.

(934–B) **(S&F, pp. 2036–2037, 2039)**

Perforated peptic ulcer (predominantly duodenal ulcer) is responsible for 40% of cases of surgical peritonitis, whereas appendicitis accounts for 20% of cases. Both are associated with a greater than 90% survival. Peritonitis due to gangrene of the bowel or gallbladder and postoperative peritonitis are less common but more morbid. Survival in such cases is approximately 50%.

(935–C) **(S&F, p. 180)**

Metabolic disorders that induce constipation include diabetes, acidosis, porphyria, amyloid neuropathy, uremia, and hypokalemia. Hypercalcemia from hyperparathyroidism, sarcoidosis, or bony metastasis can induce severe constipation that often disappears when the serum calcium concentration returns to normal. Constipation may be the presenting symptom of hypothyroidism; hyperthyroidism, in contrast, usually presents as diarrhea.

(936–A) **(S&F, pp. 332–333)**

In adults, a food bolus lodged above a mechanical lesion is the most common cause of esophageal foreign body obstruction. The lesion is typically a stricture or lower esophageal ring but may rarely be a tumor or diverticulum. The use of papain for enzymatic dissolution of an impacted meat bolus is not recommended because of published reports of complications and death. When removing a pointed foreign body, the sharp end should always be trailing to minimize mucosal trauma on removal. Glucagon has not been found to be useful in this situation.

(937–D) **(S&F, pp. 332–333)**

Lying in the left lateral decubitus position allows gastric contents to settle in the fundus. This may prevent the object from escaping through the pylorus.

(938–B) **(S&F, p. 179)**

Anismus is a common mechanism of functional outlet obstruction. Patients with anismus experience abnormal contraction of the external anal sphincter when they strain to defecate. Anismus is predominantly a problem of young boys and adult women but occasionally occurs in adult males. It is common in patients who have been sexually abused. The only successful treatment has been biofeedback.

(939–1-C, 2-B, 3-D, 4-A) **(S&F, p. 239)**

Chromium is important in promoting insulin action in peripheral tissues. Deficiency of this trace element may cause glucose intolerance similar to clinical diabetes. Zinc deficiency may produce acrodermatitis enteropathica, a syndrome of scaly, red, desquamating lesions involving the nasolabial folds and hands. Copper deficiency leads to reduced levels of ceruloplasmin, an iron oxidase that aids in transfer of iron from tissue stores to transferrin. Iron in cells is believed to be reduced to the ferrous form to cross the cell membrane and must therefore be reoxidized to the ferric form to bind to transferrin. Therefore, copper deficiency results in conditioned iron deficiency. Selenium is an antioxidant. Long-term parenteral nutrition without added selenium has been associated with muscle pain and cardiomyopathy.

(940–C) **(S&F, p. 83)**

Acute appendicitis characteristically presents as the gradual onset of periumbilical aching pain that progresses to a localized, right lower quadrant, moderately severe pain. Truly sudden onset of pain, as in minutes, suggests an acute event such as a ruptured ectopic pregnancy, a perforated ulcer, or mesenteric ischemia.

(941–C) **(S&F, p. 402)**

Non-Hodgkin's lymphomas in patients with the acquired immunodeficiency syndrome (AIDS) are almost exclusively B-cell neoplasms that display a diffuse architecture. Among AIDS patients developing lymphoma, the gastrointestinal and hepatobiliary tracts are involved in about half of all cases. The prognosis is determined mainly by the extent of the underlying immunocompromise and Karnofsky performance score, rather than by the grade of the lymphoma.

(942–1-D, 2-C, 3-E, 4-B, 5-A) **(S&F, pp. 444–448)**

Peutz-Jeghers syndrome is pigmented macules on the lips, mouth, hands, and feet associated with multiple gastrointestinal hamartomas. Acanthosis nigricans is a velvety hyperplasia and hyperpigmentation of the skin of the neck and axillae, often with multiple skin tags. Abdominal adenocarcinoma is seen in over 85% of the associated malignancies, with gastric carcinoma being most frequent. Necrolytic migratory erythema is the characteristic skin finding in glucagonoma. Gardner syndrome, or familial polyposis, is characterized by numerous adenomatous polyps; epidermoid cysts of the face, scalp, and extremities; osteomas; fibromas; and desmoid tumors. The polyps involve the colon (and often the periampullary duodenum) and will virtually always develop into adenocarcinoma. Blue rubber bleb nevus syndrome is a rare disorder. Patients develop blue subcutaneous compressible nodules on the skin. Gastrointestinal vascular malformations with mucosal cavernous hemangiomas are common, and bleeding is a frequent feature.

(943–B) **(S&F, p. 2011)**

Over 75% of patients with acute mesenteric ischemia have acute abdominal pain at the time of presentation. A similar proportion of patients have occult blood in the stool and leukocytosis. By contrast, abdominal tenderness is a relatively late finding and suggests the presence of infarcted bowel.

(944–D) **(S&F, pp. 239–241)**

Adipose tissue consumes less than 5% of resting metabolic rate but usually accounts for more than 20% of body weight. During starvation, energy is conserved by the reduced physical activity caused by fatigue and by a reduced resting metabolic rate. Resting metabolic rate has been found to decrease by 10% to 15% at 7 days and by 20% to 25% at 30 days of fasting. Energy expenditure remains relatively constant thereafter, despite continued starvation. When exogenous fuel is unavailable, endogenous stores are mobilized to meet energy requirements. Triglycerides in adipose tissue represent the major fuel reserve in the body.

(945–B) **(S&F, pp. 246–247)**

The refeeding syndrome was reported at the end of World War II when oral refeeding of war victims caused cardiac insufficiency and neurologic complications. Severely malnourished patients are at increased risk for developing fluid retention and congestive heart failure. Chronic undernutrition is associated with decreased cardiac mass, decreased stroke and end-diastolic volumes, bradycardia, and fragmentation of cardiac myofibrils. In addition, refeeding increases the concentration of plasma insulin, which enhances sodium and water reabsorption by the renal tubule. During starvation, phosphorus requirements are decreased because fat is the predominant fuel source. Refeeding stimulates intracellular uptake of phosphate for the production of phosphorylated intermediates of glucose metabolism. Severe hypophosphatemia, associated with muscle weakness, paresthesias, seizures, coma, cardiopulmonary decompensation, and even death, may occur within hours of refeeding. Increases in body cell mass and glycogen stores require increased intracellular potassium and magnesium. Refeeding with large amounts of carbohydrate or parenteral glucose may initially result in marked elevations in blood glucose with glucosuria, dehydration, and hyperosmolar coma. If the patient is depleted in thiamine, carbohydrate refeeding can precipitate Wernicke's encephalopathy. Starvation causes structural and functional deterioration of the gastrointestinal tract, including a decrease in the total mass and protein content of the intestinal mucosa and pancreas. Intestinal transport and absorption of free amino acids are impaired, whereas hydrolysis and absorption of peptides are better maintained. These alterations limit the ability of the gastrointestinal tract to digest and absorb food. When malnutrition is severe, oral refeeding has been associated with severe diarrhea and death.

(946–C) **(S&F, p. 215)**

Colonic diverticular bleeding frequently originates from the right side but can arise from anywhere within the colon. The only surgical option is subtotal colectomy unless the bleeding site has been specifically localized to one side of the colon by angiography, tagged red cell scanning, or colonoscopy.

(947–E) **(S&F, p. 133)**

This patient probably has self-limited diarrhea that may be due to either an infectious agent or a preformed bacterial toxin. She is improving, afebrile, and not dehydrated. No antibiotic therapy is indicated.

(948–A, B, D) **Defecation (S&F, p. 161)**
Incontinence (S&F, p. 163)

Rectal distention with gas or stool results in a reflex relaxation of the rectal vault to accommodate the added volume and a reflex relaxation of the internal anal sphincter. If defecation is to be deferred, the puborectalis muscle must contract to close the rectoanal angle, and the external anal sphincter (somatically innervated skeletal muscle) contracts to prevent passage. Diabetes is the most common medical condition associated with incontinence. Most cases of idiopathic fecal incontinence are due to denervation of the skeletal muscles of continence caused by a peripheral neuropathy. The neuropathy seems to be due to traction on the pudendal nerves most commonly caused by childbirth or straining at stool.

(949–D)   **(S&F, p. 83)**

Manifestations of perforation and consequent peritoneal irritation can include fever, abdominal wall rigidity, and abdominal pain. Visceral peritoneal irritation may be manifested by the presence of ileus and absent bowel sounds. Subcutaneous emphysema is often seen in esophageal rupture but not in duodenal perforation.

(950–A)   **(S&F, pp. 414–415)**

Unfortunately, the anticholinergic properties of phenothiazine antiemetics may worsen gastroparesis diabeticorum by further delaying gastric emptying, and their use cannot be recommended.

(951–A, D)   **(S&F, pp. 121–123)**

Hyperemesis gravidarum is defined as fluid and electrolyte disturbances or nutritional deficiency as a result of intractable vomiting early in pregnancy. It should be distinguished from the milder syndrome of nausea and vomiting of pregnancy. Patients with hyperemesis gravidarum do not have an increased incidence of toxemia, spontaneous abortion, or underweight or deformed babies. Antiemetics are not contraindicated, but the primary treatment should be directed at correction of the fluid and nutritional deficiency and supportive psychotherapy.

(952–C)   **(S&F, p. 224)**

A variety of infiltrative liver diseases can produce striking cholestasis. Granulomatous diseases of the liver include infections (e.g., tuberculosis, *Mycobacterium avium-intracellulare* infection, brucellosis, Q fever, syphilis) and systemic disorders such as sarcoidosis and lymphoma. Of these, tuberculosis and sarcoidosis most commonly produce jaundice. With the exception of parasitic diseases, fever is common. The presence of eosinophilia should heighten the suspicion of sarcoidosis, parasitic disease, or drug toxicity. Amyloidosis is a rare cause of jaundice and invariably is accompanied by marked hepatomegaly but not characteristically eosinophilia.

(953–D)   **(S&F, p. 412)**

Pinpointing the cause of diarrhea in a diabetic patient is difficult, and the cause may be multifactorial. In addition to all the causes of diarrhea in healthy individuals, diabetic patients may have additional processes that may contribute

to diarrhea. These include intestinal motor disorders due to diabetic autonomic neuropathy, pancreatic insufficiency, bacterial overgrowth, and celiac sprue. All of these conditions may play a causative role in diarrhea and need to be considered in the workup. There is no known association between Crohn's disease and diabetes.

(954–D)   **(S&F, pp. 279–280)**

Factors that may induce satiety include taste and smell; mechanical distention; hormones (gastrin, somatostatin, bombesin, cholecystokinin, secretin, neurotensin, gastric inhibitory peptide, pancreatic polypeptides, glucagon); and nutrient "appetostat" (glucose, fatty acids, amino acids). Deoxycholic acid is a secondary bile acid formed by bacterial dehydroxylation of cholate in the colon and has no known role in signaling satiety.

(955–A)   **(S&F, pp. 101–102)**

Globus is a common sensation noted in up to 46% of the population. It typically occurs as an isolated event and is not associated with dysphagia or odynophagia. Contrary to a common belief, globus sensation is not associated with histrionic or hysterical features.

(956–D)   **(S&F, p. 254)**

Enteral nutrition has many advantages compared with parenteral nutrition. First, enteral nutrition is associated with fewer serious complications. Second, the nutritional requirements for enterally processed nutrients are better known than the requirements for intravenously administered nutrients. Third, enteral nutrition can supply gut-specific fuels (glutamine and short-chain fatty acids) that are absent from commercially available parenteral formulations. Fourth, nutrients are needed in the intestinal lumen to prevent atrophy of intestinal mucosa and the pancreas, maintain mucosal protein and DNA concentrations, preserve mucosal digestive and pancreatic secretory enzyme activity, maintain IgA secretion, and prevent translocation of gut bacteria into the systemic circulation in critically ill patients. Fifth, enteral feeding prevents cholelithiasis by stimulating gallbladder motility. Finally, enteral nutrition is less expensive than parenteral nutrition.

(957–A)   **(S&F, pp. 206–207)**

Most studies indicate that the risk of rebleeding from an ulcer with a clean base is 0% to 2% and that urgent intervention for rebleeding is very unusual. If it is assumed that no other problems exist, patients with such a lesion can be discharged immediately after stabilization and institution of ulcer therapy.

(958–C, D)   **(S&F, pp. 301–306)**

Complications from gastrointestinal endoscopy are uncommon despite the increase in number of procedures performed over the past 30 years. The rate of complications ranges from 0.2% to 8% for all endoscopic procedures, with the highest rate from variceal sclerotherapy. Death attributable to endoscopic procedures is even rarer, ranging from 0.01% to 1.5% for all procedures. Bacteremia is most common with esophageal dilatation and variceal sclerotherapy, and some experts recommend prophylactic antibiotics in this setting. However, patients undergoing routine upper endoscopy do not require prophylactic antibiotics because bacteremia is uncommon. All benzodiazepines, including midazolam, have been associated with respiratory depression. This effect is significantly increased when a narcotic is also used. Although exceedingly rare, endoscopic transmission of *Salmonella* and *Pseudomonas* as well as *Helicobacter pylori* has been reported. Stringent adherence to universal precautions and careful disinfection of endoscopes have greatly reduced this problem.

(959–D) **(S&F, p. 222)**

Bilirubin is a breakdown product of heme. Excessive production of bilirubin can result from several mechanisms, including hemolysis, ineffective erythropoiesis, or resorption of hematomas. Thus, jaundice may complicate the clinical course of patients with hemolytic anemias, megaloblastic anemia, iron-deficiency anemia, sideroblastic anemia, and polycythemia vera. Jaundice may also follow massive transfusion, because the lifespan of transfused erythrocytes is relatively short, leading to excessive bilirubin production. Dubin-Johnson syndrome is characterized by impairment of canalicular secretion of certain organic anions, including bilirubin conjugates.

(960–D) **(S&F, p. 313)**

Seventy-five percent of gastric diverticula are juxtacardiac. They are typically noted on upper gastrointestinal series and are usually asymptomatic. They are most commonly found in the posterior aspect of the cardia. The other type of gastric diverticulum is the intramural or partial gastric, which represents a projection of gastric mucosa into the muscularis of the prepyloric region.

(961–B) **(S&F, pp. 388–391)**

Treatment of cryptosporidial infection in patients with the acquired immunodeficiency syndrome (AIDS) is unsatisfactory at present. Results of trials of spiramycin and virtually all other common antibiotics have been disappointing. *Salmonella, Shigella,* and *Campylobacter* all have higher rates of both bacteremia and antibiotic resistance in human immunodeficiency virus–infected individuals. Patients with AIDS are particularly susceptible to food-borne enteric infections. Mycobacterial involvement of the bowel either by *M. tuberculosis* or *M. avium-intracellulare* may lead to diarrhea, obstruction, or pain. Whereas *M. tuberculosis* infection is usually symptomatic, many patients with *M. avium-intracellulare* infection have asymptomatic infiltration.

(962–C) **(S&F, pp. 282–284)**

A balanced 1000 to 1200 kcal/day diet should be recommended for persons who want to lose 9 kg or less over two months. Despite the simplicity of this regimen, most patients fail because they underestimate their intake. Although total fasting can result in rapid and dramatic weight loss, it is dangerous and not a reasonable treatment for obesity. Prolonged fasting results in marked hypokalemia, hypophosphatemia, and profound postural hypotension. Very low–calorie diets are safe when patients are appropriately selected and supervised by trained physicians and can produce an average weight loss of 20 kg over a three-month period. However, less than 20% of patients keep the weight off. Sweeteners such as aspartame and saccharin may increase hunger and food intake and have no significant effect on body weight. Theoretically, a high-fiber intake could be helpful by prolonging mealtimes while diluting calorie-dense food items. However, fiber has not yet been shown to play a significant role in either weight loss or maintenance. Nonabsorbable fat substitutes can cause malabsorption of fat-soluble vitamins, including vitamins A, D, E, and K.

(963–B) **(S&F, pp. 285–286)**

Intestinal bypass surgeries were designed to produce iatrogenic malabsorption. Ironically, the mechanism of weight loss after these bypass operations is now believed to be decreased food intake, but many of the complications stem from the malabsorption.

(964–A) **(S&F, p. 153)**

Detailed studies of patients who complain of gas pains have shown that there is no increase in luminal gas when measured by accurate argon washout methods. In contrast, patients who perceive themselves as passing excess amounts of flatus are generally correct.

(965–B) **(S&F, pp. 387–388)**

The most common gastrointestinal symptom in acquired immunodeficiency syndrome (AIDS) is diarrhea, occurring in 50% to 90% of patients. It is often chronic and associated with weight loss and malnutrition. Although abdominal pain, nausea, and odynophagia are less frequently noted, they present an equally difficult diagnostic and management challenge.

(966–A) **(S&F, pp. 228–229)**

The sensitivity of abdominal computed tomography (CT) for detecting the cause of bile duct obstruction is 63% to 96%, whereas that of endoscopic retrograde cholangiopancreatography is 89% to 98% and percutaneous transhepatic cholangiography is 98% to 100%. When compared with ultrasonography, CT is less operator dependent and provides technically superior images in patients who are obese or in whom the biliary tree is obscured by bowel gas. Because only calcified stones can be imaged by CT, CT is not as good as ultrasonography in detecting cholelithiasis. Other considerations when using CT include its lack of portability and the need to use intravenous contrast material.

(967–D) **(S&F, pp. 255–256)**

Compliance with a low-fat diet (20 to 30 g/day) can be difficult, because fat is present in many foods and fat restriction reduces the palatability of meals. Severe fat restriction (<10 g/day) can be achieved by using low-fat, defined liquid formulas. However, these formulas are usually unpalatable and often need to be mixed with flavor packets or sherbet or must be administered through a feeding tube for adequate intake. Marked reduction in intestinal protein losses have been reported when patients were given diets containing less than 5 g of long-chain triglycerides per day. Because fat is calorically dense, a low-fat diet requires an increased intake of other nutrients, particularly carbohydrates, to prevent hypocaloric feeding. Fortunately, patients with intestinal lymphatic obstruction absorb carbohydrates normally. Carbohydrate should be given in complex form to reduce the osmotic load delivered to the small intestine. Medium-chain triglycerides (MCTs) can also be used to increase calorie intake because they are absorbed directly into the portal circulation and do not require lymphatic transport; however, MCTs are more ketogenic than long-chain triglycerides and should be avoided in patients prone to ketoacidosis.

(968–C) **(S&F, pp. 205–206, 630, 1394)**

Although previously controversial, current evidence indicates that corticosteroid use alone does not cause gastrointestinal bleeding. However, corticosteroids do appear to increase the risk of gastrointestinal bleeding caused by NSAIDs. Each of the remaining conditions is associated with an increased risk of gastrointestinal bleeding.

(969–C) **(S&F, p. 331)**

Although perforation from an ingested foreign body can occur at any level, it is more likely at anatomic sites of angulation or narrowing. Beyond the esophagus, these regions include the proximal duodenum, ileocecal region, sigmoid colon, and rectum. The ileocecal region is the most frequent site of perforation beyond the esophagus.

(970–D) **(S&F, p. 334)**

Trichobezoars are composed mostly of hair. Strands of hair may be too slippery to be propelled out of the stomach and are retained and enmeshed. The trichobezoar is denatured by gastric acid, becoming black and foul smelling owing to the decomposition of entrapped food.

(971–A) **(S&F, pp. 343–349)**

Chronic NSAID use may produce multiple superficial lesions of the stomach or intestines that cause occult bleeding and present as iron-deficiency anemia. Bleeding and perforation from gastric or duodenal ulcers can occur with parenteral NSAID administration after only a few doses, often in the absence of superficial ulceration. Superficial gastric damage may be reduced by enteric coatings, but the risk of ulceration does not appear to differ form the risk of non–enteric-coated preparations. Although most non-NSAID (i.e., *Helicobacter pylori*–related) gastric ulcers are associated with antral gastritis, gastritis is seen in only about 50% of NSAID-induced gastric ulcers. NSAIDs by themselves do not cause histologic gastritis. When gastritis is seen, *H. pylori* is probably present.

(972–1-D, 2-A, 3-C, 4-B) **(S&F, p. 225)**

The large amount of lactose in the full-liquid diet prevents its use in patients with lactose intolerance. Clear-liquid diets are incomplete diets. A severely malnourished patient who cannot tolerate more than a clear-liquid diet should be supported with parenteral nutrition. High-fiber diets are contraindicated in patients with luminal narrowing due to inflammation, diseases, or tumor. Medium-chain triglycerides (MCTs) are more ketogenic than long-chain triglycerides and should not be given to patients with diabetes, ketosis, or acidosis. The use of MCTs is also contraindicated in patients with cirrhosis, particularly those with portosystemic shunts.

(973–C) **(S&F, pp. 423–424)**

The symptoms are of fat malabsorption. The physical findings are classic for scleroderma, which is associated with bacterial overgrowth of the small bowel due to altered gut motility. Immunosuppressive agents may be indicated for the systemic condition, but antibiotics are most appropriate for the bacterial overgrowth.

(974–A) **(S&F, p. 260)**

Glutamine is not an essential amino acid because it can be synthesized by the body, yet exogenous glutamine may be necessary for normal intestinal structure and function. Glutamine supplementation enhances intestinal adaptation to massive resection, improves survival from peritonitis, and reduces intestinal damage from cytotoxic therapy such as 5-fluorouracil, methotrexate, and abdominal radiation. During catabolic states, glutamine uptake by the intestine increases markedly, supplied mostly from skeletal muscle breakdown. Glutamine production by skeletal muscle cannot match the rate of glutamine uptake, thereby causing a decrease in glutamine concentration in both plasma and muscle. Glutamine has been excluded from parenteral formulas because it is a nonessential amino acid and because it may be unstable in storage, generating ammonia and pyroglutamic acid.

(975–A) **(S&F, pp. 235–236)**

The liver, brain, kidney, and heart have the highest energy requirements per gram of tissue and collectively account for more than 70% of the resting metabolic rate. Skeletal muscle consumes 20% and remaining organs consume 10%.

(976–C) **(S&F, pp. 310–311)**

A Zenker diverticulum is believed to result from a lack of coordination between the proximal esophagus and the upper esophageal sphincter with failure of the sphincter to appropriately relax, eventually resulting in a proximal diverticulum. Epiphrenic diverticula have been associated with esophageal dysmotility and with lesions characterized by failure of lower esophageal sphincter relaxation. The midesophageal diverticulum (traction diverticulum) was once believed to arise in the setting of mediastinal inflammatory changes secondary to tuberculosis or histoplasmosis; however, more recent studies suggest esophageal motor abnormalities are more likely to blame. Schatzki's rings are congenital and are not related to abnormal esophageal motility.

(977–C)   **(S&F, p. 184)**

When evaluating fecal retention and soiling in children, the most important historical information is the association in the child's mind of defecation with pain. Two thirds of children with soiling report a long history of painful defecation, perhaps due to an anal fissure that causes pain and ultimately results in fecal retention, a dilated rectum, and a permanently lax internal anal sphincter. Although psychological support is warranted if the soiling causes behavioral maladjustments, primary focus should be on softening the stools and setting aside a daily time for rectal emptying. Consistency of the stools and dietary and exercise habits may provide clues to the etiology but are less useful.

(978–D)   **(S&F, pp. 288–289)**

Anorexia nervosa is defined as (1) refusal to maintain body weight over a minimal normal weight for age and height; (2) intense fear of gaining weight or becoming fat, even though underweight; (3) disturbance in the way one's body weight, size, or shape is experienced; and (4) in females, absence of at least three consecutive menstrual cycles when otherwise expected to occur (primary or secondary amenorrhea). Bulimia nervosa is a condition with features of anorexia nervosa and bulimia. The patient with bulimia nervosa has recurrent episodes of binge eating and feels a lack of control over eating behavior during the binges. The patient regularly engages in either self-induced vomiting, use of laxatives or diuretics, strict dieting or fasting, or vigorous exercise to prevent weight gain. Bingeing and purging are not features of anorexia nervosa.

(979–C)   **(S&F, pp. 364–367)**

If two ends of bowel are not apposed (end fistula) or there is obstruction distal to the bowel segment producing the fistula, spontaneous closure will not occur, and surgical management is indicated. Persistent drainage from the fistula despite management of all known infections, including percutaneous drainage of known abscesses, generally indicates a focus of unrecognized infection that will require surgical drainage. The rate of fistula output *per se* should not dictate the decision to perform surgery.

(980–A, C, D)   **(S&F, p. 280)**

Most dietary surveys suggest that hyperphagia is not the primary cause of obesity. Interest has recently shifted to studies of energy expenditure, consisting of physical activity, basal metabolic rate (BMR), and thermogenesis. Not only are obese patients less active, but they expend less energy when active than lean patients. The BMR of the obese is greater than that of lean subjects. This finding is not particularly surprising, because obese persons require a greater lean body mass to maintain their extra fat. Available data do not support the common opinion that obese persons are fat because of gluttony and sloth. Instead, obese persons appear inherently efficient in energy metabolism, burning fewer calories under similar circumstances than lean persons.

(981–B)   **(S&F, pp. 120, 414–415)**

Each of the conditions listed except for pernicious anemia is a known cause of gastroparesis.

(982–D)   **(S&F, pp. 333–334)**

Toddlers are especially attracted to small alkaline batteries because they are slim, round, and bright objects. Esophageal perforation is believed to be due to the local corrosive effect of these batteries, local pressure necrosis, and possibly local discharge of current. If the battery leaks, heavy metal intoxication may occur.

(983–1-B, 2-C, 3-A, 4-D, 5-E)   **(S&F, p. 132)**

Hypersecretion of gastric acid in the Zollinger-Ellison syndrome results in severe gastroesophageal reflux disease (GERD) in 25% to 40% of patients and in diarrhea in about one third of patients. Autonomic neuropathy is typical of amyloidosis. Malabsorption is found in about 5% of these patients. Malabsorption is probably multifactorial but is probably due in part to infiltration of the small bowel by amyloid fibrils. Excessive histamine release from mast cells results in flushing. Diarrhea is common in this disorder, but the etiology is unclear and is probably multifactorial (e.g., histamine may trigger gastric acid hypersecretion or mast cell infiltration). Extragastrointestinal manifestations of Whipple's disease are common and include fever, central nervous system involvement, arthritis, and lymphadenopathy. Collagenous colitis is usually found in women older than the age of 70.

(984–D)   **(S&F, pp. 2013–2014)**

Angiography is particularly helpful in demonstrating nonocclusive mesenteric ischemia. Helpful findings include superior mesenteric arterial branch narrowing, intestinal branch irregularities, spasm in the arterial arcades, and poor filling of intramural vessels. "Thumbprinting" is a late finding that suggests bowel infarction. Doppler and abdominal computed tomography are helpful in identifying mesenteric arterial and venous thromboses but provide little information in nonocclusive disease.

(985–B, D)   **(S&F, pp. 2017–2018)**

Low cardiac output is found in fewer than 25% of patients with colonic ischemia, in contrast to patients with acute mesenteric ischemia in whom circulatory derangements are common. Although passage of maroon stool or bright red blood per rectum often occurs, bleeding generally does not require transfusion. By the time of presentation, colonic blood flow is typically normal and angiography does not usually show significant occlusion. Features of inflammatory bowel disease, including ulcerations separated by normal mucosa, crypt abscesses, and strictures, can all occur.

(986–1-D, 2-B, 3-A, 4-C)   **(S&F, p. 240)**

There are two clinical syndromes of thiamine (B_1) deficiency—wet and dry beriberi. Wet beriberi occurs as high-output left ventricular heart failure. Dry beriberi is associated with neuropathy and Wernicke-Korsakoff psychosis. Clinical deficiency of niacin is called pellagra, which is a wasting disease with dermatitis of the exposed areas due to photosensitivity. Folic acid and vitamin B_{12} deficiencies cause megaloblastic anemias. Scurvy results from vitamin C deficiency.

(987–D)   **(S&F, p. 334)**

All of the factors listed have been associated with gastric bezoar formation except high-fiber diet, which may actually help prevent bezoar formation due to its stimulatory effect on the stomach.

(988–A, B)   **(S&F, pp. 235–236)**

For all practical purposes, resting metabolic rate (RMR), resting energy expenditure (REE), basal energy expenditure (BEE), and basal metabolic rate (BMR) are interchangeable terms. The Harris-Benedict equation uses age, height, weight, and sex to estimate RMR. Additions to this basal value are made for the effects of physical activity (typically 20% of RMR) and food digestion (typically 10%). The Harris-Benedict equation does not determine how these calories should be supplied.

(989–D)   **(S&F, pp. 324–326)**

The triad of pain, retching, and inability to pass a nasogastric tube should suggest the possibility of gastric volvulus. The clinical suspicion may be confirmed by either a Gastrografin upper gastrointestinal series or computed tomography of the chest and upper abdomen. The treatment is emergent surgical decompression in the event that decompression by a nasogastric tube is not feasible. The most common form of gastric volvulus is an organoaxial volvulus.

(990–B)   **(S&F, p. 358)**

Although abdominal abscess may be associated with all of the findings listed, gas within the mass is highly suggestive of an abscess. Gas may also be seen occasionally in necrotic tumors. Enhancement with an oral or rectal contrast medium is important to differentiate between a true abscess and a fluid-filled loop of bowel. Needle aspiration under computed tomographic guidance will usually confirm the diagnosis of abscess.

(991–D)   **(S&F, pp. 360–363)**

Resolution of fever with persistent drainage suggests a fistula. Resolution of drainage with persistent fever suggests an undrained fluid collection. Persistence of an abscess cavity may require repositioning of the drainage catheter. If all criteria are met, operative intervention can usually be avoided.

(992–A)   **(S&F, pp. 154–156)**

Anaerobic bacterial metabolism of malabsorbed carbohydrate may produce hydrogen, methane, and carbon dioxide. Hydrogen is useful diagnostically because it is not produced by normal body processes and is rapidly excreted via the lungs, where it can be measured with a breath hydrogen analyzer. Methane and carbon dioxide are also produced by bacteria fermenting carbohydrates; however, methane production depends on the type of bacteria present. Nitric oxide is not produced in the lumen of the intestine in any appreciable quantity. Nitrogen appears in colonic gas by two mechanisms. The first is by swallowed air, and the second is by diffusion into the duodenum and proximal jejunum, where there is a high partial pressure of carbon dioxide.

(993–B)   **(S&F, p. 237)**

During fasting, nitrogen is excreted in proportion to the metabolic rate (about 2 mg nitrogen lost/kcal/day). This is referred to as the obligatory nitrogen loss. When a person who has fasted is refed protein, nitrogen excretion does not rise in proportion to the intake, so there is a net gain of body nitrogen, most of which is due to rapid accumulation of nitrogen in the liver.

(994–C)   **(S&F, p. 413)**

Myxedema is associated with disturbances of esophageal peristalsis and gastroesophageal sphincter dysfunction, resulting in reflux esophagitis. It is also associated with gastric hypomotility and formation of phytobezoars. Impaired colonic motility in hypothyroidism may cause constipation, impaction, pseudo-obstruction, or rarely megacolon. Gastric acid secretion is increased, probably because of diminished adrenergic inhibition of acid secretion. Hypomotility of the gallbladder in hypothyroidism might be expected to cause an increased incidence of gallstones; however, no such finding has been documented.

(995–1-C, 2-D, 3-B, 4-A)   **(S&F, pp. 393–394)**

Erythromycin, a macrolide antibiotic, mimics the gastrointestinal effects of motilin. Metoclopramide acts as a central and peripheral antidopaminergic agent. Its 20% to 50% incidence of side effects prodded the development of other prokinetic agents. Unlike metoclopramide, cisapride does not act via the dopaminergic pathways; rather, it works by enhancing the release of acetylcholine from the myenteric plexus. Ondansetron along with granisetron are selective 5-hydroxytryptamine (serotonin) receptor antagonists and act in both the central nervous system and gastrointestinal tract.

(996–A)   **(S&F, pp. 422–423)**

The "E" in CREST stands for esophageal involvement, usually manifesting as dysphagia from either aperistalsis or a gastroesophageal reflux disease–induced peptic stricture. It is true that 38% of patients with progressive systemic sclerosis with dysphagia have Barrett's metaplasia, but the incidence of adenocarcinoma does not seem to be increased.

(997–C)   **(S&F, pp. 370–371)**

Bacterial overgrowth, Whipple's disease, eosinophilic gastroenteritis, and sprue are all associated with a visually normal mucosa. To identify these diseases, biopsies must be performed. In contrast, graft-versus-host disease is usually associated with a visually abnormal and frequently ulcerated mucosa and may therefore be diagnosed on routine endoscopy in an appropriate clinical setting.

(998–B)   **(S&F, p. 101)**

One third of patients with Barrett's esophagus are insensitive to acid. This may help explain the insidious development of significant complications such as stricture, bleeding, or carcinoma in patients with a paucity of antecedent symptoms.

(999–D)   **(S&F, p. 365)**

Young, well-nourished patients with long fistulous tracts arising from an anastomotic breakdown and draining small quantities are likely to experience spontaneous closure of their fistulas. Older, malnourished patients with malignancy or inflammatory bowel disease as a cause of the fistula generally require surgical closure. Obstruction distal to the fistula must be relieved before the fistula will close.

(1000–C)   **(S&F, pp. 411–412)**

Hypermotility of the small bowel is believed to be the major factor in the pathogenesis of diarrhea and steatorrhea in hyperthyroidism. Thyroid hormone can increase enterocyte cyclic adenosine monophosphate and induce intestinal secretion. The small bowel mucosa in thyrotoxicosis can show inflammation, but the villi are normal in structure and function as assessed by D-xylose absorption.

(1001–D)   **(S&F, p. 93)**

Evidence of organic disease (e.g., anemia, weight loss) argues against the diagnosis of a functional disorder.

(1002–D)   **(S&F, pp. 99–100)**

Common causes of odynophagia include pill esophagitis, caustic ingestion, and infectious esophagitis. Gastroesophageal reflux complicated by severe ulcerative esophagitis may present as odynophagia, whereas it is rare for esophageal carcinoma to present in this fashion.

(1003–C)   **(S&F, p. 447)**

Dermatitis herpetiformis is a pruritic skin disorder consisting of urticarial, vesicular, or bullous lesions localized to the lower back, buttocks, shoulders, elbows, knees, and scalp. Skin biopsy reveals deposition of IgA1 in the dermal papillae. When examined endoscopically, many patients will have an enteropathy indistinguishable from celiac sprue, yet only about 5% of patients have symptomatic gastrointestinal disease. A gluten-free diet reverses both the intestinal disease and the skin lesions.

(1004–A, D)   **(S&F, p. 145)**

Melanosis coli occurs after as little as four months of anthracene (e.g., senna, cascara) laxative abuse. Although the entire colon can be involved, it mainly affects the cecum and rectosigmoid region. The pigment is lipofuscin, which is found in macrophages that have migrated to the lamina propria.

(1005–B, C)   **(S&F, pp. 241–243)**

Arm circumference and triceps skin fold measurements are easy to perform and can be used to calculate arm muscle circumference. However, the coefficient of variation among observers is too large for these measurements to be useful in the observation of a single patient. If malnutrition were diagnosed by the presence of at least one abnormal anthropometric parameter, 20% to 30% of the population would be classified as malnourished. Albumin correlates well with disease and complications but may be affected by other factors and thus is not an index of nutrition *per se*. Whereas immune competence as measured by delayed cutaneous hypersensitivity is often reduced in malnutrition, several diseases and drugs may influence this measurement, making it a poor predictor of malnutrition in sick patients.

(1006–1-D, 2-E, 3-A, 4-C, 5-B)   **(S&F, p. 176)**

Irritable bowel syndrome may present as painful constipation, often influenced by stress or diet. Slow colonic transit results in infrequent bowel movements and never loose stools, whereas stool frequency in outlet delay may be normal with straining as the hallmark. Fecal impaction often causes soilage from liquid stool getting around the hard, impacted stool, and distention and occasional emesis are characteristic of pseudo-obstruction.

(1007–A)   ***EST and EVL (S&F, p. 1297)***
                    Medical therapy (S&F, p. 1299)

Active variceal bleeding stops spontaneously in about 60% of patients. Infusion of intravenous vasopressin and nitroglycerin for variceal bleeding has an efficacy of only about 50%. Intravenous octreotide is slightly more effective than vasopressin, but neither of these medical therapies is as effective as transjugular intrahepatic portosystemic shunt, sclerotherapy, and variceal band ligation, which can control active esophageal variceal bleeding in 85% to 95% of patients.

(1008–D) *(S&F, p. 358)*

Most abdominal abscesses occur by perforation of the gut or through infection of an intra-abdominal organ, and most of the responsible organisms are gut flora. *Staphylococcus,* along with *Candida,* is more common in hospitalized patients in a critical care unit who have been exposed to antibiotics.

(1009–C) *(S&F, pp. 178–197)*

The first three statements are true. Normal defecation can occur without intact connections to the brain. Defecation is organized in the lumbosacral spinal cord and can occur as a coordinated response even in paraplegics.

(1010–C) *(S&F, p. 171)*

Fecal incontinence complicates the course of diabetes in approximately one in five diabetics. It seems to reflect reduced anal sphincter pressure and impaired sensation. Coexisting diarrhea may complicate the incontinence but is not usually the cause. Biofeedback training may sometimes be helpful in regaining control of the sphincter.

(1011–D) *(S&F, p. 158)*

Excess flatus commonly reflects gas produced in the colon. The amount of gas produced in the duodenum is fairly consistent from patient to patient. Air swallowing is an important cause of intestinal gas in normal persons but does not account for excess flatus in most cases. Whereas bacteria colonizing the small bowel may increase gas production, this mechanism is a relatively uncommon cause of excess flatus.

(1012–A) *(S&F, p. 446)*

Tylosis is adult-onset diffuse hyperkeratosis of the palms and soles that has been described in association with esophageal carcinoma in several kindreds in England (Howel-Evans syndrome). The skin lesions appear in adolescence or early adulthood, and the carcinomas appear at the average age of 45 years.

(1013–D) *(S&F, pp. 339–340)*

Esophageal cancer is a late complication of caustic ingestion with squamous cell tumors most common. The incidence is 1000 to 3000 times greater than in the general population. Other gastrointestinal malignancies are not associated with caustic ingestion.

(1014–D) *(S&F, pp. 358–360)*

Although chest radiography and abdominal films will not definitively demonstrate the presence of an abscess, they provide valuable clues with respect to the presence of fluid collections and extraluminal gas. Both abdominal ultrasonography and computed tomography are quite useful because they permit image-guided aspiration of suspicious fluid collections. In contrast, magnetic resonance imaging is significantly more expensive and cannot be used for directing fine-needle aspiration.

(1015–B) *(S&F, pp. 265–266)*

Administering fat-free parenteral nutrition can cause biochemical evidence of essential fatty acid deficiency within two weeks. The optimal percentage of calories that should be infused as fat is not known. A minimum of about 5% of total calories as a lipid emulsion is necessary to prevent essential fatty acid deficiency. Parenteral nutrition can cause biochemical evidence of essential fatty acid deficiency within two weeks because the resulting increase in plasma insulin suppresses release of essential fatty acids from endogenous fat stores. Complications are more common when intravenous lipid emulsions are provided in excess of 1.0 kcal/kg/hr. Thus, 25% to 50% of daily caloric intake should be in the form of lipid emulsions unless contraindicated, and the infusion rate should not exceed 0.7 kcal/kg/hr.

(1016–C) *(S&F, pp. 180–181)*

Constipation is common in Parkinson's disease and may be due to dopamine depletion in enteric neurons or failure of relaxation of striated muscle in the pelvic floor (a localized form of the extrapyramidal manifestations affecting all skeletal muscles in this disease). Patients with multiple sclerosis commonly report constipation, and the symptom correlates with the duration of the disease. Patients with high or low spinal cord lesions are often severely constipated, and many develop fecal impactions. Those with cervical and thoracic lesions tend to have proximal impactions, and those with lumbosacral lesions tend to have rectal impactions. Subacute combined degeneration, a spinal cord lesion due to cobalamin deficiency, can cause loss of sphincter control but rarely causes constipation.

(1017–C, D) *(S&F, pp. 2041–2042)*

Most peritoneal tumors are metastatic cancers, including adenocarcinomas and lymphomas. Mesothelioma is an unusual peritoneal tumor. Only 10% of ascitic samples associated with peritoneal tumors are bloody. Although a variety of treatments, including intravenous and intraperitoneal chemotherapy, radiation therapy, surgical debulking, and therapeutic paracentesis have been applied to the management of malignant ascites, diuretics are ineffective and may cause intravascular volume depletion. Peritoneal malignancies are generally associated with a very poor prognosis. However, pseudomyxoma peritonei is an exception, with a five-year survival of approximately 50%.

(1018–C, D) *(S&F, p. 414)*

Almost 60% of all long-standing diabetics have symptoms resulting from disturbed gastric emptying. Although observed or measured motility disturbances are common, they do not correlate well with actual symptoms. This suggests that other manifestations of diabetic autonomic neuropathy may play a role. Clinical symptoms are more common in patients with long-standing diabetes, increased age, poor glucose control, and symptoms of cardiovascular or peripheral neuropathy. Because gastric emptying of solids is impaired but emptying of liquids may be normal, a saline load is not accurate for the diagnosis of diabetic gastroparesis.

(1019–D)   **(S&F, p. 205)**

Only 7% of patients with a flat pigmented spot in the ulcer bed will rebleed. All of the other lesions have a 40% or greater risk of further bleeding.

(1020–A)   **(S&F, p. 2042)**

Most cases of mesothelioma are malignant. Asbestos workers and members of their households are at risk, but the interval between exposure and diagnosis is long. Although surgical resection has been advocated by some, the best results are obtained by radiation therapy in combination with systemic and intraperitoneal chemotherapy.

(1021–D)   **(S&F, p. 413)**

The incidence of peptic ulcer has been reported in hyperparathyroidism to range from 5% to 15%. Whereas part of this association reflects the effects of calcium on acid secretion, a major part is due to patients whose hyperparathyroidism is associated with a functioning gastrinoma (multiple endocrine neoplasia–1 syndrome).

(1022–A)   **(S&F, pp. 278–279)**

The term *obesity* means the excessive accumulation of body fat. In general, men in whom more than 25% and women in whom more than 35% of body weight is fat are considered obese. In contrast, the term *overweight* refers to persons whose body weight is greater than an ideal standard. Because it ignores the composition of the body, nonobese persons with muscular bodies may be classified as overweight. The National Center for Health Statistics defines obesity as a body mass index of 27.8 or more, determined by weight in kilograms divided by estimated surface area in meters squared. Defining obesity in terms of usual or ideal body weight for a given height incorrectly assumes a strong correlation between weight and adiposity. Other problems with widespread use of height–weight tables include variations in skeletal mass, bone density, and the definition of ideal body weight.

(1023–B)   **(S&F, pp. 335–337)**

Solid agents are difficult to swallow, adhering to mucus membranes in the oropharynx; however, the absence of oropharyngeal injury does not exclude severe esophageal or gastric injury. The most common site of esophageal stricture after caustic ingestion is in the proximal esophagus at the level of the cricopharyngeus or the aortic arch. Stridor and hoarseness suggest airway injury and should be evaluated before endoscopic examination of the gastrointestinal tract to ensure airway safety.

(1024–A, B, C, D)   **(S&F, p. 144)**

Collagenous colitis is a disease that affects mostly women in their fifth and sixth decades. The most frequent presenting symptom is watery diarrhea, sometimes up to 2 L/day. Barium studies and even the colonoscopic appearance are usually normal. Appropriate evaluation includes tests to rule out other causes of chronic diarrhea. Diagnosis is made by mucosal biopsy specimens showing characteristic intraepithelial lymphocytes and an infiltrate in the lamina propria of excess inflammatory cells, mostly plasma cells. A collagenous band beneath the surface of the epithelium more than 15 mm (normal, 2 to 6 mm) is often seen in women with the disorder, in which case the term *collagenous colitis* may be used, although a better term would be *microscopic colitis with collagen table thickening*. Treatment consists of antidiarrheal measures. Sulfasalazine, corticosteroids, and mesalamine–containing drugs may also be useful.

(1025–C)   **(S&F, p. 318)**

Routine radiographic studies demonstrate a 60% incidence of hiatal hernia in unselected elderly patients, the most common type being a sliding hiatal hernia.

(1026–C)   **(S&F, pp. 230–231)**

In patients with biliary obstruction, therapy is typically directed at mechanical relief of obstruction. In cholestatic liver disease, treatment is directed toward reversing the underlying metabolic defect. Pruritus is a potentially disabling symptom of cholestatic hepatobiliary disease. Bile acid–binding resins such as cholestyramine have been of some benefit in treating this disorder. Naloxone, rifampin, and ursodiol have also been used with some success. Omeprazole has no known value in cholestasis.

(1027–A)   **(S&F, p. 360)**

Percutaneous abscess drainage requires that a safe access route be available that avoids traversing bowel and is not adjacent to major vascular structures, owing to the risk of perforation or hemorrhage.

(1028–E)   **(S&F, p. 207)**

Propranolol may reduce mortality in patients with large esophageal varices by preventing an initial bleeding episode, but none of these agents reduces mortality in patients with acute variceal bleeding.

■■■■ **Reference**

Pagliaro, C., D'Amio, G., Sorensen, T., et al. Prevention of first bleeding in cirrhosis: A meta-analysis of randomized trials of nonsurgical treatment. Ann. Intern. Med. *117*:59, 1992.

(1029–D)   **(S&F, pp. 165–166)**

Rectal balloon manometry can provide information about several physiologic functions. By inflating the rectal balloon with increasing volumes of air or water, the threshold for conscious sensation of rectal distention can be estimated. Normally, as little as 10 mL of rectal distention can be detected. By monitoring pressures in the upper anal canal during rectal distention, one can evaluate the rectoanal inhibitory reflex. The threshold amount of rectal distention required to elicit reflex relaxation of the internal anal sphincter averages about 20 mL in normal subjects. It is usually higher than the threshold for conscious sensation. The increase in pressure in the lower anal canal after rectal distention reflects contractile activity in the external anal sphincter and is called the rectoanal contractile response. Absence of this response can be due to interruption of the afferent or efferent extrinsic nerves, weakness of the external anal sphincter, or forgetting this learned response. Finally, rectal balloon manometry can be used to estimate rectal compliance.

(1030–B)   **(S&F, p. 2038)**

The presence on peritoneal lavage of a white blood cell count greater than 500 cells/mm³, a bilirubin or amylase level greater than the serum value, or bacteria on Gram stain is associated with a more than 90% chance that peritonitis is present. Albumin levels have no value in this setting.

(1031–C)   **(S&F, pp. 417–418)**

Tumors may involve the gut by direct invasion from adjacent organs, by intraperitoneal seeding, or by hematogenous or lymphatic spread. About 20% of all patients with non–gastrointestinal tract cancers have metastasis to the gastrointestinal tract, among which breast, lung, and ovarian cancer and malignant melanoma are the most common. Patterns of metastasis are not random but reflect the location and histologic type of the primary tumor. They typically develop in the serosa or submucosa and produce intraluminal lesions that may lead to obstruction, bleeding, or a polypoid mass. Thyroid cancer uncommonly spreads to the gastrointestinal tract.

(1032–D)   **(S&F, p. 180)**

Laboratory tests used to evaluate constipation should be selected based on the clinical evaluation. Thyroid and parathyroid function should be investigated routinely. Hypokalemia and hypercalcemia are also common causes of constipation. Constipation may reflect autonomic neuropathy due to long-standing diabetes. There is no reported association between serum gastrin levels and constipation.

(1033–C)   **(S&F, pp. 239–241)**

The duration of survival during starvation depends on the stores of body fuels available. People of normal weight can survive for about two months when ingesting only water. Death in Irish hunger strikers generally occurred after they had lost about 35% of their body weight and is common after loss of 40%. In contrast, obese people have undergone therapeutic fasts for more than one year without adverse consequences, surviving only on water, vitamins, and minerals.

(1034–C)   **(S&F, p. 83)**

Sudden severe pain has an abrupt and instantaneous onset. The principal causes are viscus perforation or rupture, abdominal vascular accidents, or passage of a kidney stone. Boerhaave's syndrome is esophageal perforation with an associated pleural effusion, often with sudden onset of chest pain. Uncomplicated cholecystitis may have a rapid onset of pain (15–30 minutes), but pain is not sudden.

(1035–B)   **(S&F, pp. 444–445)**

Hereditary hemorrhagic telangiectasia (Osler-Weber-Rendu disease) is characterized by vascular lesions of the skin and internal organs. Epistaxis and later gastrointestinal, pulmonary, and even cerebral hemorrhage are common complications. Identical skin and oral lesions can be seen in CREST syndrome, but epistaxis is uncommon.

(1036–B)   **(S&F, pp. 445–446)**

Gardner's syndrome, or familial polyposis, is an inherited autosomal dominant disease. Individuals invariably have multiple adenomatous polyps of the colon and a high incidence of periampullary polyps of the duodenum. Cutaneous features occur in over 50% of patients and include epidermoid cysts, osteomas, fibromas, and desmoid tumors.

(1037–C)   **(S&F, pp. 310–311)**

Small Zenker's diverticula are typically asymptomatic and generally do not increase in size with time. The indications for surgery in this setting are typically dysphagia and/or aspiration. Although carcinoma can occur in the diverticulum, it is extremely rare (i.e., 4 cases in 1249) and should not be used as an indication for surgery in an asymptomatic patient.

(1038–A)   **(S&F, p. 373)**

All available tests used to identify protein-losing enteropathy have deficiencies. Endoscopic visualization and biopsies are rarely helpful because they do not answer functional questions. The iodinated albumin clearance test has proven to be quite unreliable, whereas the chromium test is difficult to perform because the strong gamma radioactivity requires special precautions. The α_1-antitrypsin clearance test has a high sensitivity with some loss of specificity depending on values used for normal subjects but is clearly the best simple test.

(1039–C)   **(S&F, pp. 267–268)**

Administration of parenteral nutrition through peripheral veins (PPN) should be considered in well-nourished patients who have enteral nutrition interrupted for seven to ten days. Although attractive in principle because it avoids the dangers of a central venous catheter, PPN is more difficult to maintain than central parenteral nutrition because of frequent subcutaneous infiltrations and superficial phlebitis. Phlebitis affects up to 90% of patients, but the incidence can be reduced by placing a glycerol trinitrate patch over the catheter and adding small doses of heparin (600 U/L) and hydrocortisone (6 mg/L) into the PPN bag.

(1040–C) *(S&F, pp. 164–165)*

Anal manometry can provide a direct measure of the pressure sensation in the anal canal under basal conditions and with squeezing. As a group, patients with fecal incontinence have significantly lower basal squeeze pressures than age- and sex-matched controls. Manometry is most valuable when it demonstrates abnormally low pressures and thus confirms the presence of a sphincter defect.

(1041–D) *(S&F, pp. 239–240)*

The ability of stored triglyceride to act as a fuel is limited. Certain tissues, such as bone marrow, erythrocytes, leukocytes, renal medulla, eye tissues, and peripheral nerve cannot oxidize lipid and require about 40 g of glucose per day for their energy supply. Under conditions of starvation, the brain can get 70% of its energy requirements from ketone bodies, which are indirect products of lipid oxidation.

(1042–A) *(S&F, pp. 372–373)*

Any disease that causes high right atrial pressures will cause a secondary increase in lymphatic pressure that may lead to protein-losing enteropathy. Although cirrhosis causes high portal vein pressures, it does not produce high lymphatic pressures in the intestine.

(1043–C) *(S&F, p. 168)*

The only two drugs that have been systematically studied for an effect on fecal continence are Lomotil (a combined product of diphenoxylate and atropine) and loperamide. Lomotil reduced stool frequency and weight. It had no effect on sphincter pressure or on tests for incontinence for solids or rectally infused saline. Loperamide at a dose of 4 mg three times a day significantly reduced the frequency of incontinence episodes and urgency, increased basal anal sphincter pressure slightly, and improved continence for rectally infused saline.

(1044–C) *(S&F, p. 2040)*

The diagnosis of peritoneal tuberculosis is suggested by an elevated lymphocyte count in the peritoneal fluid and negative cytology. Fever is present in the majority of patients. Peritoneal fluid smears stained for acid-fast bacilli are rarely positive. By contrast, histology and culture of the peritoneum obtained by laparoscopic biopsy are virtually always diagnostic.

(1045–B) *(S&F, p. 441)*

Aphthous ulcers are painful, shallow ulcers often covered with a grayish white exudate and an erythematous margin. They appear exclusively on unkeratinized mucosal surfaces. Aphthae occur in about 25% of the general population and are not infectious. A variety of conditions have been associated with aphthous ulcers, including inflammatory bowel disease, Behçet's syndrome, pernicious anemia, and any condition leading to prolonged fever. Oral thrush may ulcerate but does not cause aphthous ulceration.

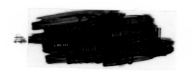

Date Due

RECD MAY 1 6 2001			
FEB 1 4 2011			
FEB 0 3 2011			